Introductory Biostatistics for the Health Sciences
Modern Applications Including Bootstrap

MICHAEL R. CHERNICK
Novo Nordisk Pharmaceuticals, Inc.
Princeton, New Jersey

ROBERT H. FRIIS
California State University
Long Beach, California

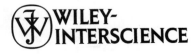

A JOHN WILEY & SONS PUBLICATION

Library of Congress Cataloging-in-Publication Data is available.

ISBN 0-471-41137-X

Printed in the United States of America.

10 9 8 7 6 5 4 3 2 1

*Michael Chernick dedicates this book to his wife Ann
and his children Nicholas, Daniel, and Kenneth.*

Robert Friis dedicates it to his wife Carol.

Contents

9. Tests of Hypotheses   182

10. Inferences Regarding Proportions   217

Preface

Statistics has evolved into a very important discipline that is applied in many fields. In the modern age of computing, both statistical methodology and its applications are expanding greatly. Among the many areas of application, we (Friis and Chernick) have direct experience in the use of statistical methods to military problems, space surveillance, experimental design, data validation, forecasting workloads, predicting the cost and duration of insurance claims, quality assurance, the design and analysis of clinical trials, and epidemiologic studies.

The idea for this book came to each of us independently when we taught an introductory course in statistics for undergraduate health science majors at California State University at Long Beach. Before Michael Chernick came to Long Beach, Robert Friis first taught Health Science 403 and 503 and developed the requirements for the latter course in the department. The Health Science 403 course gives the student an appreciation for statistical methods and provides a foundation for applications in medical research, health education, program evaluation, and courses in epidemiology.

A few years later, Michael Chernick was recruited to teach Health Science 403 on a part-time basis. The text that we preferred for the course was a little too advanced; other texts that we chose, though at the right level, contained several annoying errors and did not provide some of the latest developments and real-world applications. We wanted to provide our students with an introduction to recent statistical advances such as bootstrapping and give them real examples from our collective experience at two medical device companies, and in statistical consulting and epidemiologic research.

For the resulting course we chose the text with the annoying errors and included a few excerpts from the bootstrap book by one of the authors (Chernick) as well as reference material from a third text. A better alternative would have been a single text that incorporates the best aspects of all three texts along with examples from our work, so we wrote the present text, which is intended for an introductory course in statistical methods that emphasizes the methods most commonly used in the health sciences. The level of the course is for undergraduate health science students (juniors or seniors) who have had high school algebra, but not necessarily calculus, as well as for public health graduate students, nursing and medical students, and medical residents.

A previous statistics course may be helpful but is not required. In our experience, students who have taken a previous statistics course are probably rusty and could benefit from the reinforcement that the present text provides.

The material in the first 11 chapters (through categorical data and chi-square tests) can be used as the basis for a one-semester course. The instructor might even find time to include all or part of either Chapter 12 (correlation and regression) or Chapter 13 (one-way analysis of variance). One alternative to this suggestion is to omit Chapter 11 and include the contents of Chapter 14 (nonparametric methods) or 15 (survival analysis). Chapter 16 on statistical software packages is a must for all students and can be covered in one lecture at the end of the course. It is not commonly seen in books at this level.

This course could be taught in the suggested order with the following options:

1. Chapter 1 → Chapter 2 → Chapter 3 → Chapter 4 → Chapter 5 → Chapter 6 → Chapter 7 → Chapter 8 → Chapter 9 → Chapter 10 → Chapter 11 → Chapter 12 (at least 12.1–12.7) → Chapter 16.
2. Chapter 1 → Chapter 2 → Chapter 3 → Chapter 4 → Chapter 5 → Chapter 6 → Chapter 7 → Chapter 8 → Chapter 9 → Chapter 10 → Chapter 11 → Chapter 13 → Chapter 16.
3. Chapter 1 → Chapter 2 → Chapter 3 → Chapter 4 → Chapter 5 → Chapter 6 → Chapter 7 → Chapter 8 → Chapter 9 → Chapter 10 → Chapter 12 (at least 12.1–12.7) → Chapter 14 → Chapter 16.
4. Chapter 1 → Chapter 2 → Chapter 3 → Chapter 4 → Chapter 5 → Chapter 6 → Chapter 7 → Chapter 8 → Chapter 9 → Chapter 10 → Chapter 12 (at least 12.1–12.7) → Chapter 15 → Chapter 16.
5. Chapter 1 → Chapter 2 → Chapter 3 → Chapter 4 → Chapter 5 → Chapter 6 → Chapter 7 → Chapter 8 → Chapter 9 → Chapter 10 → Chapter 13 → Chapter 14 → Chapter 16.
6. Chapter 1 → Chapter 2 → Chapter 3 → Chapter 4 → Chapter 5 → Chapter 6 → Chapter 7 → Chapter 8 → Chapter 9 → Chapter 10 → Chapter 13 → Chapter 15 → Chapter 16.

For graduate students who have had a good introductory statistics course, a course could begin with Chapter 8 (estimating population means) and cover all the material in Chapters 9–15. At Long Beach, Health Science 503 is such a course. Topics not commonly covered in other texts include bootstrap, meta-analysis, outlier detection methods, pharmacoeconomics, epidemiology, logistic regression, and Bayesian methods. Although we touch on some modern and advanced topics, the main emphasis in the text is the classical parametric approach found in most introductory statistics courses. Some of the topics are advanced and can be skipped in an undergraduate course without affecting understanding of the rest of the text. These sections are followed by an asterisk and include Sections 9.15 through 9.18 among others.

At the beginning of each chapter, we have a statistical quote with author and reference. While the particular quote was carefully chosen to fit the theme of the chapter, it was not as difficult a task as one might at first think. We were aided by the excellent dictionary of statistical terms, "Statistically Speaking," by Gaither and Cavazos-Gaither.

A full citation for quotes used in the book is given in the additional reading section of Chapter 1. The sources for these quotes are playwrights, poets, physicists, politicians, nurses, and even some statisticians. Although many of the quotes and their authors are famous, not all are. But as Gaither and Cavazos-Gaither say, "Some quotes are profound, others are wise, some are witty but none are frivolous." It is useful to go back and think about the chapter quote after reading the chapter.

ACKNOWLEDGMENTS

We would like to thank Stephen Quigley and Heather Haselkorn of John Wiley & Sons for their hard work in helping to bring this project to fruition. We would also like to thank the various anonymous Wiley referees for their valuable comments in reviewing drafts of part of the manuscript. We also especially thank Dr. Patrick Rojas for kindly reviewing parts of the manuscript with his usual thoroughness. He made many helpful suggestions to improve the accuracy and clarity of the exposition and to correct many of the errors that invariably appear in such large manuscripts. Any remaining errors are solely the responsibility of the authors. We would very much appreciate hearing about them from our readers and students. We would also like to thank Carol Friis, who assisted with one phase of manuscript editing. Drs. Javier Lopez-Zetina and Alan Safer provided helpful comments. We would also like to add to the acknowledgments Dr. Ezra Levy, who helped with the preparation of figures and tables.

CHAPTER 1

What is Statistics? How Is It Applied to the Health Sciences?

Statistics are the food of love.
—Roger Angell, *Late Innings: A Baseball Companion.* Chapter 1 p. 9

All of us are familiar with statistics in everyday life. Very often, we read about sports statistics; for example, predictions of which country is favored to win the World Cup in soccer, baseball batting averages, standings of professional football teams, and tables of golf scores.

Other examples of statistics are the data collected by forms from the decennial U.S. census, which attempts to enumerate every U.S. resident. The U.S. Bureau of the Census publishes reports on the demographic characteristics of the U.S. population. Such reports describe the overall population in terms of gender, age, and income distributions; state and local reports are also available, as well as other levels of aggregation and disaggregation. One of the interesting types of census data that often appears in newspaper articles is regional economic status classified according to standardized metropolitan areas. Finally, census data are instrumental in determining rates for mortality and diseases in geographic areas of the United States.

A widely recognized use of statistics is for public opinion polls that predict the outcome of elections of government officials. For example, a local newspaper article reports that two candidates are in a dead heat with one garnering 45% of the votes, the other garnering 47% percent, and the remaining 8% of voters undecided. The article also qualifies these results by reporting a margin of error of ±4%; the margin of error is an expression of the statistical uncertainty associated with the sample. You will understand the meaning of the concept of statistical uncertainty when we cover the binomial distribution and its associated statistical inference. We will see that the binomial distribution is a probability model for independent repeated tests with events that have two mutually exclusive outcomes, such as "heads" or "tails" in coin tossing experiments or "alive" or "dead" for patients in a medical study.

Regarding the health applications of statistics, the popular media carry articles on the latest drugs to control cancer or new vaccines for HIV. These popular articles restate statistical findings to the lay audience based on complex analyses reported in

Introductory Biostatistics for the Health Sciences, by Michael R. Chernick
and Robert H. Friis. ISBN 0-471-41137-X. Copyright © 2003 Wiley-Interscience.

scientific journals. In recent years, the health sciences have become increasingly quantitative. Some of the health science disciplines that are particularly noteworthy in their use of statistics include public health (biostatistics, epidemiology, health education, environmental health); medicine (biometry, preventive medicine, clinical trials); nursing (nursing research); and health care administration (operations research, needs assessment), to give a few illustrations. Not only does the study of statistics help one to perform one's job more effectively by providing a set of valuable skills, but also a knowledge of statistics helps one to be a more effective consumer of the statistical information that bombards us incessantly.

1.1   DEFINITIONS OF STATISTICS AND STATISTICIANS

One use of statistics is to summarize and portray the characteristics of the contents of a data set or to identify patterns in a data set. This field is known as descriptive statistics or exploratory data analysis, defined as the branch of statistics that describes the contents of data or makes a picture based on the data. Sometimes researchers use statistics to draw conclusions about the world or to test formal hypotheses. The latter application is known as inferential statistics or confirmatory data analysis.

   The field of statistics, which is relatively young, traces its origins to questions about games of chance. The foundation of statistics rests on the theory of probability, a subject with origins many centuries ago in the mathematics of gambling. Motivated by gambling questions, famous mathematicians such as DeMoivre and Laplace developed probability theory. Gauss derived least squares estimation (a technique used prominently in modern regression analysis) as a method to fit the orbits of planets. The field of statistics was advanced in the late 19th century by the following developments: (1) Galton's discovery of regression (a topic we will cover in Chapter 12); (2) Karl Pearson's work on parametric fitting of probability distributions (models for probability distributions that depend on a few unknown constants that can be estimated from data); and (3) the discovery of the chi-square approximation (an approximation to the distribution of test statistics used in contingency tables and goodness of fit problems, to be covered in Chapter 11). Applications in agriculture, biology, and genetics also motivated early statistical work.

   Subsequently, ideas of statistical inference evolved in the 20th century, with the important notions being developed from the 1890s to the 1950s. The leaders in statistics at the beginning of the 20th century were Karl Pearson, Egon Pearson (Karl Pearson's son), Harold Cramer, Ronald Fisher, and Jerzy Neyman. They developed early statistical methodology and foundational theory. Later applications arose in engineering and the military (particularly during World War II).

   Abraham Wald and his statistical research group at Columbia University developed sequential analysis (a technique that allows sampling to stop or continue based on current results) and statistical decision theory (methods for making decisions in the face of uncertainty based on optimizing cost or utility functions). Utility functions are functions that numerically place a value on decisions, so that choices can be compared; the "best" decision is the one that has the highest or maximum utility.

The University of North Carolina and the University of California at Berkeley also were major centers for statistics. Harold Hotelling and Gertrude Cox initiated statistics departments in North Carolina. Jerzy Neyman came to California and formed a strong statistical research center at the University of California, Berkeley.

Statistical quality control developed at Bell Labs, starting with the work of Walter Shewhart. An American statistician, Ed Deming, took the statistical quality control techniques to Japan along with his management philosophy; in Japan, he nurtured a high standard of excellence, which currently is being emulated successfully in the United States.

John Tukey at Princeton University and Bell Labs developed many important statistical ideas, including:

- Methods of spectral estimation (a decomposition of time dependent data in terms of trigonometric functions with different frequencies) in time series
- The fast Fourier transform (also used in the spectral analysis of time series)
- Robust estimation procedures (methods of estimation that work well for a variety of probability distributions)
- The concept of exploratory data analysis
- Many of the tools for exploratory analysis, including: (a) PRIM9, an early graphical tool for rotating high-dimensional data on a computer screen. By high-dimensional data we mean that the number of variables that we are considering is large (even a total of five to nine variables can be considered large when we are looking for complex relationships). (b) box-and-whisker and stem-and-leaf plots (to be covered in Chapter 3).

Given the widespread applications of statistics, it is not surprising that statisticians can be found at all major universities in a variety of departments including statistics, biostatistics, mathematics, public health, management science, economics, and the social sciences. The federal government employs statisticians at the National Institute of Standards and Technology, the U.S. Bureau of the Census, the U.S. Department of Energy, the Bureau of Labor Statistics, the U.S. Food and Drug Administration, and the National Laboratories, among other agencies. In the private sector, statisticians are prominent in research groups at AT&T, General Electric, General Motors, and many Fortune 500 companies, particularly in medical device and pharmaceutical companies.

1.2 WHY STUDY STATISTICS?

Technological advances continually make new disease prevention and treatment possibilities available for health care. Consequently, a substantial body of medical research explores alternative methods for treating diseases or injuries. Because outcomes vary from one patient to another, researchers use statistical methods to quantify uncertainty in the outcomes, summarize and make sense of data, and compare the effectiveness of different treatments. Federal government agencies and private companies rely heavily on statisticians' input.

The U.S. Food and Drug Administration (FDA) requires manufacturers of new drugs and medical devices to demonstrate the effectiveness and safety of their products when compared to current alternative treatments and devices. Because this process requires a great deal of statistical work, these industries employ many statisticians to design studies and analyze the results. Controlled clinical trials, described later in this chapter, provide a commonly used method for assessing product efficacy and safety. These trials are conducted to meet regulatory requirements for the market release of the products. The FDA considers such trials to be the gold standard among the study approaches that we will cover in this text.

Medical device and pharmaceutical company employees—clinical investigators and managers, quality engineers, research and development engineers, clinical research associates, database managers, as well as professional statisticians—need to have basic statistical knowledge and an understanding of statistical terms. When you consider the following situations that actually occurred at a medical device company, you will understand why a basic knowledge of statistical methods and terminology is important.

Situation 1: You are the clinical coordinator for a clinical trial of an ablation catheter (a catheter that is placed in the heart to burn tissue in order to eliminate an electrical circuit that causes an arrhythmia). You are enrolling patients at five sites and want to add a new site. In order to add a new site, a local review board called an institution review board (IRB) must review and approve your trial protocol.

A member of the board asks you what your stopping rule is. You do not know what a stopping rule is and cannot answer the question. Even worse, you do not even know who can help you. If you had taken a statistics course, you might know that many trials are constructed using group sequential statistical methods. These methods allow for the data to be compared at various times during the trial. Thresholds that vary from stage to stage determine whether the trial can be stopped early to declare the device safe and/or effective. They also enable the company to recognize the futility of continuing the trial (for example, because of safety concerns or because it is clear that the device will not meet the requirements for efficacy). The sequence of such thresholds is called the stopping rule.

The IRB has taken for granted that you know this terminology. However, group sequential methods are more common in pharmaceutical trials than in medical device trials. The correct answer to the IRB is that you are running a fixed-sample-size trial and, therefore, no stopping rule is in effect. After studying the material in this book, you will be aware of what group sequential methods are and know what stopping rules are.

Situation 2: As a regulatory affairs associate at a medical device company that has completed a clinical trial of an ablation catheter, you have submitted a regulatory report called a premarket approval application (PMA). In the PMA, your statistician has provided statistical analyses for the study endpoints (performance measures used to demonstrate safety or effectiveness).

The reviewers at the Food and Drug Administration (FDA) send you a letter with questions and concerns about deficiencies that must be addressed before they will approve the device for marketing. One of the questions is: "Why did you use the Greenwood approximation instead of Peto's method?" The FDA prefers Peto's method and would like you to compute the results by using that method.

You recognize that the foregoing example involves a statistical question but have no idea what the Greenwood and Peto methods are. You consult your statistician, who tells you that she conducted a survival analysis (a study of treatment failure as a function of time across the patients enrolled in the study). In the survival analysis, time to recurrence of the arrhythmia is recorded for each patient. As most patients never have a recurrence, they are treated as having a right-censored recurrence time (their time to event is cut off at the end of the trial or the time of the analysis).

Based on the data, a Kaplan–Meier curve, the common nonparametric estimate for the survival curve, is generated. The survival curve provides the probability that a patient will not have a recurrence by time t. It is plotted as a function of t and decreases from 1 at time 0. The Kaplan–Meier curve is an estimate of this survival curve based on the trial data (survival analysis is covered in Chapter 15).

You will learn that the uncertainty in the Kaplan–Meier curve, a statistical estimate, can be quantified in a confidence interval (covered in general terms in Chapter 8). The Greenwood and Peto methods are two approximate methods for placing confidence intervals on the survival curve at specified times t. Statistical research has shown that the Greenwood method often provides a lower confidence bound estimate that is too high. In contrast, the Peto method gives a lower and possibly better estimate for the lower bound, particularly when t is large. The FDA prefers the bound obtained by the Peto method because for large t, most of the cases have been right-censored. However, both methods are approximations and neither one is "correct."

From the present text, you will learn about confidence bounds and survival distributions; eventually, you will be able to compute both the Greenwood and Peto bounds. (You already know enough to respond to the FDA question, "Why did you use the Greenwood approximation . . . ?" by asking a statistician to provide the Peto lower bound in addition to the Greenwood.)

Situation 3: Again, you are a regulatory affairs associate and are reviewing an FDA letter about a PMA submission. The FDA wants to know if you can present your results on the primary endpoints in terms of confidence intervals instead of just reporting p-values (the p-value provides a summary of the strength of evidence against the null hypothesis and will be covered in Chapter 9). Again, you recognize that the FDA's question involves statistical issues.

When you ask for help, the statistician tells you that the p-value is a summary of the results of a hypothesis test. Because the statistician is familiar with the test and the value of the test statistic, he can use the critical value(s) for the test to generate a confidence bound or confidence bounds for the hypothesized parameter value. Consequently, you can tell the FDA that you are able to provide them with the information they want.

The present text will teach you about the one-to-one correspondence between hypothesis tests and confidence intervals (Chapter 9) so that you can construct a hypothesis test based on a given confidence interval or construct the confidence bounds based on the results of the hypothesis test.

Situation 4: You are a clinical research associate (CRA) in the middle of a clinical trial. Based on data provided by your statistics group, you are able to change your chronic endpoint from a six-month follow-up result to a three-month follow-up result. This change is exciting because it may mean that you can finish the trial much sooner than you anticipated. However, there is a problem: the original protocol required follow-ups only at two weeks and at six months after the procedure, whereas a three-month follow-up was optional.

Some of the sites opt not to have a three-month follow-up. Your clinical manager wants you to ask the investigators to have the patients who are past three months postprocedure but not near the six-month follow-up come in for an unscheduled follow-up. When the investigator and a nurse associate hear about this request, they are reluctant to go to the trouble of bringing in the patients. How do you convince them to comply?

You ask your statistician to explain the need for an unscheduled follow-up. She says that the trial started with a six-month endpoint because the FDA viewed six months to be a sufficient duration for the trial. However, an investigation of Kaplan–Meier curves for similar studies showed that there was very little decrease in the survival probability in the period from three to six months. This finding convinced the FDA that the three-month endpoint would provide sufficient information to determine the long-term survival probability.

The statistician tells the investigator that we could not have put this requirement into the original protocol because the information to convince the FDA did not exist then. However, now that the FDA has changed its position, we must have the three-month information on as many patients as possible. By going to the trouble of bringing in these patients, we will obtain the information that we need for an early approval. The early approval will allow the company to market the product much faster and allow the site to use the device sooner. As you learn about survival curves in this text, you will appreciate how greatly survival analyses impact the success of a clinical trial.

Situation 5: You are the Vice President of the Clinical and Regulatory Affairs Department at a medical device company. Your company hired a contract research organization (CRO) to run a randomized controlled clinical trial (described in Section 1.3.5, Clinical Trials). A CRO was selected in order to maintain complete objectivity and to guarantee that the trial would remain blinded throughout. Blinding is a procedure of coding the allocation of patients so that neither they nor the investigators know to which treatment the patients were assigned in the trial.

You will learn that blinding is important to prevent bias in the study. The trial has been running for two years. You have no idea how your product is doing. The CRO is nearing completion of the analysis and is getting ready to present the report and unblind the study (i.e., let others know the treatment group assignments for the patients). You are very anxious to know if the trial will be successful. A successful trial will provide a big financial boost for your company, which will be able to market this device that provides a new method of treatment for a particular type of heart disease.

The CRO shows you their report because you are the only one allowed to see it until the announcement, two weeks hence. Your company's two expert statisticians are not even allowed to see the report. You have limited statistical knowledge, but you are accustomed to seeing results reported in terms of p-values for tests. You see a demographic analysis comparing patients by age and gender in the treatment and the control groups. As the p-value is 0.56, you are alarmed, for you are used to seeing small p-values. You know that, generally, the FDA requires p-values below 0.05 for acceptance of a device for marketing. There is nothing you can do but worry for the next two weeks.

If you had a little more statistical training or if you had a chance to speak to your statistician, you may have heard the following: Generally, hypothesis tests are set up so that the null hypothesis states that there is no difference among groups; you want to reject the null hypothesis to show that results are better for the treatment group than for the control group. A low p-value (0.05 is usually the threshold) indicates that the results favor the treatment group in comparison to the control group. Conversely, a high p-value (above 0.05) indicates no significant improvement.

However, for the demographic analysis, we want to show no difference in outcome between groups by demographic characteristics. We want the difference in the value for primary endpoints (in this case, length of time the patient is able to exercise on a treadmill three months after the procedure) to be attributed to a difference in treatment. If there are demographic differences between groups, we cannot determine whether a statistically significant difference in performance between the two groups is attributable to the device being tested or simply to the demographic differences. So when comparing demographics, we are not interested in rejecting the null hypothesis; therefore, high p-values provide good news for us.

From the preceding situations, you can see that many employees at medical device companies who are not statisticians have to deal with statistical issues and terminology frequently in their everyday work. As students in the health sciences, you may aspire to career positions that involve responsibilities and issues that are similar to those in the foregoing examples. Also, the medical literature is replete with research articles that include statistical analyses or at least provide p-values for certain hypothesis tests. If you need to study the medical literature, you will need to evaluate some of these statistical results. This text will help you become statistically literate. You will have a basic understanding of statistical techniques and the assumptions necessary for their application.

We noted previously that in recent years, medically related research papers have included more and increasingly sophisticated statistical analyses. However, some medical journals have tended to have a poor track record, publishing papers that contain various errors in their statistical applications. See Altman (1991), Chapter 16, for examples.

Another group that requires statistical expertise in many situations is comprised of public health workers. For example, they may be asked to investigate a disease outbreak (such as a food-borne disease outbreak). There are five steps (using statistics) required to investigate the outbreak: First, collect information about the persons involved in the outbreak, deciding which types of data are most appropriate. Second, identify possible sources of the outbreak, for example, contaminated or improperly stored food or unsafe food handling practices. Third, formulate hypotheses about modes of disease transmission. Fourth, from the collected data, develop a descriptive display of quantitative information (see Chapter 3), e.g., bar charts of cases of occurrence by day of outbreak. Fifth, assess the risks associated with certain types of exposure (see Chapter 11).

Health education is another public health discipline that relies on statistics. A central concern of health education is program evaluation, which is necessary to demonstrate program efficacy. In conjunction with program evaluation, health educators decide on alternative statistical tests, including (but not limited to) independent groups or paired groups (paired t-tests or nonparametric analogues) chi-square tests, or one-way analyses of variance. In designing a needs assessment protocol, health educators conduct a power analysis for sample surveys. Not to be minimized is the need to be familiar with the plethora of statistical techniques employed in contemporary health education and public health literature.

The field of statistics not only has gained importance in medicine and closely related disciplines, as we have described in the preceding examples, but it has become the method of choice in almost all scientific investigations. Salsburg's recent book "The Lady Tasting Tea" (Salsburg, 2001) explains eloquently why this is so and provides a glimpse at the development of statistical methodology in the 20th century, along with the many famous probabilists and statisticians who developed the discipline during that period. Salsburg's book also provides insight as to why (possibly in some changing form) the discipline will continue to be important in the 21st century. Random variation just will not go away, even though deterministic theories (i.e., those not based on chance factors) continue to develop.

The examples described in this section are intended to give you an overview of the importance of statistics in all areas of medically related disciplines. The examples also highlight why all employees in the medical field can benefit from a basic understanding of statistics. However, in certain positions a deeper knowledge of statistics is required. These examples were intended to give you an understanding of the importance of statistics in realistic situations. We have pointed out in each situation the specific chapters in which you will learn more details about the relevant statistical topics. At this point, you are not expected to understand all the details regarding the examples, but by the completion of the text, you will be able to review and reread them in order to develop a deeper appreciation of the issues involved.

1.3   TYPES OF STUDIES

Statisticians use data from a variety of sources: observational data are from cross-sectional, retrospective, and prospective studies; experimental data are derived from planned experiments and clinical trials. What are some illustrations of the types of data from each of these sources? Sometimes, observational data have been collected from naturally or routinely occurring situations. Other times, they are collected for administrative purposes; examples are data from medical records, government agencies, or surveys. Experimental data include the results that have been collected from formal intervention studies or clinical trials; some examples are survival data, the proportion of patients who recover from a medical procedure, and relapse rates after taking a new medication.

Most study designs contain one or more outcome variables that are specified explicitly. (Sometimes, a study design may not have an explicitly defined outcome variable but, rather, the outcome is implicit; however, the use of an implicit outcome variable is not a desirable practice.) Study outcome variables may range from counts of the number of cases of illness or the number of deaths to responses to an attitude questionnaire. In some disciplines, outcome variables are called dependent variables. The researcher may wish to relate these outcomes to disease risk factors such as exposure to toxic chemicals, electromagnetic radiation, or particular medications, or to some other factor that is thought to be associated with a particular health outcome.

In addition to outcome variables, study designs assess exposure factors. For example, exposure factors may include toxic chemicals and substances, ionizing radiation, and air pollution. Other types of exposure factors, more formally known as risk factors, include a lack of exercise, a high-fat diet, and smoking. In other disciplines, exposure factors sometimes are called independent variables. However, epidemiologists prefer to use the term exposure factor.

One important issue pertains to the time frame for collection of data, whether information about exposure and outcome factors is referenced about a single point in time or whether it involves looking backward or forward in time. These distinctions are important because, as we will learn, they affect both the types of analyses that we can perform and our confidence about inferences that we can make from the analyses. The following illustrations will clarify this issue.

1.3.1   Surveys and Cross-Sectional Studies

A cross-sectional study is referenced about a single point in time—now. That is, the reference point for both the exposure and outcome variables is the present time. Most surveys represent cross-sectional studies. For example, researchers who want to know about the present health characteristics of a population might administer a survey to answer the following kinds of questions: How many students smoke at a college campus? Do men and women differ in their current levels of smoking?

Other varieties of surveys might ask subjects for self-reports of health characteristics and then link the responses to physical health assessments. Survey research might ascertain whether current weight is related to systolic blood pressure levels or whether subgroups of populations differ from one another in health characteristics; e.g., do Latinos in comparison to non-Latinos differ in rates of diabetes? Thus, it is apparent that although the term "cross-sectional study" may seem confusing at first, it is actually quite simple. Cross-sectional studies, which typically involve descriptive statistics, are useful for generating hypotheses that may be explored in future research. These studies are not appropriate for making cause and effect assertions. Examples of statistical methods appropriate for analysis of cross-sectional data include cross-tabulations, correlation and regression, and tests of differences between or among groups as long as time is not an important factor in the inference.

1.3.2   Retrospective Studies

A retrospective study is one in which the focus upon the risk factor or exposure factor for the outcome is in the past. One type of retrospective study is the case-control study, in which patients who have a disease of interest to the researchers are asked about their prior exposure to a hypothesized risk factor for the disease. These patients represent the case data that are matched to patients without the disease but with similar demographic characteristics.

Health researchers employ case-control studies frequently when rapid and inexpensive answers to a question are required. Investigations of food-borne illness require a speedy response to stop the outbreak. In the hypothetical investigation of a suspected outbreak of *E. coli*-associated food-borne illness, public health officials would try to identify all of the cases of illness that occurred in the outbreak and administer a standardized questionnaire to the victims in order to determine which foods they consumed. In case-control studies, statisticians evaluate associations and learn about risk factors and health outcomes through the use of odds ratios (see Chapter 11).

1.3.3   Prospective Studies

Prospective studies follow subjects from the present into the future. In the health sciences, one example is called a prospective cohort study, which begins with individuals who are free from disease, but who have an exposure factor. An example would be a study that follows a group of young persons who are initiating smoking and who are free from tobacco-related diseases. Researchers might follow these youths into the future in order to note their development of lung cancer or emphysema. Because many chronic, noninfectious diseases have a long latency period and low incidence (occurrence of new cases) in the population, cohort studies are time-consuming and expensive in comparison to other methodologies. In cohort studies, epidemiologists often use relative risk (RR) as a measure of association between risk exposure and disease. The term relative risk is explained in Chapter 11.

1.3.4   Experimental Studies and Quality Control

An experimental study is one in which there is a study group and a control group as well as an independent (causal) variable and a dependent (outcome) variable. Subjects who participate in the study are assigned randomly to either the study or control conditions. The investigator manipulates the independent variable and observes its influence upon the dependent variable. This study design is similar to those that the reader may have heard about in a psychology course. Experimental designs also are related to clinical trials, which were described earlier in this chapter.

Experimental studies are used extensively in product quality control. The manufacturing and agricultural industries have pioneered the application of statistical design methods to the production of first-rate, competitive products. These methods also are used for continuous process improvement. The following statistical methods have been the key tools in this success:

- Design of Experiments (DOE, methods for varying conditions to look at the effects of certain variables on the output)
- Response Surface Methodology (RSM, methods for changing the experimental conditions to move quickly toward optimal experimental conditions)
- Statistical Process Control (SPC, procedures that involve the plotting of data over time to track performance and identify changes that indicate possible problems)
- Evolutionary Operation (EVOP, methods to adjust processes to reach optimal conditions as processes change or evolve over time)

Data from such experiments are often analyzed using linear or nonlinear statistical models. The simplest of these models (simple linear regression and the one-way analysis of variance) are covered in Chapters 12 and 13, respectively, of this text. However, we do not cover the more general models, nor do we cover the methods of experimental design and quality control. Good references for DOE are Montgomery (1997) and Wu and Hamada (2000). Montgomery (1997) also covers EVOP. Myers and Montgomery (1995) is a good source for information on RSM. Ryan (1989) and Vardeman and Jobe (1999) are good sources for SPC and other quality assurance methods.

In the mid-1920s, quality control methods in the United States began with the work of Shewhart at Bell Laboratories and continued through the 1960s. In general, the concept of quality control involves a method for maximizing the quality of goods produced or a manufacturing process. Quality control entails planning, ongoing inspections, and taking corrective actions, if necessary, to maintain high standards. This methodology is applicable to many settings that need to maintain high operating standards. For example, the U.S. space program depends on highly redundant systems that use the best concepts from the field of reliability, an aspect of quality control.

Somehow, the U.S. manufacturing industry in the 1970s lost its knowledge of quality controls. The Japanese learned these ideas from Ed Deming and others and quickly surpassed the U.S. in quality production, especially in the automobile industry in the late 1980s. Recently, by incorporating DOE and SPC methods, US manufacturing has made a comeback. Many companies have made dramatic improvements in their production processes through a formalized training program called Six Sigma. A detailed picture of all these quality control methods can be found in Juran and Godfrey (1999).

Quality control is important in engineering and manufacturing, but why would a student in the health sciences be interested in it? One answer comes from the growing medical device industry. Companies now produce catheters that can be used for ablation of arrhythmias and diagnosis of heart ailments and also experimentally for injection of drugs to improve the cardiovascular system of a patient. Firms also produce stents for angioplasty, implantable pacemakers to correct bradycardia (slow heart rate that causes fatigue and can lead to fainting), and implantable defibrillators that can prevent ventricular fibrillation, which can lead to sudden death. These devices already have had a big impact on improving and prolonging life. Their use and value to the health care industry will continue to grow.

Because these medical devices can be critical to the lives of patients, their safety and effectiveness must be demonstrated to regulatory bodies. In the United States, the governing regulatory body is the FDA. Profitable marketing of a device generally occurs after a company has conducted a successful clinical trial of the device. These devices must be reliable; quality control procedures are necessary to ensure that the manufacturing process continues to work properly.

Similar arguments can be made for the control of processes at pharmaceutical plants, which produce prescription drugs that are important for maintaining the health of patients under treatment. Tablets, serums, and other drug regimens must be of consistently high quality and contain the correct dose as described on the label.

1.3.5 Clinical Trials

A clinical trial is defined as ". . . an experiment performed by a health care organization or professional to evaluate the effect of an intervention or treatment against a control in a clinical environment. It is a prospective study to identify outcome measures that are influenced by the intervention. A clinical trial is designed to maintain health, prevent diseases, or treat diseased subjects. The safety, efficacy, pharmacological, pharmacokinetic, quality-of-life, health economics, or biochemical effects are measured in a clinical trial." (Chow, 2000, p. 110).

Clinical trials are conducted with human subjects (who are usually patients). Before the patients can be enrolled in the trial, they must be informed about the perceived benefits and risks. The process of apprising the patients about benefits and risks is accomplished by using an informed consent form that the patient must sign. Each year in the United States, many companies perform clinical trials. The impetus for these trials is the development of new drugs or medical devices that the companies wish to bring to market. A primary objective of these clinical trials is to demonstrate the safety and effectiveness of the products to the FDA.

Clinical trials take many forms. In a randomized, controlled clinical trial, patients are randomized into treatment and control groups. Sometimes, only a single treatment group and a historical control group are used. This procedure may be followed when the use of a concurrent control group would be expensive or would expose patients in the control group to undue risks. In the medical device industry, the control also can be replaced by an objective performance criterion (OPC). Established standards for current forms of available treatments can be used to determine these OPCs. Patients who undergo the current forms of available treatment thus constitute a control group. Generally, a large amount of historical data is needed to establish an OPC.

Concurrent randomized controls are often preferred to historical controls because the investigators want to have a sound basis for attributing observed differences between the treatment and control groups to treatment effects. If the trial is conducted without concurrent randomized controls, statisticians can argue that any differences shown could be due to differences among the study patient populations rather than to differences in the treatment. As an example, in a hypothetical study conducted in Southern California, a suitable historical control group might consist of Hispanic women. However, if the treatment were intended for males as well as females (including both genders from many other races), a historical control group comprised of Hispanic women would be inappropriate. In addition, if we then were to use a diverse population of males and females of all races for the treatment group only, how would we know that any observed effect was due to the treatment and not simply to the fact that males respond differently from females or that racial differences are playing a role in the response? Thus, the use of a concurrent control group would overcome the difficulties produced by a historical control group.

In addition, in order to avoid potential bias, patients are often blinded as to study conditions (i.e., treatment or control group), when such blinding is possible. It is also preferable to blind the investigator to the study conditions to prevent bias that could invalidate the study conclusions. When both the investigator and the patient are blinded, the trial is called double-blinded. Double-blinding often is possible in drug treatment studies but rarely is possible in medical device trials. In device trials, the patient sometimes can be blinded but the attending physician cannot be.

To illustrate the scientific value of randomized, blinded, controlled, clinical trials, we will describe a real trial that was sponsored by a medical device company that produces and markets catheters. The trial was designed to determine the safety and efficacy of direct myocardial revascularization (DMR). DMR is a clinical procedure designed to improve cardiac circulation (also called perfusion). The medical procedure involves the placement of a catheter in the patient's heart. A small laser on the tip of the catheter is fired to produce channels in the heart muscle that theoretically promote cardiac perfusion. The end result should be improved heart function in those patients who are suffering from severe symptomatic coronary artery disease.

In order to determine if this theory works in practice, clinical trials were required. Some studies were conducted in which patients were given treadmill tests before and after treatment in order to demonstrate increased cardiac output. Other measures of improved heart function also were considered in these studies. Results indicated promise for the treatment.

However, critics charged that because these trials did not have randomized controls, a placebo effect (i.e., patients improve because of a perceived benefit from knowing that they received a treatment) could not be ruled out. In the DMR DIRECT trial, patients were randomized to a treatment group and a sham control group. The sham is a procedure used to keep the patient blinded to the treatment. In all cases the laser catheter was placed in the heart. The laser was fired in the patients randomized to the DMR treatment group but not in the patients randomized to the control group. This was a single-blinded trial; i.e., none of the patients knew whether or not they received the treatment. Obviously, the physician conducting the procedure had to know which patients were in the treatment and control groups. The patients, who were advised of the possibility of the sham treatment in the informed consent form, of course received standard care for their illness.

At the follow-up tests, everyone involved, including the physicians, was blinded to the group associated with the laser treatment. For a certain period after the data were analyzed, the results were known only to the independent group of statisticians who had designed the trial and then analyzed the data.

These results were released and made public in October 2000. Quoting the press release, "Preliminary analysis of the data shows that patients who received this laser-based therapy did not experience a statistically significant increase in exercise times or a decrease in the frequency and severity of angina versus the control group of patients who were treated medically. An improvement across all study groups may suggest a possible placebo effect."

As a result of this trial, the potential benefit of DMR was found not to be significant and not worth the added risk to the patient. Companies and physicians looking for effective treatments for these patients must now consider alternative therapies. The trial saved the sponsor, its competitors, the patients, and the physicians from further use of an ineffective and highly invasive treatment.

1.3.6 Epidemiological Studies

As seen in the foregoing section, clinical trials illustrate one field that requires much biostatistical expertise. Epidemiology is another such field. Epidemiology is defined as the study of the distribution and determinants of health and disease in populations.

Although experimental methods including clinical trials are used in epidemiology, a major group of epidemiological studies use observational techniques that were formalized during the mid-19th century. In his classic work, John Snow reported on attempts to investigate the source of a cholera outbreak that plagued London in 1849. Snow hypothesized that the outbreak was associated with polluted water drawn from the Thames River. Both the Lambeth Company and the Southwark and Vauxhall Company provided water inside the city limits of London. At first, both the Lambeth Company and the Southwark and Vauxhall Company took water from a heavily polluted section of the Thames River.

The Broad Street area of London provided an excellent opportunity to test this hypothesis because households in the same neighborhood were served by interdigitating water supplies from the two different companies. That is, households in the same geographic area (even adjacent houses) received water from the two companies. This observation by Snow made it possible to link cholera outbreaks in a particular household with one of the two water sources.

Subsequently, the Lambeth Company relocated its water source to a less contaminated section of the river. During the cholera outbreak of 1854, Snow demonstrated that a much greater proportion of residents who used water from the more polluted source contracted cholera than those who used water from the less polluted source. Snow's method, still in use today, came to be known as a natural experiment [see Friis and Sellers (1999) for more details].

Snow's investigation of the cholera outbreak illustrates one of the main approaches of epidemiology—use of observational studies. These observational study designs encompass two major categories: descriptive and analytic. Descriptive studies attempt to classify the extent and distribution of disease in populations. In contrast, analytic studies are concerned with causes of disease. Descriptive studies rely on a variety of techniques: (1) case reports, (2) astute clinical observations, and (3) use of statistical methods of description, e.g., showing how disease frequency varies in the population according to demographic variables such as age, sex, race, and socioeconomic status.

For example; *Morbidity and Mortality Reports,* published by the Centers for Disease Control (CDC) in Atlanta, periodically issues data on persons diagnosed with acquired immune deficiency syndrome (AIDS) classified according to demographic subgroups within the United State. With respect to HIV and AIDS, these descriptive studies are vitally important for showing the nation's progress in controlling the AIDS epidemic, identifying groups at high risk, and suggesting needed health care services and interventions. Descriptive studies also set the stage for analytic studies by suggesting hypotheses to be explored in further research.

Snow's natural experiment provides an excellent example of both descriptive and analytic methodology. The reader can probably think of many other examples that would interest statisticians. Many natural experiments are the consequences of government policies. To illustrate, California has introduced many innovative laws to control tobacco use. One of these, the Smoke-free Bars Law, has provided an excellent opportunity to investigate the health effects of prohibiting smoking in alcohol-serving establishments. Natural experiments create a scenario for researchers to test causal hypotheses. Examples of analytic research designs include ecological, case-control, and cohort studies.

We previously defined case-control (Section 1.3.2, Retrospective Studies) and cohort studies (Section 1.3.3, Prospective Studies). Case-control studies have been used in such diverse naturally occurring situations as exploring the causes of toxic shock syndrome among tampon users and investigating diethylstibesterol as a possible cause of birth defects. Cohort studies such as the famous Framingham Study have been used in the investigation of cardiovascular risk factors.

Finally, ecologic studies involve the study of groups, rather than the individual, as the unit of analysis. Examples are comparisons of national variations in coronary heart disease mortality or variations in mortality at the census tract level. In the former example, a country is the "group," whereas in the latter, a census tract is the group. Ecologic studies have linked high fat diets to high levels of coronary heart disease mortality. Other ecologic studies have suggested that congenital malformations may be associated with concentrations of hazardous wastes.

1.3.7   Pharmacoeconomic Studies and Quality of Life

Pharmacoeconomics examines the tradeoff of cost versus benefit for new drugs. The high cost of medical care has caused HMOs, other health insurers, and even some regulatory bodies to consider the economic aspects of drug development and marketing. Cost control became an important discipline in the development and marketing of drugs in the 1990s and will continue to grow in importance during the current century. Pharmaceutical companies are becoming increasingly aware of the need to gain expertise in pharmacoeconomics as they start to implement cost control techniques in clinical trials as part of winning regulatory approvals and, more importantly, convincing pharmacies of the value of stocking their products. The ever-increasing cost of medical care has led manufacturers of medical devices and pharmaceuticals to recognize the need to evaluate products in terms of cost versus effectiveness in addition to the usual efficacy and safety criteria that are standard for regulatory approvals. The regulatory authorities in many countries also see the need for these studies.

Predicting the cost versus benefit of a newly developed drug involves an element of uncertainty. Consequently, statistical methods play an important role in such analyses. Currently, there are many articles and books on projecting the costs versus benefits in new drug development. A good starting point is Bootman (1996). One of the interesting and important messages from Bootman's book is the need to consider a perspective for the analysis. The perceptions of cost/benefit tradeoffs differ depending on whether they are seen from the patient's perspective, the physician's perspective, society's perspective, an HMO's perspective, or a pharmacy's perspective. The perspective has an important effect on which drug-related costs should be included, what comparisons should be made between alternative formulations, and which type of analysis is needed. Further discussion of cost/benefit tradeoffs is beyond the scope of this text. Nevertheless, it is important for health scientists to be aware of such tradeoffs.

Quality of life has played an increasing role in the study of medical treatments for patients. Physicians, medical device companies, and pharmaceutical firms have started to recognize that the patient's own feeling of well-being after a treatment is as important or more important than some clinically measurable efficacy parameters. Also, in comparing alternative treatments, providers need to realize that many products are basically equivalent in terms of the traditional safety and efficacy measures and that what might set one treatment apart from the others could be an increase in the quality of a patient's life. In the medical research literature, you will see many terms that all basically deal with the patients' view of the quality of their life. These terms and acronyms are quality of life (QoL), health related quality of life (HRQoL), outcomes research, and patient reported outcomes (PRO).

Quality of life usually is measured through specific survey questionnaires. Researchers have developed and validated many questionnaires for use in clinical trials to establish improvements in aspects of patients' quality of life. These questionnaires, which are employed to assess quality of life issues, generate qualitative data.

In Chapter 12, we will introduce you to research that involves the use of statistical analysis measures for qualitative data. The survey instruments, their validation and analysis are worthy topics for an entire book. For example, Fayers and Machin (2000) give an excellent introduction to this subject matter.

In conclusion, Chapter 1 has presented introductory material regarding the field of statistics. This chapter has illustrated how statistics are important in everyday life and, in particular, has demonstrated how statistics are used in the health sciences. In addition, the chapter has reviewed major job roles for statisticians. Finally, information was presented on major categories of study designs and sources of health data that statisticians may encounter. Tables 1.1 through 1.3 review and summarize the key points presented in this chapter regarding the uses of statistics, job roles for statisticians, and sources of health data.

Table 1.1. Uses of Statistics in Health Sciences

1. Interpret research studies
   Example: Validity of findings of health education and medical research
2. Evaluate statistics used every day
   Examples: Hospital mortality rates, prevalence of infectious diseases
3. Presentation of data to audiences
   Effective arrangement and grouping of information and graphical display of data
4. Illustrate central tendency and variability
5. Formulate and test hypotheses
   Generalize from a sample to the population.

Table 1.2. What Do Statisticians Do?

1. Guide design of an experiment, clinical trial, or survey
2. Formulate statistical hypotheses and determine appropriate methodology
3. Analyze data
4. Present and interpret results

Table 1.3. Sources of Health Data.

1. Archival and vital statistics records
2. Experiments
3. Medical research studies
   Retrospective—case control
   Prospective—cohort study
4. Descriptive surveys
5. Clinical trials

1.4 EXERCISES

1.1   What is your current job or future career objective? How can an understanding of statistics be helpful in your career?

1.2   What are some job roles for statisticians in the health field?

1.3   Compare and contrast descriptive and inferential statistics. How are they related?

1.4   Explain the major difference between prospective and retrospective studies. Does one have advantages over the other?

1.5   What is the difference between observational and experimental studies? Why do we conduct experimental studies? What is the purpose of observational studies?

1.6   What are cross-sectional studies? What types of questions can they address?

1.7   Why are quality control methods important to manufacturers? List at least three quality control methods discussed in the chapter.

1.8   Clinical trials play a vital role in testing and development of new drugs and medical devices.
   a. What are clinical trials?
   b. Explain the difference between controlled and uncontrolled trials.
   c. Why are controls important?
   d. What are single and double blinding? How is blinding used in a clinical trial?
   e. What types of outcomes for patients are measured through the use of clinical trials? Name at least four.

1.9   Epidemiology, a fundamental discipline in public health, has many applications in the health sciences.
   a. Name three types of epidemiologic study designs.
   b. What types of problems can we address with them?

1.10   Suppose a health research institute is conducting an experiment to determine whether a computerized, self-instructional module can aid in smoking cessation.
   a. Propose a research question that would be relevant to this experiment.
   b. Is there an independent variable (exposure factor) in the institute's experiment?
   c. How should the subjects be assigned to the treatment and control groups in order to minimize bias?

1.11 A pharmaceutical company wishes to develop and market a new medication to control blood sugar in diabetic patients. Suggest a clinical trial for evaluating the efficacy of this new medication.

    a. Describe the criteria you would use to select cases or patients.

    b. Is there a treatment to compare with a competing treatment or against a placebo?

    c. How do you measure effectiveness?

    d. Do you need to address the safety aspects of the treatment?

    e. Have you planned an early stopping rule for the trial if the treatment appears to be unsafe?

    f. Are you using blinding in the trial? If so, how are you implementing it? What problems does blinding help you avoid?

1.12 Search the Web for a media account that involves statistical information. For example, you may be able to locate a report on a disease, a clinical trial, or a new medical device. Alternatively, if you do not have access to the Web, newspaper articles may cover similar topics. Sometimes advertisements for medicines present statistics. Select one media account and answer the following questions:

    a. How were the data obtained?

    b. Based on the information presented, do you think that the investigators used a descriptive or inferential approach?

    c. If inferences are being drawn, what is the main question being addressed?

    d. How was the sample selected? To what groups can the results be generalized?

    e. Could the results be biased? If so, what are the potential sources of bias?

    f. Were conclusions presented? If so, do you think they were warranted? Why or why not?

1.13 Public interest groups and funding organizations are demanding that clinical trials include diverse study populations—from the standpoint of age, gender, and ethnicity. What do you think is the reasoning behind this demand? Based on what you have read in this chapter as well as your own experiences, what are the advantages and disadvantages of using diverse study groups in clinical trials?

1.5   ADDITIONAL READING

Included here is a list of many references that the student might find helpful. Many pertain to the material in this chapter and all are relevant to the material in this text as a whole. Some also were referenced in the chapter. In addition, the quotes in the present text come from the book of statistical quotations, "Statistically Speaking," by Gaither and Cavazos-Gaither, as we mentioned in the Preface. The student is encouraged to look through the other quotes in that book.

They may be particularly meaningful after you have completed reading this textbook.

Senn (reference #32) covers important and subtle issues in drug development, including issues that involve the design and analysis of experiments, epidemiological studies, and clinical trials. We already have alluded to some of these issues in this chapter. Chow and Shao (reference #11) presents the gamut of statistical methodologies in the various stages of drug development. The present text provides basic methods and a few advanced techniques but does not cover issues such as clinical relevance, development objectives, and regulatory objectives that the student might find interesting. Senn's book (reference #32) and Chow and Shao (reference #11) both provide this insight at a level that the student can appreciate, especially after completing this text.

1. Altman, D. G. (1991). *Practical Statistics for Medical Research*. Chapman and Hall, London.

2. Anderson, M. J. and Fienberg, S. E. (2000). *Who Counts? The Politics of Census-Taking in Contemporary America*. Russell Sage Foundation, New York.

3. Bland, M. (2000). *An Introduction to Medical Statistics. Third Edition*. Oxford University Press, Oxford.

4. Bootman, J. L. (Ed.) (1996). *Principles of Pharmacoeconomics*. Harvey Whitney Books, Cincinnati.

5. Box, G. E. P. and Draper, N. R. (1969). *Evolutionary Operation*. Wiley, New York.

6. Box, G. E. P. and Draper, N. R. (1987). *Empirical Model-Building and Response Surfaces*. Wiley, New York.

7. Box, G. E. P., Hunter, W. G. and Hunter, J. S. (1978). *Statistics for Experimenters*. Wiley, New York.

8. Box, J. F. (1978). *R. A. Fisher: The Life of a Scientist*. Wiley, New York.

9. Chernick, M. R. (1999). *Bootstrap Methods: A Practitioner's Guide*. Wiley, New York.

10. Chow, S.-C. (2000). *Encyclopedia of Biopharmaceutical Statistics*. Marcel Dekker, New York.

11. Chow, S.-C. and Shao, J. (2002). *Statistics in Drug Research: Methodologies and Recent Developments*. Marcel Dekker, New York.

12. Fayers, P. M. and Machin, D. (2000). *Quality of Life: Assessment, Analysis and Interpretation*. Wiley, New York.

13. Friis, R. H. and Sellers, T. A. (1999). *Epidemiology for Public Health Practice*, Second Edition. Aspen Publishers, Inc., Gaithersburg, Maryland.

14. Gaither, C. C. and Cavazos-Gaither, A. E. (1996). *"Statistically Speaking": A Dictionary of Quotations*. Institute of Physics Publishing, Bristol, United Kingdom.

15. Hald, A. (1990). *A History of Probability and Statistics and Their Applications before 1750*. Wiley, New York.

16. Hald, A. (1998). *A History of Mathematical Statistics from 1750 to 1930*. Wiley, New York.

17. Jennison, C and Turnbull, B. W. (2000). *Group Sequential Methods with Applications to Clinical Trials*. Chapman and Hall/CRC, Boca Raton, Florida.

18. Juran, J. M. and Godfrey, A. B. (Eds.) (1999). *Juran's Quality Handbook,* Fifth Edition. McGraw-Hill, New York.

19. Kuzma, J. W. (1998). *Basic Statistics for the Health Sciences,* Third Edition. Mayfield Publishing Company, Mountain View, California.

20. Kuzma, J. W. and Bohnenblust, S. E. (2001). *Basic Statistics for the Health Sciences,* Fourth Edition. Mayfield Publishing Company, Mountain View, California.

21. Lachin, J. M. (2000). *Biostatistical Methods: The Assessment of Relative Risks.* Wiley, New York.

22. Montgomery, D. C. (1997). *Design and Analysis of Experiments,* Fourth Edition. Wiley, New York.

23. Mosteller, F. and Tukey, J. W. (1977). *Data Analysis and Regression: A Second Course in Statistics.* Addison-Wesley, Reading, Massachusetts.

24. Myers, R. H. and Montgomery, D. C. (1995). *Response Surface Methodology: Process and Product Optimization Using Designed Experiments.* Wiley, New York.

25. Motulsky, H. (1995). *Intuitive Biostatistics.* Oxford University Press, New York.

26. Orkin, M. (2000). *What are the Odds? Chance in Everyday Life.* W. H. Freeman, New York.

27. Piantadosi, S. (1997). *Clinical Trials: A Methodologic Perspective.* Wiley, New York.

28. Porter, T. M. (1986). *The Rise of Statistical Thinking.* Princeton University Press, Princeton, New Jersey.

29. Riffenburgh, R. H. (1999). *Statistics in Medicine.* Academic Press, San Diego.

30. Ryan, T. P. (1989). *Statistical Methods for Quality Improvement.* Wiley, New York.

31. Salsburg, D. (2001). *The Lady Tasting Tea: How Statistics Revolutionized Science in the Twentieth Century.* W. H. Freeman and Company, New York.

32. Senn, S. (1997). *Statistical Issues in Drug Development.* Wiley, Chichester, United Kingdom.

33. Shumway, R. H. and Stoffer, D. S. (2000). *Time Series Analysis and Its Applications.* Springer-Verlag, New York.

34. Sokal, R. R. and Rohlf, F. J. (1981). *Biometry,* Second Edition. W. H. Freeman, New York.

35. Stigler, S. M. (1986). *The History of Statistics: The Measurement of Uncertainty before 1900.* Harvard University Press, Cambridge, Massachusetts.

36. Stigler, S. M. (1999). *Statistics on the Table.* Harvard University Press, Cambridge, Massachusetts.

37. Tukey, J. W. (1977). *Exploratory Data Analysis.* Addison-Wesley, Reading, Massachusetts.

38. Vardeman, S. B. and Jobe, J. M. (1999). *Statistical Quality Assurance Methods for Engineers.* Wiley, New York.

39. Wu, C. F. J. and Hamada, M. (2000). *Experiments: Planning, Analysis, and Parameter Design Optimization.* Wiley, New York.

CHAPTER 2

Defining Populations
and Selecting Samples

*After painstaking and careful analysis of a sample, you are always
told that it is the wrong sample and doesn't apply to the problem.*
—Arthur Bloch, *Murphy's Law.* Fourth Law of Revision, p. 48

Chapter 1 provided an introduction to the field of biostatistics. We discussed applications of statistics, study designs, as well as descriptive statistics, or exploratory
data analysis, and inferential statistics, or confirmatory data analysis. Now we will
consider in more detail an aspect of inferential statistics—sample selection—that
relates directly to our ability to make inferences about a population.

In this chapter, we define the terms population and sample and present several
methods for selecting samples. We present a rationale for selecting samples and
give examples of several types of samples: simple random, convenience, systematic, stratified random, and cluster. In addition, we discuss bootstrap sampling because of its similarity to simple random sampling. Bootstrap sampling is a procedure for generating bootstrap estimates of parameters, as we will demonstrate in
later chapters. Detailed instructions for selecting simple random and bootstrap samples will be provided. The chapter concludes with a discussion of an important
property of random sampling, namely, unbiasedness.

2.1 WHAT ARE POPULATIONS AND SAMPLES?

The term population refers to a collection of people or objects that share common
observable characteristics. For example, a population could be all of the people who
live in your city, all of the students enrolled in a particular university, or all of the
people who are afflicted by a certain disease (e.g., all women diagnosed with breast
cancer during the last five years). Generally, researchers are interested in particular
characteristics of a population, not the characteristics that define the population but
rather such attributes as height, weight, gender, age, heart rate, and systolic or diastolic blood pressure.

Introductory Biostatistics for the Health Sciences, by Michael R. Chernick
and Robert H. Friis. ISBN 0-471-41137-X. Copyright © 2003 Wiley-Interscience.

Recall the approaches of statistics (descriptive and inferential) discussed in Chapter 1. In making inferences about populations we use samples. A sample is a subset of the population.

In this chapter we will discuss techniques for selecting samples from populations. You will see that various forms of random sampling are preferable to nonrandom sampling because random sample designs allow us to apply statistical methods to make inferences about population characteristics based on data collected from samples.

When describing the attributes of populations, statisticians use the term parameter. In this text, the symbol μ will be used to denote a population parameter for the average (also called the mean or expected value). The corresponding estimate from a sample is called a statistic. For the sample estimate, the mean is denoted by $\overline{X}$.

Thus, it is possible to refer to the average height or age of a population (the parameter) as well as the average height of a sample (a statistic). In fact, we need inferential statistics because we are unable to determine the values of the population parameters and must use the sample statistics in their place. Using the sample statistic in place of the population parameter is called estimation.

2.2   WHY SELECT A SAMPLE?

Often, it is too expensive or impossible to collect information on an entire population. For appropriately chosen samples, accurate statistical estimates of population parameters are possible. Even when we are required to count the entire population as in a U.S. decennial census, sampling can be used to improve estimates for important subpopulations (e.g., states, counties, cities, or precincts).

In the most recent national election, we learned that the outcome of a presidential election in a single state (Florida) was close enough to be in doubt as a consequence of various types of counting errors or exclusion rules. So even when we think we are counting every vote accurately we may not be; surprisingly, a sample estimate may be more accurate than a "complete" count.

As an example of a U.S. government agency that uses sampling, consider the Internal Revenue Service (IRS). The IRS does not have the manpower necessary to review every tax return for mistakes or misrepresentation; instead, the IRS chooses a selected sample of returns. The IRS applies statistical methods to make it more likely that those returns prone to error or fraud are selected in the sample.

A second example arises from reliability studies, which may use destructive testing procedures. To illustrate, a medical device company often tests the peel strength of its packaging material. The company wants the material to peel when suitable force is applied but does not want the seal to come open upon normal handling and shipping. The purpose of the seal is to maintain sterility for medical products, such as catheters, contained in the packages. Because these catheters will be placed inside patients' hearts to treat arrhythmias, maintenance of sterility in order to prevent infection is very important. When performing reliability tests, it is feasible to peel only a small percentage of the packages, because it is costly to waste good packaging. On the other hand, accurate statistical inference requires selecting sufficiently large samples.

One of the main challenges of statistics is to select a sample in an efficient, appropriate way; the goal of sample selection is to be as accurate as possible in order to draw a meaningful inference about population characteristics from results of the sample. At this point, it may not be obvious to you that the method of drawing a sample is important. However, history has taught us that it is very easy to draw incorrect inferences because samples were chosen inappropriately.

We often see the results of inappropriate sampling in television and radio polls. This subtle problem is known as a selection bias. Often we are interested in a wider target population but the poll is based only on those individuals who listened to a particular TV or radio program and chose to answer the questions. For instance, if there is a political question and the program has a Republican commentator, the audience may be more heavily Republican than the general target population. Consequently, the survey results will not reflect the target population. In this example, we are assuming that the response rate was sufficiently high to produce reliable results had the sample been random.

Statisticians also call this type of sampling error response bias. This bias often occurs when volunteers are asked to respond to a poll. Even if the listeners of a particular radio or TV program are representative of the target population, those who respond to the poll may not be. Consequently, reputable poll organizations such as Gallup or Harris use well-established statistical procedures to ensure that the sample is representative of the population.

A classic example of failure to select a representative sample of voters arose from the *Literary Digest* Poll of 1936. In that year, the *Literary Digest* mailed out some 10 million ballots asking individuals to provide their preference for the upcoming election between Franklin Roosevelt and Alfred Landon. Based on the survey results derived from the return of 2.3 million ballots, the *Literary Digest* predicted that Landon would be a big winner.

In fact, Roosevelt won the election with a handy 62% majority. This single poll destroyed the credibility of the *Literary Digest* and soon caused it to cease publication. Subsequent analysis of their sampling technique showed that the list of 10 million persons was taken primarily from telephone directories and motor vehicle registration lists. In more recent surveys of voters, public opinion organizations have found random digit dialed telephone surveys, as well as surveys of drivers, to be acceptable, because almost every home in the United States has a telephone and almost all citizens of voting age own or lease automobiles and hence have drivers licenses. The requirement for the pollsters is not that the list be exhaustive but rather that it be representative of the entire population and thus not capable of producing a large response or selection bias. However, in 1936, mostly Americans with high incomes had phones or owned cars.

The *Literary Digest* poll selected a much larger proportion of high-income families than are typical in the voting population. Also, the high-income families were more likely to vote Republican than the lower-income families. Consequently, the poll favored the Republican, Alf Landon, whereas the target population, which contained a much larger proportion of low-income Democrats than were in the survey, strongly favored the Democrat, Franklin Roosevelt. Had these economic groups been sampled in the appropriate proportions, the poll would have correctly predicted the outcome of the election.

2.3   HOW SAMPLES CAN BE SELECTED

2.3.1   Simple Random Sampling

Statisticians have found that one of the easiest and most convenient methods for achieving reliable inferences about a population is to take a simple random sample. Random sampling ensures unbiased estimates of population parameters. Unbiased means that the average of the sample estimates over all possible samples is equal to the population parameter. Unbiasedness is a statistical property based on probability theory and can be proven mathematically through the definition of a simple random sample.

The concept of simple random sampling involves the selection of a sample of size n from a population of size N. Later in this text, we will show, through combinatorial mathematics, the total number of possible ways (say Z) to select a sample of size n out of a population of size N. Simple random sampling provides a mechanism that gives an equal chance $1/Z$ of selecting any one of these Z samples. This statement implies that each individual in the population has an equal chance of selection into the sample.

In Section 2.4, we will show you a method based on random number tables for selecting random samples. Suppose we want to estimate the mean of a population (a parameter) by using the mean of a sample (a statistic). Remember that we are not saying that the individual sample estimate will equal the population parameter. If we were to select all possible samples of a fixed size (n) from the parent population, when all possible means are averaged we would obtain the population parameter. The relationship between the mean of all possible sample means and the population parameter is a conceptual issue specified by the central limit theorem (discussed in Chapter 7). For now, it is sufficient to say that in most applications we do not generate all possible samples of size n. In practice, we select only one sample to estimate the parameter. The unbiasedness property of sample means does not even guarantee that individual estimates will be accurate (i.e., close to the parameter value).

2.3.2   Convenience Sampling

Convenience sampling is just what the name suggests: the patients or samples are selected by an arbitrary method that is easy to carry out. Some researchers refer to these types of samples as "grab bag" samples.

A desirable feature of samples is that they be representative of the population, i.e., that they mirror the underlying characteristics of the population from which they were selected. Unfortunately, there is no guarantee of the representativeness of convenience samples; thus, estimates based on these samples are likely to be biased.

However, convenience samples have been used when it is very difficult or impossible to draw a random sample. Results of studies based on convenience samples are descriptive and may be used to suggest future research, but they should not be used to draw inferences about the population under study.

As a final point, we note that while random sampling does produce unbiased estimates of population parameters, it does not *guarantee* balance in any particular sample drawn at random. In random sampling, all samples of size n out of a population of size N are equally possible. While many of these samples are balanced with respect to demographic characteristics, some are not.

Extreme examples of nonrepresentative samples are (1) the sample containing the n smallest values for the population parameter and (2) the sample containing the n largest values. Because neither of these samples is balanced, both can give poor estimates.

For example (regarding point 2), suppose a catheter ablation treatment is known to have a 95% chance of success. That means that we expect only about one failure in a sample of size 20. However, even though the probability is very small, it is possible that we could select a random sample of 20 individuals with the outcome that all 20 individuals have failed ablation procedures.

2.3.3 Systematic Sampling

Often, systematic sampling is used when a sampling frame (a complete list of people or objects constituting the population) is available. The procedure is to go to the top of the list and select the first person or start at an arbitrary but specified initial point in the table. The choice of the first point really does not matter, but merely starts the process and must be specified to make the procedure repeatable. Then we skip the next n people on the list and select the $n + 2$ person. We continue to skip n people and select the next one after n people are skipped. We continue this process until we have exhausted the list.

Here is an example of systematic sampling: suppose a researcher needs to select 30 patients from a list of 5000 names (as stated previously, the list is called the sampling frame and conveniently defines the population from which we are sampling). The researcher would select the first patient on the list, skip to the thirty-second name on the list, select that name, and then skip the next 30 names and select the next name after that, repeating this process until a total of 30 names has been selected. In this example, the sampling interval (i.e., number of skipped cases) is 30.

In the foregoing procedure, we designated the sampling interval first. As we would go through only slightly more than 800 of the 5000 names, we would not exhaust the list. Alternatively, we could select a certain percentage of patients, for example, 1%. That would be a sample size of 50 for a list of 5000. Although the choice of the number of names to skip is arbitrary, suppose we skip 100 names on the list; the first patient will be 1, the second 102, the third 203, the fourth 304, the fifth 405, and so on until we reach the final one, the fiftieth number, 4950. In this case, we nearly exhaust the list, and the samples are evenly selected throughout the list.

As you can see, systematic sampling is easy and convenient when such a complete list exists. If there is no relationship between the order of the people on the list and the characteristics that we are measuring, it is a perfectly acceptable sampling method. In some applications, we may be able to convince ourselves that this situation is true.

However, there are situations in which systematic sampling can be disastrous. Suppose, for example, that one of the population characteristics we are interested in is age. Now let us assume that the population consists of 50 communities in Southern California. Each community contains 100 people.

We construct our sampling frame by sorting each member according to age, from the youngest to the oldest in each community, and then arranging the communities in some order one after another, such as in alphabetical order by community name. Here $N = 5,000$ and we want $n = 50$. One way to choose a systematic sample would be to select the first member from each community.

We could have obtained the sample by selecting the first person on the list and then skipping the next 99. But, thereby, we would select the youngest member from each community, thus providing a severely biased estimate (on the low side) of the average age in the population. Similarly, if we were to skip the first 99 people and always take the hundreth, we would be biased on the high side, as we would select only the oldest person in each community.

Systematic sampling can lead to difficulties when the variable of interest is periodic (with period n) in the sequence order of the sampling frame. The term periodic refers to the situation in which groups of elements appear in a cyclical pattern in the list instead of being uniformly distributed throughout the list. We can consider the sections of the list in which these elements are concentrated to be peaks, and the sections in which they are absent to be troughs. If we skip n people in the sequence and start at a peak value, we will select only the peak values. The same result would happen for troughs. For the scenario in which we select the peaks, our estimate will be biased on the high side; for the trough scenario, we will be biased on the low side.

Here is an example of the foregoing source of sampling error, called a periodic or list effect. If we used a very long list such as a telephone directory for our sampling frame and needed to sample only a few names using a short sampling interval, it is possible that we could select by accident a sample from a portion of the list in which a certain ethnic group is concentrated. The resulting sample would not be very representative of the population. If the characteristics of interest to us varied considerably by ethnic group, our estimate of the population parameter could be very biased.

To realize that the foregoing situation could happen easily, recall that many Caucasians have the surnames Jones and Smith, whereas many Chinese are named Liu, and many Vietnamese are named Nguyen. So if we happened to start near Smith we would obtain mostly Caucasian subjects and mostly Chinese subjects if we started at Liu!

2.3.4   Stratified Random Sampling

Stratified random sampling is a modification of simple random sampling that is used when we want to ensure that each stratum (subgroup) constitutes an appropriate proportion or representation in the sample. Stratified random sampling also can be used to improve the accuracy of sample estimates when it is known that the variability in the data is not constant across the subgroups.

The method of stratified random sampling is very simple. We define m subgroups or strata. For the ith subgroup, we select a simple random sample of size n_i. We follow this procedure for each subgroup. The total sample size n is then $\Sigma_{i=1}^n n_i$.

The notation Σ stands for the summation of the individual n_i's. For example, if there are three groups, then $\Sigma_{i=1}^3 n_i = n_1 + n_2 + n_3$. Generally we have a total sample size "n" in mind.

Statistical theory can demonstrate that in many situations, stratified random sampling produces an unbiased estimate of the population mean with better precision than does simple random sampling with the same total sample size n. Precision of the estimate is improved when we choose large values of n_i for the subgroups with the largest variability and small values for the subgroups with the least variability.

2.3.5   Cluster Sampling

As an alternative to the foregoing sampling methods, statisticians sometimes select cluster samples. Cluster sampling refers to a method of sampling in which the element selected is a group (as distinguished from an individual), called a cluster. For example, the clusters could be city blocks. Often, the U.S. Bureau of the Census finds cluster sampling to be a convenient way of sampling.

The Bureau might conduct a survey by selecting city blocks at random from a list of city blocks in a particular city. The Bureau would interview a head of household from every household in each city block selected. Often, this method will be more economically feasible than other ways to sample, particularly if the Census Bureau has to send employees out to the communities to conduct the interviews in person.

Cluster sampling often works very well. Since the clusters are selected at random, the samples can be representative of the population; unbiased estimates of the population total or mean value for a particular parameter can be obtained. Sometimes, there is loss of precision for the estimate relative to simple random sampling; however, this disadvantage can be offset by the reduction in cost of the data collection.

See Chapter 9 of Cochran (1977) for a more detailed discussion and some mathematical results about cluster sampling. Further discussion can be found in Lohr (1999) and Kish (1965). While clusters can be of equal or unequal size, the mathematics is simpler for equal size. The three aforementioned texts develop the theory for equal cluster sizes first and then go on to deal with the more complicated case of unequal cluster sizes.

Thus far in Section 2.3, we have presented a brief description of sampling techniques used in surveys. For a more complete discussion see Scheaffer, Mendenhall, and Ott (1979), Kish (1965), Cochran (1977), or Lohr (1999).

2.3.6   Bootstrap Sampling

Throughout this text, we will discuss both parametric and nonparametric methods of statistical inference. One such nonparametric technique is the bootstrap, a statistical technique in which inferences are made without reliance on parametric models for the population distribution. Other nonparametric techniques are covered in Chapter 14. Nonparametric methods provide a means for obtaining sample estimates or testing hypotheses without making parametric assumptions about the distribution being sampled.

The account of the bootstrap in this book is very elementary and brief. A more thorough treatment can be obtained from the following books: Efron and Tibshirani (1993), Davison and Hinkley (1997), and Chernick (1999). An elementary and abbreviated account can be found in the monograph by Mooney and Duval (1993).

Before considering the bootstrap in more detail, let us review sampling with replacement and sampling without replacement. Suppose we are selecting items in sequence from our population. If, after we select the first item from our population, we allow that item to remain on the list of eligible items for subsequent selection and we continue selecting in this way, we are performing sampling with replacement. Simple random sampling differs from sampling with replacement in that we remove each item from the list of possible subsequent selections. So in simple random sampling, no observations are repeated. Simple random sampling uses sampling without replacement.

The bootstrap procedure can be approximated by using a Monte Carlo (random sampling) method. This approximation makes the bootstrap a practical, though computationally intensive, procedure. The bootstrap sampling procedure takes a random sample with replacement from the original sample. That is, we take samples from a sample (i.e., we resample).

In Section 2.4, we describe a mechanism for generating a simple random sample (sampling without replacement from the population). Because bootstrap sampling is so similar to simple random sampling, Section 2.5 will describe the procedure for generating bootstrap samples.

The differences between bootstrap sampling and simple random sampling are first, that instead of sampling from a population, a bootstrap sample is generated by sampling from a sample, and, second, that the sampling is done with replacement instead of without replacement. These differences will be made clear in Section 2.5.

2.4   HOW TO SELECT A SIMPLE RANDOM SAMPLE

Simple random sampling can be defined as sampling without replacement from a population. In Section 5.5, when we cover permutations and combinations, you will learn that there are $C(N, n) = N!/[(N - n)! \, n!]$ distinct samples of size n out of a population of size N, where $n!$ is factorial notation and stands for the product $n(n - 1)$ $(n - 2) \ldots 3\ 2\ 1$. The notation $C(N, n)$ is just a symbol for the number of ways of selecting a subgroup of size n out of a larger group of size N, where the order of selecting the elements is not considered.

Simple random sampling has the property that each of these $C(N, n)$ samples has the same probability of selection. One way, but not a common way, to generate a simple random sample is to order these samples from 1 all the way to $C(N, n)$ and then randomly generate (using a uniform random number generator, which will be described shortly) an integer between 1 and $C(N, n)$. You then choose the sample that corresponds to a chosen index.

Let us illustrate this method of generating a simple random sample with the following example. We have six patients whom we have labeled alphabetically. So the population of patients is the set {A, B, C, D, E, F}. Suppose that we want our sample size to be four. The number of possible samples will be $C(6, 4) = 6!/[4! \, 2!] = 6 \times 5 \times 4 \times 3 \times 2 \times 1/[(4 \times 3 \times 2 \times 1)(2 \times 1)]$; after reducing the fraction, we obtain $3 \times 5 = 15$ possible samples.

We enumerate the samples as follows:

  1. {A, B, C, D}
  2. {A, B, C, E}
  3. {A, B, C, F}
  4. {A, B, D, E}
  5. {A, B, D, F}
  6. {A, B, E, F}
  7. {A, C, D, E}
  8. {A, C, D, F}
  9. {A, C, E, F}
 10. {A, D, E, F}
 11. {B, C, D, E}
 12. {B, C, D, F}
 13. {B, C, E, F}
 14. {B, D, E, F}
 15. {C, D, E, F}.

We then use a table of uniform random numbers or a computerized pseudorandom number generator. A pseudorandom number generator is a computer algorithm that generates a sequence of numbers that behave like uniform random numbers.

Uniform random numbers and their associated uniform probability distribution will be explained in Chapter 5. To assign a random index, we take the interval [0, 1] and divide it into 15 equal parts that do not overlap. This means that the first interval will be from 0 to 1/15, the second from 1/15 to 2/15, and so on. A decimal approximation to 1/15 is 0.0667. So the assigned index (we will call it an index rule) depends on the uniform random number U as follows:

If $0 \leq U < 0.0667$, then the index is 1.
If $0.0667 \leq U < 0.1333$, then the index is 2.
If $0.1333 \leq U < 0.2000$, then the index is 3.
If $0.2000 \leq U < 0.2667$, then the index is 4.
If $0.2667 \leq U < 0.3333$, then the index is 5.
If $0.3333 \leq U < 0.4000$, then the index is 6.
If $0.4000 \leq U < 0.4667$, then the index is 7.
If $0.4667 \leq U < 0.5333$, then the index is 8.
If $0.5333 \leq U < 0.6000$, then the index is 9.
If $0.6000 \leq U < 0.6667$, then the index is 10.
If $0.6667 \leq U < 0.7333$, then the index is 11.
If $0.7333 \leq U < 0.8000$, then the index is 12.
If $0.8000 \leq U < 0.8667$, then the index is 13.
If $0.8667 \leq U < 0.9333$, then the index is 14.
If $0.9333 \leq U < 1.0$, then the index is 15.

Now suppose that we consulted a table of uniform random numbers, (refer to Table 2.1). We see that this table consists of five-digit numbers. Let us arbitrarily select the number in column 7, row 19. We see that this number is 24057.

To convert 24057 to a number between 0 and 1, we simply place a decimal point in front of the first digit. Our uniform random number is then 0.24057. From the index rule described previously, we see that $U = 0.24057$. Since $0.2000 \leq U < 0.2667$, the index is 4. We now refer back to our enumeration of samples and see that the index 4 corresponds to the sample $\{A, B, D, E\}$. So patients A, B, D, and E are selected as our sample of four patients from the set of six patients.

A more common way to generate a simple random sample is to choose four random numbers to select individual patients. This procedure is accomplished by sampling without replacement. First we order the patients as follows:

1. A
2. B
3. C
4. D
5. E
6. F

TABLE 2.1. Five Digit Uniform Random Numbers (350)

Col./Row	1	2	3	4	5	6	7	8	9	10
1	00439	60176	48503	14559	18274	45809	09748	19716	15081	84704
2	29676	37909	95673	66757	04164	94000	19939	55374	26109	58722
3	69386	71708	88608	67251	22512	00169	02887	84072	91832	97489
4	68381	61725	49122	75836	15368	52551	58711	43014	95376	57402
5	69158	38683	41374	17028	09304	10834	10332	07534	79067	27126
6	00858	04352	17833	41105	46569	90109	32335	65895	64362	01431
7	86972	51707	58242	16035	94887	83510	53124	85750	98015	00038
8	30606	45225	30161	07973	03034	82983	61369	65913	65478	62319
9	93864	49044	57169	43125	11703	87009	06219	28040	10050	05974
10	61937	90217	56708	35351	60820	90729	28489	88186	74006	18320
11	94551	69538	52924	08530	79302	34981	60530	96317	29918	16918
12	79385	49498	48569	57888	70564	17660	68930	39693	87372	09600
13	86232	01398	50258	22868	71052	10127	48729	67613	59400	65886
14	04912	01051	33687	03296	17112	23843	16796	22332	91570	47197
15	15455	88237	91026	36454	18765	97891	11022	98774	00321	10386
16	88430	09861	45098	66176	59598	98527	11059	31626	10798	50313
17	48849	11583	63654	55670	89474	75232	14186	52377	19129	67166
18	33659	59617	40920	30295	07463	79923	83393	77120	38862	75503
19	60198	41729	19897	04805	09351	76734	24057	87776	36947	88618
20	55868	53145	66232	52007	81206	89543	66226	45709	37114	78075
21	22011	71396	95174	43043	68304	36773	83931	43631	50995	68130
22	90301	54934	08008	00565	67790	84760	82229	64147	28031	11609
23	07586	90936	21021	54066	87281	63574	41155	01740	29025	19909
24	09973	76136	87904	54419	34370	75071	56201	16768	61934	12083
25	59750	42528	19864	31595	72097	17005	24682	43560	74423	59197
26	74492	19327	17812	63897	65708	07709	13817	95943	07909	75504
27	69042	57646	38606	30549	34351	21432	50312	10566	43842	70046
28	16054	32268	29828	73413	53819	39324	13581	71841	94894	64223
29	17930	78622	70578	23048	73730	73507	69602	77174	32593	45565
30	46812	93896	65639	73905	45396	71653	01490	33674	16888	53434
31	04590	07459	04096	15216	56633	69845	85550	15141	56349	56117
32	99618	63788	86396	37564	12962	96090	70358	23378	63441	36828
33	34545	32273	45427	30693	49369	27427	28362	17307	45092	08302
34	04337	00565	27718	67942	19284	69126	51649	03469	88009	41916
35	73810	70135	72055	90111	71202	08210	76424	66364	63081	37784

Source: Adapted from Kuzma (1998), p. 15.

Then we divide [0, 1] into six equal intervals to assign the index. We choose a uniform random number U and assign the indices as follows:

If $0 \le U < 0.1667$, then the index is 1.
If $0.1667 \le U < 0.3333$, then the index is 2.
If $0.3333 \le U < 0.5000$, then the index is 3.
If $0.5000 \le U < 0.6667$, then the index is 4.

If $0.6667 \leq U < 0.8333$, then the index is 5
If $0.8333 \leq U < 1.0$, then the index is 6.

Refer back to Table 2.1. We will use the first four numbers in column 1 as our set of uniform random numbers for this sample. The resulting numbers are 00439, 29676, 69386, and 68381. For the first patient we have the uniform random number (U) 0.00439. Since $0 \leq U < 0.1667$, the index is 1. Hence, our first selection is patient A.

Now we select the second patient at random but without replacement. Therefore, A must be removed. We are left with only five indices. So we must revise our scheme. The patient order is now as follows:

1. B
2. C
3. D
4. E
5. F

The uniform random number must be divided into five equal parts, so the index assignment is as follows:

If $0 \leq U < 0.2000$, then the index is 1.
If $0.2000 \leq U < 0.4000$, then the index is 2.
If $0.4000 \leq U < 0.6000$, then the index is 3.
If $0.6000 \leq U < 0.8000$, then the index is 4.
If $0.8000 \leq U < 1.0$, then the index is 5.

The second uniform number is 29676, so our uniform number U in [0, 1] is 0.29676. Since $0.2000 \leq U < 0.4000$, the index is 2. We see that the index 2 corresponds to patient C.

We continue to sample without replacement. Now we have only four indices left, which are assigned as follows:

1. B
2. D
3. E
4. F

The interval from [0, 1] must be divided into four equal parts with U assigned as follows:

If $0 \leq U < 0.2500$, then the index is 1.
If $0.2500 \leq U < 0.5000$, then the index is 2.

If $0.5000 \leq U < 0.7500$, then the index is 3.
If $0.7500 \leq U < 1.0$, then the index is 4.

Since our third uniform number is 69386, $U = 0.69386$. Since $0.5000 \leq U < 0.7500$, the index is 3. We see that the index 3 corresponds to patient E.

We have one more patient to select and are left with only three patients to choose from. The new ordering of patients is as follows:

1. B
2. D
3. F

We now divide $[0, 1]$ into three equal intervals as follows:

If $0 \leq U < 0.3333$, then the index is 1.
If $0.3333 \leq U < 0.6667$, then the index is 2.
If $0.6667 \leq U < 1.0$, then the index is 3.
The final uniform number is 68381. Therefore, $U = 0.68381$.

From the assignment above, we see that index 3 is selected and corresponds to patient F. The four patients selected are A, C, E, and F. The foregoing approach, in which patients are selected at random without replacement, is another legitimate way to generate a random sample of size 4 from a population of size 6. (When we do bootstrap sampling, which requires sampling with replacement, the methodology will be simpler than the foregoing approach.)

The second approach was simpler, in one respect, than the first approach. We did not have to identify and order all 15 possible samples of size 4. When the population size is larger than in the given example, the number of possible samples can become extremely large, making it difficult and time-consuming to enumerate them.

On the other hand, the first approach required the generation of only a single uniform random number, whereas the second approach required the generation of four. However, we have large tables and fast pseudorandom number generator algorithms at our disposal. So generating four times as many random numbers is not a serious problem.

It may not seem obvious that the two methods are equivalent. The equivalence can be proved mathematically by using probability methods. The proof of this equivalence is beyond the scope of this text. The sampling without replacement approach is not ideal because each time we select a patient we have to revise our index schemes, both the mapping of patients to indices and the choice of the index based on the uniform random number.

The use of a rejection-sampling scheme can speed up the process of sample selection considerably. In rejection sampling, we reject a uniform random number if it corresponds to an index that we have already picked. In this way, we can begin with the original indexing scheme and not change it. The trade-off is that we may need to generate a few more uniform random numbers in order to complete the sample. Because random number generation is fast, this trade-off is worthwhile.

Let us illustrate a rejection-sampling scheme with the same set of six patients as before, again selecting a random sample of size 4. This time, we will start in the second row, first column and move across the row. Our indexing schemes are fixed as described in the next paragraphs.

First we order the patients as follows:

1. A
2. B
3. C
4. D
5. E
6. F

Then we divide [0, 1] into six equal intervals to assign the index. We choose a uniform random number U and assign the indices as follows:

If $0 \le U < 0.1667$, then the index is 1.
If $0.1667 \le U < 0.3333$, then the index is 2.
If $0.3333 \le U < 0.5000$, then the index is 3.
If $0.5000 \le U < 0.6667$, then the index is 4.
If $0.6667 \le U < 0.8333$, then the index is 5
If $0.8333 \le U < 1.0$, then the index is 6.

The first uniform number is 29676, so $U = 0.29676$. The index is 2, and the corresponding patient is B. Our second uniform number is 37909, so $U = 0.37909$. The index is 3, and the corresponding patient is C. Our third uniform number is 95673, so $U = 0.95673$. The index is 6, and this corresponds to patient F. The fourth uniform number is 66757, so $U = 0.6676$ and the index is 5; this corresponds to patient E.

Through the foregoing process we have selected patients B, C, E, and F for our sample. Thus, we see that this approach was much faster than previous approaches. We were somewhat lucky in that no index repeated; thus, we did not have to reject any samples. Usually one or more samples will be rejected due to repetition.

To show what happens when we have repeated index numbers, suppose we had started in column 1 and simply gone down the column as we did when we used the sampling without replacement approach. The first random number is 00439, corresponding to $U = 0.00439$. The resulting index is 1, corresponding to patient A. The second random number is 29676, corresponding to $U = 0.29676$. The resulting index is 2, corresponding to patient B. The third random number is 69386, corresponding to $U = 0.69386$. The resulting index is 5, corresponding to patient E. The fourth random number is 68381, corresponding to $U = 0.68381$.

Again this process yields index 5 and corresponds to patient E. Since we cannot repeat patient E, we reject this number and proceed to the next uniform random number in our sequence. The number turns out to be 69158, corresponding to $U = 0.69158$, and index 5 is repeated again. So this number must be rejected also. The next random number is 00858, corresponding to $U = 0.00858$, and an index of 1, corresponding to patient A.

Now patient A already has been selected, so again we must reject the number and continue. The next uniform random number is 86972, corresponding to $U = 0.86972$; this corresponds to the index 6 and patient F. Because patient F has not been selected already, we accept this number and have completed the sample.

Recall the random number sequence 00439 $\rightarrow$ patient A, 29676 $\rightarrow$ patient B, 69386 $\rightarrow$ patient E, 68381 $\rightarrow$ patient E (repeat, so reject), 69158 $\rightarrow$ patient E (repeat, so reject), 00858 $\rightarrow$ patient A (repeat, so reject), and 86972 $\rightarrow$ patient F. Because we now have a sample of four patients, we are finished. The random sample is A, B, E, and F.

We have illustrated three methods for generating simple random samples and repeated the rejection method with a second sequence of uniform random numbers. Although the procedures are quite different from one another, it can be shown mathematically that samples generated by any of these three methods have the properties of simple random samples.

This result is important for you to remember, even though we are not showing you the mathematical proof. In our examples, the samples turned out to be different from one another. The first method led to A, B, D, E, the second to A, C, E, F, and the third to B, C, E, F, using the first sequence; and A, B, E, F when using the second sequence.

Differences occurred because of differences in the methods and differences in the sequence of uniform random numbers. But note also that even when different methods are used or different uniform random number sequences are used, it is possible to repeat a particular random sample.

Once the sample has been selected, we generally are interested in a characteristic of the patient population that we estimate from the sample. In our example, let us suppose that age is the characteristic of the population and that the six patients in the population have the following ages:

A. 26 years old
B. 17 years old
C. 45 years old
D. 70 years old
E. 32 years old
F. 9 years old

Although we generally refer to the sample as the set of patients, often the value of their characteristic is referred to as the sample. Because two patients can have the same age, it is possible to obtain repeat values in a simple random sample. The point to remember is that the individual patients selected cannot be repeated but the value of their characteristic may be repeated if it is the same for another patient.

A population parameter of interest might be the average age of the patients in the population. Because our population consists of only six patients, it is easy for us to calculate the population parameter in this instance. The mean age is defined as the sum of the ages divided by the number of patients. In this case, the population mean $\mu = (26 + 17 + 45 + 70 + 32 + 9)/6 = 199/6 = 33.1667$.

$$\mu = \frac{\sum_{i=1}^{N} X_i}{N} \qquad (2.1)$$

where X_i is the value for patient i and N is the population size.

Recall that a simple random sample has the property that the sample mean is an unbiased estimate of the population mean. This does not imply that the sample mean equals the population mean. It means only that the average of the sample means taken over all possible simple random samples equals the population mean.

This is a desirable statistical property and is one of the reasons why simple random sampling is used. Consider the population of six ages given previously. Suppose we choose a random sample of size 4. Suppose that the sample consists of patients B, C, E, and F. Then the sample mean $\overline{X} = (17 + 45 + 32 + 9)/4 = 19.5$.

$$\overline{X} = \frac{\sum_{i=1}^{n} X_i}{n} \qquad (2.2)$$

where X_i is the value for patient i in the sample and n is the sample size.

Now let us look at the four random samples that we generated previously and calculate the mean age in each case. In the first case, we chose A, B, D, E with ages 26, 17, 70, and 32, respectively. The sample mean $\overline{X} = (26 + 17 + 70 + 32)/4$ (the sum of the ages of the sample patients divided by the total sample size). In this case $\overline{X} = 36.2500$, which is slightly higher than the population mean of 33.1667.

Now consider case 2 with patients A, C, E, and F and corresponding ages 26, 45, 32, and 9. In this instance, $\overline{X} = (26 + 45 + 32 + 9)/4 = 28.0000$, producing a sample mean that is lower than the population mean of 33.1667.

In case 3, the sample consists of patients B, C, E, and F with ages 17, 45, 32, and 9, respectively, and a corresponding sample mean, $\overline{X} = 25.7500$. In case 4, the sample consists of patients A, B, E, and F with ages 26, 17, 32, and 9, respectively, and a corresponding sample mean, $\overline{X} = 21.0000$. Thus, we see that the sample means from samples selected from the same population can differ substantially. However, the unbiasedness property still holds and has nothing to do with the variability.

What is the unbiasedness property and how do we demonstrate it? For simple random sampling, each of the $C(N, n)$ samples has a probability of $1/C(N, n)$ of being selected. (Chapter 5 provides the necessary background to cover this point in more detail.) In our case, each of the 15 possible samples has a probability of 1/15 of being selected.

The unbiasedness property means that if we compute all 15 sample means, sum them, and divide by 15, we will obtain the population mean. The following example will verify the unbiasedness property of sample means. Recall that the 15 samples with their respective sample means are as follows:

1. $\{A, B, C, D\}, \overline{X} = (26 + 17 + 45 + 70)/4 = 39.5000$
2. $\{A, B, C, E\}, \overline{X} = (26 + 17 + 45 + 32)/4 = 30.0000$
3. $\{A, B, C, F\}, \overline{X} = (26 + 17 + 45 + 9)/4 = 24.2500$
4. $\{A, B, D, E\}, \overline{X} = (26 + 17 + 70 + 32)/4 = 36.2500$
5. $\{A, B, D, F\}, \overline{X} = (26 + 17 + 70 + 9)/4 = 30.5000$
6. $\{A, B, E, F\}, \overline{X} = (26 + 17 + 32 + 9)/4 = 21.0000$
7. $\{A, C, D, E\}, \overline{X} = (26 + 45 + 70 + 32)/4 = 43.2500$
8. $\{A, C, D, F\}, \overline{X} = (26 + 45 + 70 + 9)/4 = 37.5000$
9. $\{A, C, E, F\}, \overline{X} = (26 + 45 + 32 + 9)/4 = 28.0000$
10. $\{A, D, E, F\}, \overline{X} = (26 + 70 + 32 + 9)/4 = 34.2500$
11. $\{B, C, D, E\}, \overline{X} = (17 + 45 + 70 + 32)/4 = 41.0000$
12. $\{B, C, D, F\}, \overline{X} = (17 + 45 + 70 + 9)/4 = 35.2500$
13. $\{B, C, E, F\}, \overline{X} = (17 + 45 + 32 + 9)/4 = 25.7500$
14. $\{B, D, E, F\}, \overline{X} = (17 + 70 + 32 + 9)/4 = 32.0000$
15. $\{C, D, E, F\}, \overline{X} = (45 + 70 + 32 + 9)/4 = 39.0000$

Notice that the largest mean is 43.2500, the smallest is 21.0000, and the closest to the population mean is 34.2500. The average of the 15 sample means is called the expected value of the sample mean, denoted by the symbol E.

The property of unbiasedness states that the expected value of the estimate equals the population parameter [i.e., $E(\overline{X}) = \mu$]. In this case, the population parameter is the population mean, and its value is 33.1667 (rounded to four decimal places).

To calculate the expected value of the sample mean, we average the 15 values of sample means (computed previously). The average yields $E(\overline{X}) = (39.5 + 30.0 + 24.25 + 36.25 + 30.5 + 21.0 + 43.25 + 37.5 + 28.0 + 34.25 + 41.0 + 35.25 + 25.75 + 32.0 + 39.0)/15 = 497.5/15 = 33.1667$. Consequently, we have demonstrated the unbiasedness property in this case. As we have mentioned previously, this statistical property of simple random samples can be proven mathematically. Sample estimates of other parameters can also be unbiased and the unbiasedness of these estimates for simple random samples can also be proven mathematically. But it is important to note that not all estimates of parameters are unbiased. For example, ratio estimates obtained by taking the ratio of unbiased estimates for both the numerator and denominator are biased. The interested reader may consult Cochran (1977) for a mathematical proof that the sample mean is an unbiased estimate of a finite population mean [Cochran (1977), page 22, Theorem 2.1] and the sample variance is an unbiased estimate of the finite population variance [as defined by Cochran (1977); see Theorem 2.4 page 26].

2.5   HOW TO SELECT A BOOTSTRAP SAMPLE

The bootstrap method and its use in statistical inference will be covered more extensively in Chapter 8 when we discuss its application in estimation and contrast it to parametric methods. In most applications, a sampling procedure is used to approximate the bootstrap method. That sampling procedure generates what are called bootstrap samples, which are obtained by sampling with replacement. Because sampling with replacement is a general sampling technique that is similar to random sampling, we introduce it here.

In general, we can choose a random sample of size n with replacement from a population of size N. In our applications of the bootstrap, the population for bootstrap sampling will not be the actual population of interest but rather a given, presumably random, sample from the population.

In the first stage of selecting a bootstrap sample, we take the interval [0, 1] and divide it into N equal parts. Then, for uniform random number U, we assign index 1 if $0 \leq U < 1/N$, and index 2 if $1/N \leq U < 2/N$, and so on until we assign index N if $(N-1)/N \leq U < 1$. We generate n such indices by generating n consecutive uniform random numbers. The procedure is identical to our rejection sampling scheme except that none of the samples is rejected because repeated indices are allowed.

Bootstrap sampling is a special case of sampling with replacement. In ordinary bootstrap sampling, $n = N$. Remember, for bootstrap sampling the population size N is actually the size of the original random sample; the true population is replaced by that sample.

Let us consider the population of six patients described previously in Section 2.4. Again, age is the variable of interest. We will generate 10 bootstrap samples of size six for the ages of the patients. For the first sample we will use row 3 from Table 2.1. The second sample will be generated using row 4, and so on for samples 3 through 10.

The first six uniform random numbers in row 3 are 69386, 71708, 88608, 67251, 22512, and 00169. The corresponding indices are 5, 5, 6, 5, 2, and 1. The corresponding patients are E, E, F, E, B, and A, and the sampled ages are 32, 32, 9, 32, 17, and 26. The average age for this bootstrap sample is 24.6667.

There are $6^6 = 46,656$ possible bootstrap samples of size six. In practice, we sample only a small number, such as 50 to 100, when the total number of possible samples is so large. A random selection of 100 samples provides a good estimate of the bootstrap mean obtained from averaging the 46,656 bootstrap samples.

It is also true that the bootstrap sample mean is an unbiased estimate of the population mean for the following reason: For any random sample, the bootstrap sample estimate is an unbiased estimate of the mean of the random sample, and the mean of the random sample is an unbiased estimate of the population mean.

We will determine all ten bootstrap samples, calculate their sample means, and see how close the average of the ten bootstrap sample means is to the population mean age. Note that although the bootstrap provides an unbiased estimate of the population mean, we can demonstrate this result only by averaging all 46,656 bootstrap samples. Obviously, this calculation is difficult, so we will approximate only the mean of the original sample by averaging the ten bootstrap samples. We expect the result to be close to the mean of the original sample.

The 10 bootstrap samples are as follows:

1. 69386, 71708, 88608, 67251, 22512, and 00169 corresponding to patients E, E, F, E, B, and A and ages 32, 32, 9, 32, 17, and 26 with mean $\bar{X}$ = 24.6667.

2. 68381, 61725, 49122, 75836, 15368, and 52551 corresponding to patients E, D, C, E, A, and D, corresponding to ages 32, 70, 45, 32, 26, and 70 with mean $\bar{X}$ = 45.8333.

3. 69158, 38683, 41374, 17028, 09304, and 10834 corresponding to patients E, C, C, B, A, and A, corresponding to ages 32, 45, 45, 17, 26, and 26 with mean $\bar{X}$ = 31.8333.

4. 00858, 04352, 17833, 41105, 46569, and 90109 corresponding to patients A, A, B, C, C, and F, corresponding to ages 26, 26, 17, 45, 45, and 9 with mean $\bar{X}$ = 28.0.

5. 86972, 51707, 58242, 16035, 94887, and 83510 corresponding to patients F, D, D, A, F, and F, corresponding to ages 9, 70, 70, 26, 9, and 9 with mean $\bar{X}$ = 32.1667.

6. 30606, 45225, 30161, 07973, 03034, and 82983 corresponding to patients B, C, B, A, A, and E, corresponding to ages 17, 45, 17, 26, 26, and 32 with mean $\bar{X}$ = 27.1667.

7. 93864, 49044, 57169, 43125, 11703, and 87009 corresponding to patients F, C, D, C, A, and F, corresponding to ages 9, 45, 70, 45, 26, and 9 with mean $\bar{X}$ = 34.0.

8. 61937, 90217, 56708, 35351, 60820, and 90729 corresponding to patients D, F, D, C, D, and F, corresponding to ages 70, 9, 70, 45, 70, and 9 with mean $\bar{X}$ = 45.5.

9. 94551, 69538, 52924, 08530, 79302, and 34981 corresponding to patients F, E, D, A, D, and C, corresponding to ages 9, 32, 70, 26, 70, and 45 with mean $\bar{X}$ = 42.0

10. 79385, 49498, 48569, 57888, 70564, and 17660 corresponding to patients E, C, C, D, E, and B, corresponding to ages 32, 45, 45, 70, and 17 with mean $\bar{X}$ = 34.8333.

The bootstrap mean is (24.6667 + 45.8333 + 31.8333 + 28.0 + 32.1667 + 27.1667 + 34.0 + 45.5 + 42.0 + 34.8333)/10 = 31.8833. This is to be compared to the original sample mean of 33.1667. Recall from Section 2.4 that the population consisting of patients A, B, C, D, E, and F represents our original sample for the bootstrap. We determined that the mean age for that sample was 33.1667. We would have obtained greater accuracy if we had generated 50 to 100 bootstrap samples rather than just 10. Had we generated all 46,656 possible distinct bootstrap samples, we would have calculated the sample mean exactly.

2.6   WHY DOES RANDOM SAMPLING WORK?

We have illustrated an important property of simple random sampling, namely, that estimates of population averages are unbiased. Under certain conditions, appropriately chosen stratified random samples can produce unbiased estimates with better accuracy than simple random samples (see Cochran, 1977).

A quantity that provides a description of the accuracy of the estimate of a population mean is called the variance of the mean, and its square root is called the standard error of the mean. The symbol σ^2 is used to denote the population variance. (Chapter 4 will provide the formulas for σ^2.) When the population size N is very large, the sampling variance of the sample mean is known to be approximately σ^2/n for a sample size of n.

In fact, as Cochran (1977) has shown, the exact value of this sample variance is slightly smaller than the population variance due to the finite number N for the population. To correct for this slightly smaller estimate, a correction factor is applied (see Chapter 4). If n is small relative to N, this correction factor can be ignored. The fact that the variance of the sample mean is approximately σ^2/n tells us that since the variance of the sample mean becomes small as n becomes large, individual sample means will be highly accurate.

Kuzma illustrated the phenomenon that large sample sizes produce highly accurate estimates of the population mean with his Honolulu Heart Study data (Kuzma, 1998; Kuzma and Bohnenblust, 2001). For his data, the population size for the male patients was $N = 7683$ (a relatively large number).

Kuzma determined that the population mean for his data was 54.36. Taking repeated samples of $n = 100$, Kuzma examined the mean age of the male patients. Choosing five simple random samples of size $n = 100$, he obtained sample means of 54.85, 54.31, 54.32, 54.67, and 54.02. All these estimates were within one-half year of the population mean. In Kuzma's example, the variance of the sample means was small and n was large. Consequently, all sample estimates were close to one another and to the population mean. Thus, in general we can say that the larger the n, the more closely the sample estimate of the mean approaches the population mean.

2.7   EXERCISES

2.1   Why does the field of inferential statistics need to be concerned about samples? Give in your own words the definitions of the following terms that pertain to sample selection:

    a. Sample
    b. Census
    c. Parameter
    d. Statistic
    e. Representativeness
    f. Sampling frame
    g. Periodic effect

2.2 Describe the following types of sample designs, noting their similarities and differences. State also when it is appropriate to use each type of sample design.
    a. Random sample
    b. Simple random samples
    c. Convenience/grab bag samples
    d. Systematic samples
    e. Stratified
    f. Cluster
    g. Bootstrap

2.3 Explain what is meant by the term parameter estimation.

2.4 How can bias affect a sample design? Explain by using the terms selection bias, response bias, and periodic effects.

2.5 How is sampling with replacement different from sampling without replacement?

2.6 Under what circumstances is it appropriate to use rejection sampling methods?

2.7 Why would a convenience sample of college students on vacation in Fort Lauderdale, Florida, not be representative of the students at a particular college or university?

2.8 What role does sample size play in the accuracy of statistical inference? Why is the method of selecting the sample even more important than the size of the sample?

Exercises 2.9 to 2.13 will help you acquire familiarity with sample selection. These exercises use data from Table 2.2.

2.9 By using the random number table (Table 2.1), draw a sample of 10 height measurements from Table 2.2. This sample is said to have size 10, or $n = 10$. The rows and columns in Table 2.2 have numbers, which in combination are the "addresses" of specific height measurements. For example, the number

TABLE 2.2. Heights in Inches of 400 Female Clinic Patients

Col./Row	1	2	3	4	5	6	7	8
1	61	55	52	59	62	66	59	66
2	61	62	73	63	64	65	63	60
3	63	61	69	57	65	59	67	64
4	58	61	61	61	63	61	65	63
5	63	67	58	60	63	58	67	63
6	63	63	61	63	65	62	65	63
7	61	61	62	59	61	59	71	58
8	59	66	63	60	65	65	62	65
9	61	63	65	61	70	61	65	63
10	66	63	62	66	63	59	61	57
11	63	62	64	67	64	58	63	62
12	59	60	63	67	57	63	67	70
13	60	61	62	65	60	61	62	68
14	61	62	70	67	67	62	67	67
15	57	61	64	61	59	63	67	58
16	63	61	64	54	63	57	71	64
17	59	62	63	59	59	64	67	64
18	62	63	61	63	63	72	63	64
19	64	63	65	65	64	67	72	65
20	61	61	60	64	68	61	71	68
21	64	63	63	61	60	62	59	43
22	62	61	69	64	65	59	67	68
23	58	62	47	60	63	66	65	71
24	63	63	67	59	63	65	60	63
25	64	63	59	60	61	69	55	59
26	64	61	67	63	65	62	65	61
27	62	59	66	57	64	63	67	66
28	58	62	67	61	59	64	67	66
29	62	64	64	59	66	64	65	59
30	63	55	63	64	63	60	61	66
31	61	59	58	60	68	67	58	66
32	66	61	60	67	55	57	69	62
33	63	61	63	59	63	69	57	62
34	63	62	63	59	65	62	58	62
35	61	61	56	63	66	61	68	62
36	58	62	59	64	61	61	65	64
37	47	61	58	66	63	64	71	62
38	59	59	72	58	61	58	71	58
39	59	60	59	62	66	67	65	63
40	61	60	60	61	60	60	63	64
41	60	61	60	61	59	63	63	68
42	62	60	55	64	63	64	71	66
43	63	63	59	59	65	67	71	61
44	64	60	55	67	61	63	65	70
45	62	63	68	61	67	65	64	66

(*continued*)

TABLE 2.2. *Continued*

Col./Row	1	2	3	4	5	6	7	8
46	59	62	55	67	58	63	64	59
47	64	60	65	63	62	63	71	58
48	62	66	61	66	57	65	61	70
49	66	66	63	67	61	65	62	63
50	59	60	61	59	56	65	61	62

Source: Robert Friis.

defined by row 15, column 4 denotes the 154th height measurement, or 61. Use two indices based on numbers from Table 2.1. Draw one random number to select the row between 1 and 50 and another to choose the column between 1 and 8. Use the rejection method. List the ten values you have selected by this process. What name is given to the kind of sample you have selected?

2.10 Again use Table 2.2 to select a sample, but this time select only one random number from Table 2.1. Start in the row determined by the index for that random number. Choose the first value from the first column in that row; then skip the next seven columns and select the second value from column 8. Continue skipping seven consecutive values before selecting the next value. When you come to the end of the row, continue the procedure on the next row. What kind of sampling procedure is this? Can bias be introduced when you sample in this way?

2.11 From the 400 height measurements in Table 2.2, we will take a sample of ten distinct values by taking the first six values in row 1 and the two values in the last two columns in row 2 and the last two columns in row 3. Let these ten values comprise the sample. Draw a sample of size 10 by sampling with replacement from these 10 measurements.
   a. List the original sample and the sample generated by sampling with replacement from it.
   b. What do we call the sample generated by sampling with replacement?

2.12 Repeat the procedure of Exercise 2.11 five times. List all five samples. How do they differ from the original sample?

2.13 Describe the population and the sample for:
   a. Exercise 2.9
   b. The bootstrap sampling plan in Exercise 2.11

2.14 Suppose you selected a sample from Table 2.2 by starting with the number in row 1, column 2. You then proceed across the row, skipping the next five numbers and take the sixth number. You continue in this way, skipping five numbers and taking the sixth, going to the leftmost element in the next row when all the elements in a row are exhausted, until you have exhausted the table.

a. What is such a sample selection scheme called?

b. Could any possible sources of bias arise from using this scheme?

2.8   ADDITIONAL READING

1. Chernick, M. R. (1999). *Bootstrap Methods: A Practitioner's Guide.* Wiley, New York.

2. Cochran, W. G. (1977). *Sampling Techniques.* Wiley, New York.

3. Davison, A. C. and Hinkley D. V. (1997). *Bootstrap Methods and their Applications.* Cambridge University Press, Cambridge, England.

4. Dunn, O. J. (1977). *Basic Statistics: A Primer for the Biomedical Sciences,* 2nd Edition. Wiley, New York.

5. Efron, B. and Tibshirani, R. (1993). *An Introduction to the Bootstrap.* Chapman and Hall, London.

6. Lohr, S. L. (1999). *Sampling: Design and Analysis.* Duxbury Press, Pacific Grove, California.

7. Kish, L. (1965). *Survey Sampling.* Wiley, New York.

8. Kuzma, J. W. (1998). *Basic Statistics for the Health Sciences,* 3rd Edition. Mayfield, Mountain View, California.

9. Kuzma, J. W. and Bohnenblust, S. E. (2001). *Basic Statistics for the Health Sciences,* 4th Edition. Mayfield, Mountain View, California.

10. Mooney, C. Z. and Duval, R. D. (1993). *Bootstrapping: A Nonparametric Approach to Statistical Inference.* Sage, Newbury Park, California.

11. Scheaffer, R. L., Mendenhall, W. and Ott, L. (1979). *Elementary Survey Sampling,* 2nd Edition. Duxbury Press, Boston.

CHAPTER 3

Systematic Organization and Display of Data

The preliminary examination of most data is facilitated by the use of diagrams. Diagrams prove nothing, but bring outstanding features readily to the eye; they are therefore no substitutes for such critical tests as may be applied to the data, but are valuable in suggesting such tests, and in explaining the conclusions founded upon them.
—Sir Ronald Alymer Fisher, *Statistical Methods for Research Workers*, p. 27

This chapter covers methods for organizing and displaying data. Such methods provide summary information about a data set and may be used to conduct exploratory data analyses. We will discuss types of data used in biostatistics, methods for describing how data are distributed (e.g., frequency tables and histograms), and methods for displaying data graphically. The methods for providing summary information are essential to the development of hypotheses and to establishing the groundwork for more complex statistical analyses. Chapter 4 will cover specific summary statistics: e.g., the mean, mode, and standard deviation.

3.1 TYPES OF DATA

The methods for displaying and analyzing data depend upon the type of data being used. In this section, we will define and provide examples of the two major types of data: qualitative and quantitative. Quantitative data can be continuous or discrete. Chapter 11 will give more information about the related topic of measurement systems. We collect data to characterize populations and to estimate parameters, which are numerical or categorical characteristics of a population probability distribution.

In order to describe types of data, we need to be familiar with the concept of variables. The term "variable" is used to describe a quantity that can vary (i.e., take on various values), such as age, height, weight, or sex. Variables can be characteristics of a population, such as the age of a randomly selected individual in the U.S.

Introductory Biostatistics for the Health Sciences, by Michael R. Chernick and Robert H. Friis. ISBN 0-471-41137-X. Copyright © 2003 Wiley-Interscience.

population. They can also be estimates (statistics) of population parameters such as the mean age of a random sample of 100 individuals in the U.S. population. These variables will have probability distributions associated with them and these distributions will be discussed in Chapter 5.

3.1.1   Qualitative Data

Variables that can be identified for individuals according to a quality are called qualitative variables. These variables place individuals into categories that do not have numerical values. When the observations are not ordered, they form a nominal scale. (A dichotomous scale—true/false, male/female, yes/no, dead/alive—also is a nominal scale.) Many qualitative variables cannot be ordered (as in going from worst to best). Occupation, marital status, and sex are examples of qualitative data that have no natural ordering. The term nominal refers to qualitative data that do not have a natural ordering.

Some qualitative data can be ordered in the manner of a preference scale (e.g., strongly agree, agree, disagree, strongly disagree). Levels of educational attainment can be ordered from low to moderate to high: less than a high school education might be categorized as low; education beyond high school but without a four year bachelor's degree could be considered moderate; a four year bachelor's degree might be considered high; and a degree at the masters, Ph.D., or M.D. level considered very high. Although still considered qualitative, categorical data that can be ordered are called ordinal.

Qualitative data can be summarized and displayed in pie charts and bar graphs, which describe the frequency of occurrence in the sample or the population of particular values of the characteristics. These graphical representations will be described in Section 3.3. For ordinal data with the categories ordered from lowest to highest, bar graphs might be more appropriate than pie charts. Because a pie chart is circular, it is more appropriate for nominal data.

3.1.2   Quantitative Data

Quantitative data are numerical data that have a natural order and can be continuous or discrete. Continuous data can take on any real value in an interval or over the whole real number line. Continuous data can be classified as interval. Continuous data also can be summarized with box-and-whisker plots, histograms, frequency polygons, and stem-and-leaf displays. Examples of continuous data include variables such as age, height, weight, heart rate, blood pressure, and cholesterol level.

Discrete data take on only a finite or countable (equivalent to the set of integers) number of values. Examples of discrete data are the number of children in a household, the number of visits to a doctor in a year, or the number of successful ablation treatments in a clinical trial. Often, discrete data are integers or fractions. Discrete data can be described and displayed in histograms, frequency polygons, stem-and-leaf displays, and box-and-whisker plots (see Section 3.3).

If the data can be ordered, and we can identify ratios with them, we call the data ratio data. For example, integers form a quantitative discrete set of numbers that are ratio data; we can quantify 2 as being two times 1, 4 as two times 2, and 6 as three times 2. The ability to create ratios distinguishes quantitative data from qualitative data. Qualitative ordinal data can be ordered but cannot be used to produce ratios. We cannot say, for example, that a college education is worth twice as much as a high school education.

Continuous interval data can be used to produce ratios but not all ratio data are continuous. For example, the integers form a discrete set that can produce ratios, but such data are not interval data because of the gaps between consecutive integers.

3.2   FREQUENCY TABLES AND HISTOGRAMS

A frequency table provides one of the most convenient ways to summarize or display grouped data. Before we construct such a table, let us consider the following numerical data. Table 3.1 lists 120 values of body mass index data from the 1998 National Health Interview Survey. The body mass index (BMI) is defined as [Weight (in kilograms)/Height (in meters) squared]. According to established standards, a BMI from 19 to less than 25 is considered healthy; a BMI from 25 to less than 30 is regarded as overweight; a BMI greater than or equal to 30 is defined as obese. Table 3.1 arranges the numbers in the order in which they were collected.

In constructing a frequency table for grouped data, we first determine a set of class intervals that cover the range of the data (i.e., include all the observed values). The class intervals are usually arranged from lowest numbers at the top of the table to highest numbers at the bottom of the table and are defined so as not to overlap. We then tally the number of observations that fall in each interval and present that number as a frequency, called a class frequency. Some frequency tables include a

TABLE 3.1. Body Mass Index for a Sample of 120 U.S. Adults

27.4	31.0	34.2	28.9	25.7	37.1	24.8	34.9	27.5	25.9
23.5	30.9	27.4	25.9	22.3	21.3	37.8	28.8	28.8	23.4
21.9	30.2	24.7	36.6	25.4	21.3	22.9	24.2	27.1	23.1
28.6	27.3	22.7	22.7	27.3	23.1	22.3	32.6	29.5	38.8
21.9	24.3	26.5	30.1	27.4	24.5	22.8	24.3	30.9	28.7
22.4	35.9	30.0	26.2	27.4	24.1	19.8	26.9	23.3	28.4
20.8	26.5	28.2	18.3	30.8	27.6	21.5	33.6	24.8	28.3
25.0	35.8	25.4	27.3	23.0	25.7	22.3	35.5	29.8	27.4
31.3	24.0	25.8	21.1	21.1	29.3	24.0	22.5	32.8	38.2
27.3	19.2	26.6	30.3	31.6	25.4	34.8	24.7	25.6	28.3
26.5	28.3	35.0	20.2	37.5	25.8	27.5	28.8	31.1	28.7
24.1	24.0	20.7	24.6	21.1	21.9	30.8	24.6	33.2	31.6

Source: Adapted from the National Center for Health Statistics (2000). Data File Documentation, National Health Interview Survey, 1998 (machine readable data file and documentation, CD-ROM Series 10, No 13A), National Center for Health Statistics, Hyattsville, Maryland.

column that represents the frequency as a percentage of the total number of observations; this column is called the relative frequency percentage. The completed frequency table provides a frequency distribution.

Although not required, a good first step in constructing a frequency table is to rearrange the data table, placing the smallest number in the first row of the leftmost column and then continuing to arrange the numbers in increasing order going down the first column to the top of the next row. (We can accomplish this procedure by sorting the data in ascending order.) After the first column is completed, the procedure is continued starting in the second column of the first row, and continuing until the largest observation appears in the rightmost column of the bottom row.

We call the arranged table an ordered array. It is much easier to tally the observations for a frequency table from such an ordered array of data than it is from the original data table. Table 3.2 provides a rearrangement of the body mass index data as an ordered array.

In Table 3.2, by inspection we find that the lowest and highest values are 18.3 and 38.8, respectively. We will use these numbers to help us create equally spaced intervals for tabulating frequencies of data. Although the number of intervals that one may choose for a frequency distribution is arbitrary, the actual number should depend on the range of the data and the number of cases. For a data set of 100 to 150 observations, the number chosen usually ranges from about five to ten. In the present example, the range of the data is $38.8 - 18.3 = 20.5$. Suppose we divide the data set into seven intervals. Then, we have $20.5 \div 7 = 2.93$, which rounds to 3.0. Consequently, the intervals will have a width of three. These seven intervals are as follows:

1. $18.0 - 20.9$
2. $21.0 - 23.9$
3. $24.0 - 26.9$

TABLE 3.2. Body Mass Index Data for a Sample of 120 U.S. Adults: Ordered Array (Sorted in Ascending Order)

18.3	21.9	23.0	24.3	25.4	26.6	27.5	28.8	30.9	34.8
19.2	21.9	23.1	24.3	25.6	26.9	27.5	28.8	30.9	34.9
19.8	21.9	23.1	24.5	25.7	27.1	27.6	28.9	31.0	35.0
20.2	22.3	23.3	24.6	25.7	27.3	28.2	29.3	31.1	35.5
20.7	22.3	23.4	24.6	25.8	27.3	28.3	29.5	31.3	35.8
20.8	22.3	23.5	24.7	25.8	27.3	28.3	29.8	31.6	35.9
21.1	22.4	24.0	24.7	25.9	27.3	28.3	30.0	31.6	36.6
21.1	22.5	24.0	24.8	25.9	27.4	28.4	30.1	32.6	37.1
21.1	22.7	24.0	24.8	26.2	27.4	28.6	30.2	32.8	37.5
21.3	22.7	24.1	25.0	26.5	27.4	28.7	30.3	33.2	37.8
21.3	22.8	24.1	25.4	26.5	27.4	28.7	30.8	33.6	38.2
21.5	22.9	24.2	25.4	26.5	27.4	28.8	30.8	34.2	38.8

4. 27.0 – 29.9
5. 30.0 – 32.9
6. 33.0 – 35.9
7. 36.0 – 38.9

Table 3.3 presents a frequency distribution and a relative frequency distribution (%) of the BMI data.

A cumulative frequency (%) table provides another way to display a frequency distribution. In a cumulative frequency (%) table, we list the class intervals and the cumulative relative frequency (%) in addition to the relative frequency (%). The cumulative relative frequency or cumulative percentage gives the percentage of cases less than or equal to the upper boundary of a particular class interval. The cumulative relative frequency can be obtained by summing the relative frequencies in a particular row and in all the preceding class intervals. Table 3.4 lists the relative frequencies and cumulative relative frequencies for the body mass index data.

A histogram presents the same information as a frequency table in the form of a bar graph. The endpoints of the intervals are displayed as the x-axis; on the y-axis

TABLE 3.3. Body Mass Index (BMI) Data ($n = 120$)

Class Interval for BMI Levels	Frequency (f)	Cumulative Frequency (cf)	Relative Frequency (%)
18.0–20.9	6	6	5.00
21.0–23.9	24	30	20.00
24.0–26.9	32	62	26.67
27.0–29.9	28	90	23.33
30.0–32.9	15	105	12.50
33.0–35.9	9	114	7.50
36.0–38.9	6	120	5.00
Total	120	—	100.00

TABLE 3.4. Relative Frequency Table of BMI Levels

Class Interval for BMI Levels	Relative Frequency (%)	Cumulative Relative Frequency (%)
18.0–20.9	5.00	5.00
21.0–23.9	20.00	55.00
24.0–26.9	26.67	51.67
27.0–29.9	23.33	75.00
30.0–32.9	12.50	87.50
33.0–35.9	7.50	95.00
36.0–38.9	5.00	100.00
Total	100.00	100.00

the frequency is represented, shown as a bar with the frequency as the height. We call a histogram a relative frequency histogram if we replace the frequency on the y-axis with the relative frequency expressed as a percent. Refer to Section 3.3 for examples using the body mass index.

Table 3.5 summarizes Section 3.2 by providing guidelines for creating frequency distributions of grouped data.

3.3 GRAPHICAL METHODS

A second way to display data is through the use of graphs. Graphs give the reader an overview of the essential features of the data. Generally, visual aids provided by graphs are easier to read than tables, although they do not contain all the detail that can be incorporated in a table.

Graphs are designed to provide visually an intuitive understanding of the data. Effective graphs are simple and clean: thus, it is important that the graph be self-explanatory (i.e., have a descriptive title, properly labeled axes, and an indication of the units of measurement).

Using the BMI data, we will illustrate the following seven graphical methods: histograms, frequency polygons, cumulative frequency polygons, stem-and-leaf displays, bar charts, pie charts, and box-and-whisker plots.

3.3.1 Frequency Histograms

As we mentioned previously, a frequency histogram is simply a bar graph with the class intervals listed on the x-axis and the frequency of occurrence of the values in the interval on the y-axis. Appropriate labeling is important. For the BMI data described earlier, Figure 3.1 provides an appropriate example of a frequency histogram.

Proper graphing of statistical data is an art, governed by what we would like to communicate. Several excellent books provide helpful guidelines for proper graphics. Among the most popular books are two by Edward Tufte [Tufte (1983, 1997)].

TABLE 3.5. Guidelines for Creating Frequency Distributions from Grouped Data

1. Find the range of values—the difference between the highest and lowest values.
2. Decide how many intervals to use (usually choose between 6 and 20 unless the data set is very large). The choice should be based on how much information is in the distribution you wish to display.
3. To determine the width of the interval, divide the range by the number of class intervals selected. Round this result as necessary.
4. Be sure that the class categories do not overlap!
5. Most of the time, use equally spaced intervals, which are simpler than unequally spaced intervals and avoid interpretation problems. In some cases, unequal intervals may be helpful to emphasize certain details. Sometimes wider intervals are needed where the data are sparse.

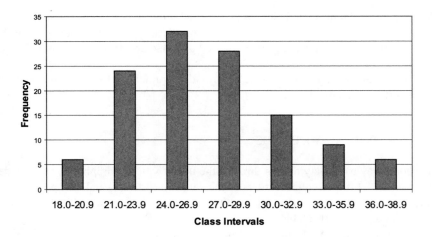

Figure 3.1. Frequency histogram of the BMI data.

Huff's (1954) popular book illustrates how playing tricks with the scales on a plot can distort information and mislead the reader. These experts provide sage guidance regarding construction of graphs.

Figure 3.2 provides a graph, called a relative frequency histogram, of the same data as in Figure 3.1 with the height of the y-axis represented by the relative frequency (%) rather than the actual frequency. By comparing Figures 3.1 and 3.2, you can see that the shapes of the graphs are similar.

Here the magnitude of the relative frequency is determined strictly by the height of the bar; the width of the bar should be ignored. For equally spaced class intervals, the height of the bar multiplied by the width of the bar (i.e., the area of the bar) also can represent the proportion of the cases in the given class.

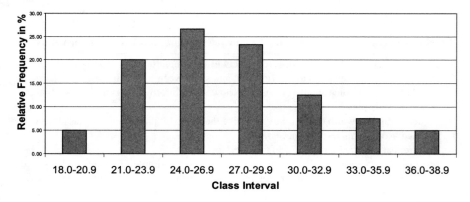

Figure 3.2. Relative frequency histogram for the BMI data.

In Chapter 5, when we discuss probability distributions, we will see that when properly defined, relative frequency histograms are useful in approximating probability distributions. In such cases, the area of the bar represents the percentage of the cases in the interval. When the class intervals have varying lengths, we need to adjust the height of the bar so that the area, not the height, is proportional to the percentage of cases. For example, if two intervals each contain 10% of the sampled cases but one has a width of 2 units and the other a width of 4 units, we would require that the intervals with width 4 units have one-half of the height of the interval with a width of 2 units.

Figure 3.3 provides a relative frequency histogram for the same BMI data except that we have combined the second and third and fifth and sixth class intervals into one interval; the resulting frequency distribution has five class intervals instead of the original seven.

The first, third, and fifth intervals all have a width of 3 units, whereas the second and fourth intervals have a width of 6 units. Consequently, the relative percentages are represented correctly by the height of the histogram but not by the area. The excessive height of the second and fourth intervals is corrected by dividing the height (i.e., frequency) of these intervals by 2. Figure 3.4 shows the adjusted histogram.

Figure 3.5 presents a cumulative frequency histogram in which the frequency in the interval is replaced by the cumulative frequency, as we demonstrated in the cumulative frequency tables. The analogous figure for cumulative relative frequency (%) is shown in Figure 3.6.

3.3.2   Frequency Polygons

Frequency polygons are very similar to frequency histograms. However, instead of placing a bar across the interval, the height of the frequency or relative frequency is

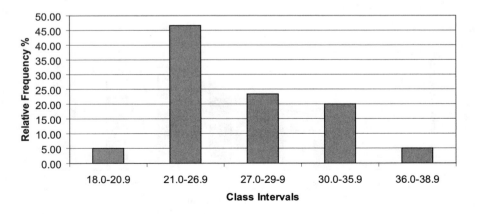

Figure 3.3. BMI data: relative frequency histogram with unequally spaced intervals.

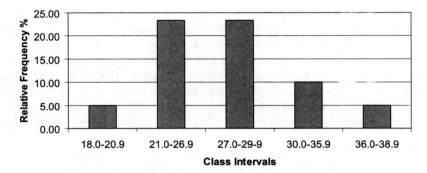

Figure 3.4. BMI data: relative frequency histogram with unequally spaced intervals (height adjusted for correct area).

plotted at the midpoint of the class interval; these points are then connected by straight lines creating a polygonal shape, hence the name frequency polygon.

Figures 3.7 and 3.8 represent, respectively, a frequency polygon and relative frequency polygon for the BMI data. These figures are analogous to the histograms presented in Figures 3.1 and 3.2, respectively.

3.3.3 Cumulative Frequency Polygon

A cumulative frequency polygon, or ogive, is similar to a cumulative frequency histogram. The height of the function represents the sum of the frequencies in all the class intervals up to and including the current one. The only differences between a cumulative frequency polygon and a cumulative frequency histogram are that the height is taken at the midpoint of the class interval and the points are connected by straight lines instead of being represented by bars. Figures 3.9 and 3.10 represent, respectively, the cumulative frequency polygon and cumulative relative frequency polygon for the BMI data.

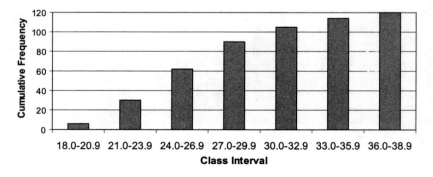

Figure 3.5. Cumulative frequency histogram for BMI data.

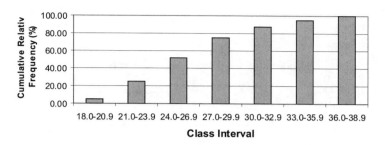

Figure 3.6. Cumulative relative frequency histogram for BMI data.

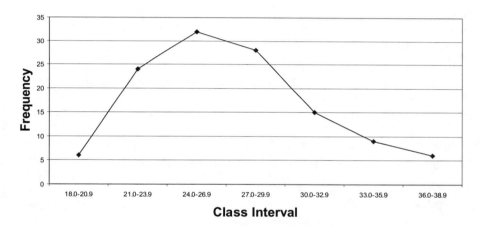

Figure 3.7. Frequency polygon for BMI data.

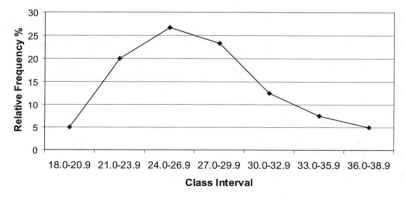

Figure 3.8. Relative frequency polygon for BMI data.

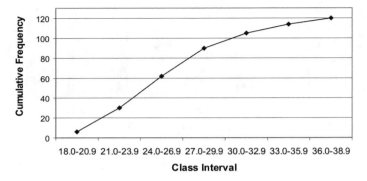

Figure 3.9. Cumulative frequency polygon (ogive) for BMI data.

3.3.4   Stem-and-Leaf Diagrams

Histograms summarize a dataset and provide an idea of the shape of the distribution of the data. However, some information is lost in the summary. We are not able to reconstruct the original data from the histogram.

John W. Tukey created an innovation in the 1970s that he termed the "stem-and-leaf diagram." Tukey (1977) elaborates on this method and other innovative exploratory data analysis techniques. The stem-and-leaf diagram not only provides the desirable features of the histogram, but also gives us a way to reconstruct the entire data set from the diagram. Consequently, we do not lose any information by constructing the plot.

The basic idea of a stem-and-leaf diagram is to construct "stems" that represent the class intervals and to have "leaves" that exhibit all the individual values. Let us demonstrate the technique with the BMI data. Recall that these data ranged from a lowest value of 18.3 to a highest value of 38.8. The class groups will be the integer part of each number; any value from 18.0 to 18.9 will belong to the first stem, from 19.0 to 19.9 to the second stem, and continuing to the highest value in the dataset.

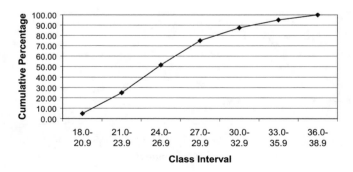

Figure 3.10. Cumulative relative frequency polygon for BMI data.

To form the leaves, we place a single digit for each observation that belongs to that class interval (stem). The value used will be the single digit that appears after the decimal point. If a particular value is repeated in the data set, we repeat that value on the leaf as many times as it appears in the data set. Usually the numbers on the leaf are placed in increasing order. In this way, we can exhibit all of the data. Intervals that include more observations than others will have longer leaves and thus produce the frequency appearance of a histogram. The display of the BMI data is:

18. 3
19. 28
20. 278
21. 111335999
22. 333457789
23. 011345
24. 000112335667788
25. 04446778899
26. 255569
27. 1333344444556
28. 233346778889
29. 358
30. 01238899
31. 01366
32. 68
33. 62
34. 289
35. 0589
36. 6
37. 158
38. 28

From this display, we are able to reach several conclusions about the frequency of cases in each interval and the shape of the distribution, and even reconstruct the original dataset, if necessary. First, it is apparent that the intervals that contain the highest and second-highest frequencies of observations are 24.0 to 24.9 and 25.0 to 25.9, respectively. Also, empty or low-frequency intervals such as 36.0 to 36.9 are recognized easily. Second, the shape of the distribution is also easy to visualize; it resembles a histogram placed sideways. The individual digits on the leaves represent all of the 120 observations.

The frequencies associated with each of the class intervals are calculated by totaling the number of digits on the corresponding leaf. Each individual value can be reconstructed by observing its stem and leaf value. For example, the 9 in the fourth row of the diagram represents the value "21.9" because 21 is the stem for that row and 9 is the leaf value. The stem represents the digits to the left of the decimal place and the leaf the digit to the right.

Table 3.5 reconstructs the stem-and-leaf diagram shown in the foregoing display. In addition, the table illustrates the class interval associated with the stem and provides the frequency counts obtained from the leaves.

3.3.5   Box-and-Whisker Plots

John W. Tukey created another scheme for data analysis, the box-and-whisker plot. The box-and-whisker plot provides a convenient and compact picture of the general shape of a data distribution. Although it contains less information than a histogram, the Box-and-Whisker plot can be very useful in comparing one distribution to other distributions. Figure 3.11 presents a box-and-whisker plot in which the distribution of weights is compared for patients diagnosed with cancer, diabetes, and coronary heart disease. From the figure, we can see that although the distributions overlap, the average weight increases for each of these diagnoses.

To define a box-and-whisker plot, we must give definitions of several terms related to the distribution of a data set; these terms are the median, α-percentile, and

TABLE 3.5. Stem-and-Leaf Display for BMI Data

Stems (Intervals)	Leaves (Observations)	Frequency
18.0–18.9	3	1
19.0–19.9	28	2
20.0–20.9	278	3
21.0–21.9	111335999	9
22.0–22.9	333457789	9
23.0–23.9	011345	6
24.0–24.9	000112335667788	15
25.0–25.9	04446778899	11
26.0–26.9	255569	6
27.0–27.9	1333344444556	13
28.0–28.9	233346778889	12
29.0–29.9	358	3
30.0–30.9	01238899	8
31.0–31.9	01366	5
32.0–32.9	68	2
33.0–33.9	62	2
34.0–34.9	289	3
35.0–35.9	0589	4
36.0–36.9	6	1
37.0–37.9	158	3
38.0–38.9	28	2
Total		120

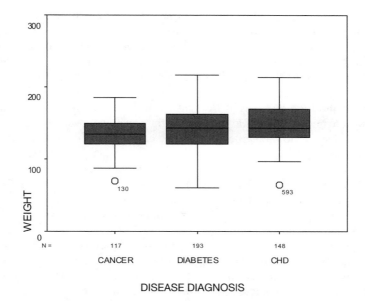

Figure 3.11. Box-and-whisker plot for female patients who have cancer, diabetes, and coronary heart disease (CHD). (Source: Robert Friis, unpublished data.)

the interquartile range. The median of a data set is the value of the observation that divides the ordered dataset in half. Essentially, the median is the observation whose value defines the midpoint of a distribution; i.e., half of the data fall above the median and half below.

A precise mathematical definition of a median is as follows: If the sample size n is odd, then $n = 2m + 1$, where m is an integer greater than or equal to zero. The median then is taken to be the value of the $m + 1$ observation ordered from smallest to largest. If the sample size n is even, then $n = 2m$ where m is an integer greater than or equal to 1. Any value between the mth and $m + 1$st values ordered from smallest to largest could be the median, as there would be m observed values below it and m observed values above it. When n is even, a convention that makes the median unique is to take the average of the mth and $m + 1$st observations (i.e., the sum of the two values divided by 2).

The α-percentile is defined as the value such that α percent of the observations have values lower than the α-percentile value; $100 - \alpha$ percent of the observations are above the α-percentile value. The quantity α is a number between 0 and 100. The median is a special case in which the $\alpha = 50$.

We use specific α-percentiles for box-and-whisker plots. We can draw these plots either horizontally, or vertically as in the case of Figure 3.11. The α-percentiles of interest are for $\alpha = 1, 5, 10, 25, 50, 75, 90, 95,$ and 99. A box-and-whisker plot, based on these percentiles, is represented by a box with lines (called whiskers) extending out of the box in both north and south directions. These lines terminate with bars perpendicular to them. The lower end of the box represents the location of the 25th percentile of the distribution. Inside the box, a line is drawn to mark the location of the median, or 50th percentile, of the distribution. The upper end of the box represents the location of the 75th percentile of the distribution.

The length of the box is called the interquartile range, the range of values that constitute the middle half of the data. Out of the upper and lower ends of the box are the lines extending to the perpendicular bars called whiskers, which represent extremes of the distribution.

While there are no consistent standards for defining the extremes, people who construct the plots need to be very specific about the meaning of these extremes. Often, these extremes correspond to the smallest and largest observations, in which case the length from the end of the whisker on the bottom to the end of the whisker on the top is the range of the data.

In many applications, the ends of the whiskers represent α-percentiles. For example, choices can be 1 for the end of the lower whisker and 99 for the end of the upper whisker, or 5 for the lower whisker and 95 for the upper whisker. The foregoing are the most common choices; however, sometimes 10 and 90 are used for the lower and upper whiskers, respectively.

Sometimes, we consider the minimum (i.e., the smallest value in the data set) and the maximum (i.e., the largest value in the data set) to be the ends of whiskers. In this text, we will assume that the endpoints of the whiskers are the minimum and maximum values of the data. If other percentiles are used, we will be careful to state their values.

The box plot is very useful for indicating the presence or absence of symmetry and for comparing spread or variability of two or more data sets. If the distribution is not symmetric, it is possible that the median will not be in the center of the box and that the whiskers will not be the same length. Looking at box plots is a very good first step to take when analyzing data.

If a box-and-whisker plot indicates the presence of symmetry, the distribution may be a normal distribution. Symmetry means that if we split the distribution (i.e., probability density function) at the median, the half to the right will be the mirror image of the half to the left. For a box-and-whisker plot that shows a symmetric distribution: (1) the median will be in the middle of the box; and (2) the right and left whiskers will have equal lengths. Regardless of the definition we choose for the ends of the whiskers, points one and two will be true.

Concluding this section, we note that Chapters 5 and 6, respectively, describe probability distributions and the normal distribution. The normal, or Gaussian, distribution is a symmetric distribution used for many applications. When the data come from a normal distribution, the sample should appear to be nearly symmetric. So for normally distributed data, we expect the box-and-whisker plot to have a median near the center of the box and whiskers of nearly equal width. Large deviations from the model of symmetry suggest that the data do not come from a normal distribution.

3.3.6   Bar Graphs and Pie Charts

Bar graphs and pie charts are useful tools for summarizing categorical data. A bar graph has the same form as a histogram. However, in a histogram the values on the x-axis represent intervals of numerically ordered data. Consequently, as we move from left to right on the x-axis, the intervals represent increasing values of the variable under study. As categorical data do not exhibit ordering, the ordering of the bars is arbitrary. Meaning is assigned only to the height of the bar, which represents the frequency or relative frequency of occurrence of cases that belong to that particular class interval. In addition, the width of the bar has no meaning.

Pie charts depict the same information as do bar graphs, but in the shape of a circle or pie. The circle is divided into wedges, one for each category of the data. The size of each wedge is determined by its angular measurement. Since a circle contains 360°, a wedge that contains 50% of the cases would have an angular measurement of 180°. In general, if the wedge is to contain α percent of the cases, then the angle for the wedge will be $360\alpha/100°$. Figure 3.12 illustrates a pie chart of categorical data. Using data from a research study of clinic patients, the figure presents the proportions of female patients who were diagnosed with cancer, diabetes, and coronary heart disease.

We can use pie charts also to represent ordinal data. Table 3.6 presents data regarding a characteristic called the Pugh level, a measure of the severity of liver disease. Figure 3.13 illustrates these data in the form of a pie chart. Based on 24 pediatric patients with liver disease, this pie chart presents ordinal data, which indicate severity of the disease. As an alternative to a pie chart, Figure 3.14 shows a bar graph for the same Pugh data presented in Table 3.6.

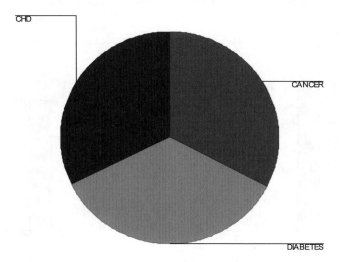

Figure 3.12. Pie chart—proportions of patients diagnosed with cancer, diabetes, and coronary heart disease (CHD). (Source: Robert Friis, unpublished data.)

TABLE 3.6. Pugh Categories and Pugh Severity Levels

Pugh Category	Pugh Severity Level
1	0
2	5
3	6
4	7
5	8
6	10
7	11

Note: For these data, the Pugh categories are 1–7, corresponding to Pugh levels 0–11.

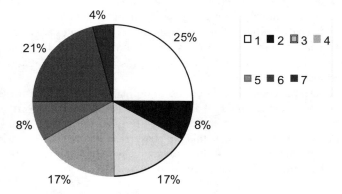

Figure 3.13. Pie chart for Pugh level for 24 children with liver disease.

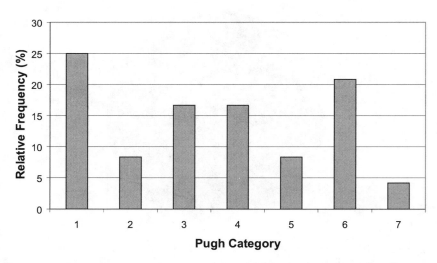

Figure 3.14. Relative frequency bar graph for Pugh categories of 24 pediatric patients with liver disease.

3.4   EXERCISES

3.1 Define the term "variable" and describe the following types of variables:
   a. Qualitative
      (1) Nominal
      (2) Ordinal
   b. Quantitative
      (1) Interval
      (2) Ratio
   c. Discrete versus continuous

3.2 The following terms relate to frequency tables. Define each term.
   a. Class interval
   b. Class frequency
   c. Relative frequency percentage
   d. Cumulative frequency
   e. Cumulative relative frequency
   f. Cumulative percentage

3.3 Define the following graphical methods and describe how they are used.
   a. Histogram
   b. Relative frequency histogram
   c. Frequency polygon
   d. Cumulative frequency polygon (ogive)

3.4 How does one construct a stem-and-leaf diagram? What are the advantages of this type of diagram?

3.5 How may the box-and-whisker plot be used to describe data? How are the following terms used in a box-and-whisker plot?
   a. Median
   b. Alpha percentile
   c. Interquartile range

3.6 Refer to the following dataset that shows the class interval (and frequency in parentheses):

{0.0–0.4 (20); 0.5–0.9 (30); 1.0–1.4 (50); 1.5–1.9 (40); 2.0–2.4 (10); 2.5–2.9 (20); 3.0–3.4 (20); 3.5–3.9 (10)}

Construct a relative frequency histogram, a cumulative frequency histogram, a relative frequency (%) histogram, a cumulative relative frequency (%) histogram, a frequency polygon, and a relative frequency polygon. Describe the shapes of these graphs. What are the midpoint and limits of the interval, 2.0–2.4?

3.7 Using the data in Table 3.7, construct a frequency table with nine intervals and then calculate the mean and median blood levels.

TABLE 3.7. Blood Levels (mg/dl) of 50 Subjects

4.9	23.3	3.9	2.5	7.6
5.5	3.9	1.0	5.0	4.2
7.6	0.7	1.6	2.2	4.0
2.3	14.1	1.0	6.1	5.4
1.2	4.3	4.8	0.7	4.8
0.7	3.9	1.5	8.0	6.5
4.1	6.9	2.9	2.1	2.8
1.5	2.0	1.1	10.6	2.0
6.7	3.2	1.6	0.7	9.0
2.1	2.7	3.5	8.2	4.4

Source: U.S. Department of Health and Human Services (DHHS). National Center for Health Statistics. Third National Health and Nutrition Examination Survey, 1988–1994, NHANES III Laboratory Data File (CD-ROM). Public Use Data File Number 76200. Hyattsville, MD: Centers for Disease Control and Prevention, 1996.

3.8 Take the data set from Exercise 3.7 and order the observations from smallest to largest. Determine the lower and the upper quartiles and generate a box-and-whiskers plot for the data using the smallest and largest observations for the whiskers.

3.9 Take the data from Exercise 3.7 and construct a stem-and-leaf plot using the integer part of the number for the stem and the digit to the right of the decimal point for the leaf.

3.10 Consider the following data set: {3, 4, 8, 5, 7, 2, 5, 6, 5, 9, 7, 8, 6, 4, 5}. Determine the median and quartiles, and the minimum and maximum values.

3.11 Using the data presented in Table 3.8, calculate the mean, median, and quartiles, and construct a box-and-whisker plot.

TABLE 3.8. Ages of Patients in a Primary Care Medical Clinic ($n = 50$)

18	14	22	34	86
105	72	44	49	64
90	98	65	26	33
88	62	70	61	57
12	17	21	101	15
22	24	51	56	27
85	81	94	93	86
83	100	104	55	66
89	56	61	50	57
53	94	58	59	99

3.12 Construct a frequency histogram and a cumulative frequency histogram with the data from Exercise 3.11 using the following class intervals: 10–19, 20–29, 30–39, 40–49, 50–59, 60–69, 70–79, 80–89, 90–99, 100–109.

3.13 Construct a stem-and-leaf plot with the data from Exercise 3.11.

3.14 Classify the following data as either (1) nominal, (2) ordinal, (3) interval, or (4) ratio.
a. The names of the patients in a clinical trial
b. A person's weight
c. A person's age in years
d. A person's blood type
e. Your top ten list of professional basketball players ranked in ascending order of preference
f. The face of a coin that lands up (a head or a tail)

3.15 The following questions (a-d) refer to the data presented in Table 3.9.
a. Construct a frequency table with the class intervals 0–1, 2–3, 4–5, 6–7, 8–9, 10–11, and 12–13.
b. Construct a frequency histogram of the weight losses.
c. Construct a frequency polygon and describe the shape of the distribution.
d. What is the most common weight loss?

3.16 The FBI gathers data on violent crimes. For 20,000 murders committed over the past few years, the following fictitious data set represents the classification of the weapon used to commit the crime.

12,500 committed with guns
2,000 with a knife
5000 with hands
500 with explosives

Construct a pie chart to describe this data.

3.17 In 1961, Roger Maris broke Babe Ruth's home run record by hitting 61 home runs. Ruth's record was 60. The following set of numbers is the consecutive list of home run totals that Ruth collected over a span of 15 seasons as a Yan-

TABLE 3.9. Weight Loss in Pounds of Individuals on a Five-Week Weight Control Program ($n = 25$)

9	5	2	1	3
11	11	10	8	9
6	4	8	10	9
12	11	7	11	13
10	11	5	4	11

kee: 54, 59, 35, 41, 46, 25, 47, 60, 54, 46, 49, 46, 41, 34, 22. Maris had a 10-year career in the American League before joining the St. Louis Cardinals in the National League at the end of his career. Here is the list of home runs Maris hit during his 10 years: 14, 28, 16, 39, 61, 33, 23, 26, 8, 13

a. Find the seasonal median number of home runs for each player.

b. For each player, determine the minimum, the first quartile, the median, the third quartile, and the maximum of their home run totals. Use these results to construct comparative box-and-whisker plots. These five numbers that highlight a box plot are called the five-number summary.

c. How do the two distributions differ based on the box plots?

3.18 In 1998, Mark McGwire broke Roger Maris' home run record of 61 by hitting 70 home runs. Incredibly, in the same year Sammy Sosa also broke the record, hitting 66. Again, in 1999 both players broke Maris' mark but did not top their 1998 results: McGwire hit 65 and Sosa 63. In 2001, another slugger, Barry Bonds, whose top home run total was 49 in 2000, broke McGwire's record with 73 home runs. Here we present the seasonal home run totals for McGwire over his major league career starting with his rookie 1987 season, along with those for Sammy Sosa, Barry Bonds and Ken Griffey Jr.

McGwire 49, 32, 33, 39, 22, 42, 9, 9, 39, 52, 58, 70, 65, 32
Sosa   4, 15, 10, 8, 33, 25, 36, 40, 36, 66, 63, 50
Bonds   16, 25, 24, 19, 33, 25, 34, 46, 37, 33, 42, 40, 37, 34, 49
Griffey 16, 22, 22, 27, 45, 40, 17, 49, 56, 56, 48, 40

McGwire's low totals of 9 in 1993 and 1994 are explained by a combination of the baseball strike that cancelled many games and some injuries he sustained. Sosa's rookie year was 1989. His home run totals were fairly high during the strike years. Bonds' rookie year was 1986. He has been a consistent home run hitter but has never before approached the total of 60 home runs.

Ken Griffey Jr. had a spectacular start during the strike season, and many thought he would have topped Maris that year had there not been a strike. Griffey's rookie year was 1989. In the strike-shortened season of 1993, Griffey hit 45 home runs; he has approached 60 twice.

a. Find the seasonal median number of home runs for each player.

b. For each player, determine the minimum, the first quartile, the median, the third quartile, and the maximum of their home run totals. Use these results to construct comparative box-and-whisker plots.

c. What are the similarities and differences among these famous sluggers?

3.19 In 2001, due to injury, McGwire hit only 29 home runs; Sosa hit 64 home runs; Bonds hit 73 home runs for a new major league record; and Griffey hit 22. Their current career home runs are as follows:

McGwire 49, 32, 33, 39, 22, 42, 9, 9, 39, 52, 58, 70, 65, 32, 29
Sosa   4, 15, 10, 8, 33, 25, 36, 40, 36, 66, 63, 50, 64

Bonds   16, 25, 24, 19, 33, 25, 34, 46, 37, 33, 42, 40, 37, 34, 49, 73
Griffey   16, 22, 22, 27, 45, 40, 17, 49, 56, 56, 48, 40, 22

a. Find the seasonal median number of home runs for each player.
b. For each player, determine the minimum, the first quartile, the median, the third quartile and the maximum of their home run totals. Use these results to construct comparative box-and-whisker plots.
c. What are the similarities and differences among these famous sluggers?
d. Did the results from 2001 change your conclusions from the previous problem? If so, how did they change and why?

3.5 ADDITIONAL READING

The books listed here provide further insight into graphical methods and exploratory data analysis. Some were referenced earlier in this chapter. The reader should be aware that Launer and Siegel (1982) and du Toit et al. (1986) are advanced texts, appropriate for those who have mastered the present text.

1. Campbell, S. K. (1974). *Flaws and Fallacies in Statistical Thinking.* Prentice Hall, Englewood Cliffs, New Jersey.
2. Chambers, J. M., Cleveland, W. S., Kleiner, B. and Tukey, P. (1983). *Graphical Methods for Data Analysis.* Wadsworth, Belmont, California.
3. Dunn, O. J. (1977). *Basic Statistics: A Primer for the Biomedical Sciences,* 2nd Edition. Wiley, New York.
4. du Toit, S. H. C., Steyn, A. G. W. and Stumpf, R. H. (1986). *Graphical Exploratory Data Analysis.* Springer-Verlag, New York.
5. Gonick, L. and Smith, W. (1993). *The Cartoon Guide to Statistics.* HarperPerennial, New York.
6. Hoaglin, D. C., Mosteller, F. and Tukey, J. W. (Editors). (1983). *Understanding Robust and Exploratory Data Analysis.* Wiley, New York.
7. Hoaglin, D. C., Mosteller, F. and Tukey, J. W. (Editors). (1985). *Exploring Data Tables, Trends and Shapes.* Wiley, New York.
8. Huff, D. (1954). *How to Lie with Statistics.* W.W. Norton and Company, New York.
9. Launer, R. L. and Siegel, A. F. editors (1982). *Modern Data Analysis.* Academic Press, New York.
10. Tufte, E. R. (1983). *The Visual Display of Quantitative Information.* Graphics Press, Cheshire, Connecticut.
11. Tufte, E. R. (1997). *Visual Explanations.* Graphics Press, Cheshire, Connecticut.
12. Tukey, J. W. (1977). *Exploratory Data Analysis.* Addison-Wesley, Reading, Massachusetts.
13. Velleman, P. F. and Hoaglin, D. C. (1981). *Applications, Basics, and Computing of Exploratory Data Analysis.* Duxbury Press, Boston.

CHAPTER 4

Summary Statistics

A want of the habit of observing and an inveterate habit of taking
averages are each of them often equally misleading.
—Florence Nightingale, *Notes on Nursing,* Chapter XIII

4.1 MEASURES OF CENTRAL TENDENCY

The previous chapter, which discussed data displays such as frequency histograms and frequency polygons, introduced the concept of the shape of distributions of data. For example, a frequency polygon illustrated the distribution of body mass index data. Chapter 4 will expand on these concepts by defining measures of central tendency and measures of dispersion.

Measures of central tendency are numbers that tell us where the majority of values in the distribution are located. Also, we may consider these measures to be the center of the probability distribution from which the data were sampled. An example is the average age in a distribution of patients' ages. Section 4.1 will cover the following measures of central tendency: arithmetic mean, median, mode, geometric mean, and harmonic mean. These measures also are called measures of location. In contrast to measures of central tendency, measures of dispersion inform us about the spread of values in a distribution. Section 4.2 will present measures of dispersion

4.1.1 The Arithmetic Mean

The arithmetic mean is the sum of the individual values in a data set divided by the number of values in the data set. We can compute a mean of both a finite population and a sample. For the mean of a finite population (denoted by the symbol μ), we sum the individual observations in the entire population and divide by the population size, N. When data are based on a sample, to calculate the sample mean (denoted by the symbol $\bar{X}$) we sum the individual observations in the sample and divide by the number of elements in the sample, n. The sample mean is the sample analog to the mean of a finite population. Formulas for the population (4.1a) and sample means (4.1b) are shown below; also see Table 4.1.

**TABLE 4.1. Calculation of Mean
(Small Population, $N = 5$)**

Index (i)	X
1	70
2	80
3	95
4	100
5	125
Σ	470

$$\mu = \frac{\sum_{i=1}^{N} X_i}{N} = \frac{470}{5} = 94$$

Population mean (μ):

$$\mu = \frac{\sum_{i=1}^{N} X_i}{N} \tag{4.1a}$$

where X_i are the individual values from a finite population of size N.
Sample mean ($\overline{X}$):

$$\overline{X} = \frac{\sum_{i=1}^{n} X_i}{n} \tag{4.1b}$$

where X_i are the individual values of a sample of size n.

The population mean (and also the population variance and standard deviation) is a parameter of a distribution. Means, variances, and standard deviations of finite populations are almost identical to their sample analogs. You will learn more about these terms and appreciate their meaning for infinite populations after we cover absolutely continuous distributions and random variables in Chapter 5. We will refer to the individual values in the data set as elements, a point that will be discussed in more detail in Chapter 5, which covers probability theory.

Statisticians generally use the arithmetic mean as a measure of central tendency for numbers that are from a ratio scale (e.g., many biological values, height, blood sugar, cholesterol), from an interval scale (e.g., Fahrenheit temperature or personality measures such as depression), or from an ordinal scale (high, medium, low). The values may be either discrete or continuous; for example, ranking on an attitude scale (discrete values) or blood cholesterol measurements (continuous).

It is important to distinguish between a continuous scale such as blood cholesterol and cholesterol measurements. While the scale is continuous, the measurements we record are discrete values. For example, when we record a cholesterol measurement of 200, we have converted a continuous variable into a discrete measurement. The speed of an automobile is also a continuous variable. As soon as we state a specific speed, for example, 60 miles or 100 kilometers per hour, we have created a discrete measurement. This example becomes clearer if we have a speedometer that gives a digital readout such as 60 miles per hour.

For large data sets (e.g., more than about 20 observations when performing calculations by hand), summing the individual numbers may be impractical, so we use grouped data. When using a computer, the number of values is not an issue at all. The procedure for calculating a mean is somewhat more involved for grouped data than for ungrouped data. First, the data need to be placed in a frequency table, as illustrated in Chapter 3. We then apply Formula 4.2, which specifies that the midpoint of each class interval (X) is multiplied by the frequency of observation in that class.

The mean using grouped data is

$$\overline{X} = \frac{\sum_{i=3}^{n} f_i X_i}{\sum_{i=1}^{n} f_i} \tag{4.2}$$

where X_i is the midpoint of the ith interval and f_i is the frequency of observations in the ith interval.

In order to perform the calculation specified by Formula 4.2, first we need to place the data from Table 4.2 in a frequency table, as shown in Table 4.3. For a review of how to construct such a table, consult Chapter 3. From Table 4.3, we can see that $\Sigma f X = 9715$, $\Sigma f = n = 100$, and that the mean is estimated as 97.2 (rounding to the nearest tenth).

4.1.2   The Median

Previously in Chapter 3, we defined the term median and illustrated its calculation for small data sets. In review, the median refers to the 50% point in a frequency dis-

TABLE 4.2. Plasma Glucose Values (mg/dl) for a Sample of 100 Adults, Aged 20–74 Years

74	82	86	88	90	91	94	97	106	123
75	82	86	89	90	92	95	98	108	124
77	82	87	89	90	92	95	99	108	128
78	83	87	89	90	92	95	99	113	132
78	83	87	89	90	92	95	99	113	134
78	83	88	89	90	93	95	99	115	140
80	83	88	89	90	93	96	100	118	151
81	85	88	89	90	94	96	101	120	153
81	86	88	89	90	94	97	104	121	156
81	86	88	90	91	94	97	105	122	164

TABLE 4.3. Calculation of a Mean from a Frequency Table (Using Data from Table 4.2)

Class Interval	Midpoint (x)	f	fx
160–169	165.5	1	165.50
150–159	155.5	3	466.50
140–149	145.5	1	145.50
130–139	134.5	2	269.00
120–129	124.5	6	747.00
110–119	114.5	4	458.00
100–109	104.5	7	731.50
90–99	94.5	37	3496.50
80–89	84.5	33	2788.50
70–79	74.5	6	447.00
		100	9715.00

$$\overline{X} = \frac{\sum_{i=1}^{n} f_i X_i}{\sum_{i=1}^{n} f_i} = \frac{9715.0}{100} = 97.15$$

tribution of a population. When data are grouped in a frequency table, the median is an estimate because we are unable to calculate it precisely. Thus, Formula 4.3 is used to estimate the median from data in a frequency table:

$$\text{median} = \text{lower limit of the interval} + i(0.50n - cf) \qquad (4.3)$$

where i = the width of the interval
  n = sample size (or N = population size)
  cf = the cumulative frequency below the interval that contains the median

The sample median (an analog to the population median) is defined in the same way as a population median. For a sample, 50% of the observations fall below and 50% fall above the median. For a population, 50% of the probability distribution is above and 50% is below the median.

In Table 4.4, the lower end of the distribution begins with the class 70–79. The column "cf" refers to the cumulative frequency of cases at and below a particular interval. For example, the cf at interval 80–89 is 39. The cf is found by adding the numbers in columns f and cf diagonally; e.g., 6 + 33 = 39. First, we must find the interval in which the median is located. There are a total of 100 cases, so one-half of them (0.50n) equals 50. By inspecting the cumulative frequency column, we find the interval in which 50% of the cases (the 50th case) fall in or below: 90–99. The lower real limit of the interval is 89.5.

Here is a point that requires discussion. Previously, we stated that the mea-

TABLE 4.4. Determining a Median from a Frequency Table

Class Interval	f	cf
160–169	1	100
150–159	3	99
140–149	1	96
130–139	2	95
120–129	6	93
110–119	4	87
100–109	7	83
90–99	37	76
80–89	33	39
70–79	6	6

surements from a continuous scale represent discrete values. The numbers placed in the frequency table were continuous numbers rounded off to the nearest unit. The real limits of the class interval are halfway between adjacent intervals. As a result, the real limits of a class interval, e.g., 90–99, are 89.5 to 99.5. The width of the interval (i) is (99.5 – 89.5), or 10. Thus, placing these values in Formula 4.3 yields

$$\text{median} = 89.5 + 10[(0.50)(100) - 39] = 97.47$$

For data that have not been grouped, the sample median also can be calculated in a reasonable amount of time on a computer. The computer orders the observations from smallest to largest and finds the middle value for the median if the sample size is odd. For an even number of observations, the sample does not have a middle value; by convention, the sample median is defined as the average of two values that fall in the middle of a distribution. The first number in the average is the largest observation below the halfway point and the second is the smallest observation above the halfway point.

Let us illustrate this definition of the median with small data sets. Although the definition applies equally to a finite population, assume we have selected a small sample. For $n = 7$, the data are {2.2, 1.7, 4.5, 6.2, 1.8, 5.5, 3.3}. Ordering the data from smallest to largest, we obtain {1.7, 1.8, 2.2, 3.3, 4.5, 5.5, 6.2}. The middle observation (median) is the fourth number in the sequence; three values fall below 3.3 and three values fall above 3.3. In this case, the median is 3.3.

Suppose $n = 8$ (the previous data set plus one more observation, 5.7). The new data set becomes {1.7, 1.8, 2.2, 3.3, 4.5, 5.5, 5.7, 6.2}. When n is even, we take the average of the two middle numbers in the data set, e.g., 3.3 and 4.5. In our example, the sample median is (3.3 + 4.5)/2 = 3.9. Note that there are three observations above and three below the two middle observations.

4.1.3   The Mode

The mode refers to the class (or midpoint of the class) that contains the highest frequency of cases. In Table 4.4, the modal class is 90–99. When a distribution is portrayed graphically, the mode is the peak in the graph. Many distributions are multimodal, referring to the fact that they may have two or more peaks. Such multimodal distributions are of interest to epidemiologists because they may indicate different causal mechanisms for biological phenomena, for example, bimodal distributions in the age of onset of diseases such as tuberculosis, Hodgkins disease, and meningococcal disease. Figure 4.1 illustrates unimodal and bimodal distributions.

4.1.4   The Geometric Mean

The geometric mean (GM) is found by multiplying a set of values and then finding their nth root. All of the values must be non-0 and greater than 1. Formula 4.4 shows how to calculate a GM.

$$GM = \sqrt[n]{X_1 X_2 X_3 \cdots X_n} = \sqrt[n]{\prod_{i=1}^{n} X_i} \qquad (4.4)$$

A GM is preferred to an arithmetic mean when several values in a data set are much higher than all of the others. These higher values would tend to inflate or distort an arithmetic mean. For example, suppose we have the following numbers: 10, 15, 5, 8, 17. The arithmetic mean is 11. Now suppose we add one more number—100—to the previous five numbers. Then the arithmetic mean is 25.8, an inflated value not very close to 11. However, the geometric mean is 14.7, a value that is closer to 11.

In practice, is it desirable to use a geometric mean? When greatly differing values within a data set occur, as in some biomedical applications, the geometric mean becomes appropriate. To illustrate, a common use for the geometric mean is to determine whether fecal coliform levels exceed a safe standard. (Fecal coliform bacteria are used as an indicator of water pollution and unsafe swimming conditions at

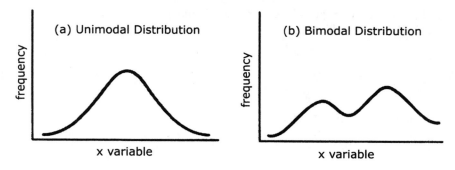

Figure 4.1. Unimodal and bimodal distribution curves. (Source: Authors.)

beaches.) For example, the standard may be set at a 30-day geometric mean of 200 fecal coliform units per 100 ml of water. When the water actually is tested, most of the individual tests may fall below 200 units. However, on a few days some of the values could be as high as 10,000 units. Consequently, the arithmetic mean would be distorted by these extreme values. By using the geometric mean, one obtains an average that is closer to the average of the lower values. To cite another example, when the sample data do not conform to a normal distribution, the geometric mean is especially useful. A log transformation of the data will produce a symmetric distribution that is normally distributed.

Review Formula 4.4 and note the nth root of the product of a set of numbers. You may wonder how to find the nth root of a number. This problem is solved by logarithms or, much more easily, by using the "geometric mean function" in a spreadsheet program.

Here is a simple calculation example of the GM. Let $X_1, X_2, X_3, \ldots, X_n$ denote our sample of n values. The geometric mean is the nth root of the product of these values, or $(X_1 X_2 X_3 \ldots X_n)^{1/n}$.

If we apply the log transformation to this geometric mean we obtain $\{\log(X_1) + \log(X_2) + \log(X_3) + \ldots + \log(X_n)\}/n$. From these calculations, we see that the GM is the arithmetic mean of the data after transforming them to a log scale. On the log scale, the data become symmetric. Consequently, the arithmetic mean is the natural parameter to use for the location of the distribution, confirming our suspicion that the geometric mean is the correct measure of central tendency on the original scale.

4.1.5 The Harmonic Mean

The harmonic mean (HM) is the final measure of location covered in this chapter. Although the HM is not used commonly, we mention it here because you may encounter it in the biomedical literature. Refer to Iman (1983) for more information about the HM, including applications and relationships with other measures of location, as well as additional references.

The HM is the reciprocal of the arithmetic average of the reciprocals of the original observations. Mathematically, we define the HM as follows: Let the original observations be denoted by $X_1, X_2, X_3, \ldots, X_n$. Consider the observations $Y_1, Y_2, Y_3, \ldots, Y_n$ obtained by reciprocal transformation, namely $Y_i = 1/X_i$ for $i = 1, 2, 3, \ldots, n$. Let Y_h denote the arithmetic average of the Y's, where

$$Y_h = \frac{\sum_{i=1}^{n} Y_i}{n}$$

The harmonic mean (HM) of the X's is $1/Y_h$:

$$HM = \frac{1}{Y_h} \tag{4.5}$$

where $Y_i = 1/X_i$ for $i = 1, 2, 3, \ldots, n$ and $Y_h = (\sum Y_i)/n$.

4.1.6 Which Measure Should You Use?

Each of the measures of central tendency has strengths and weaknesses. The mode is difficult to use when a distribution has more than one mode, especially when these modes have the same frequencies. In addition, the mode is influenced by the choice of the number and size of intervals used to make a frequency distribution.

The median is useful in describing a distribution that has extreme values at either end; common examples occur in distributions of income and selling prices of houses. Because a few extreme values at the upper end will inflate the mean, the median will give a better picture of central tendency.

Finally, the mean often is more useful for statistical inference than either the mode or the median. For example, we will see that the mean is useful in calculating an important measure of variability: variance. The mean is also the value that minimizes the sum of squared deviations (mean squared error) between the mean and the values in the data set, a point that will be discussed in later chapters (e.g., Chapter 12) and that is exceedingly valuable for statistical inference.

The choice of a particular measure of central tendency depends on the shape of the population distribution. When we are dealing with sample-based data, the distribution of the data from the sample may suggest the shape of the population distribution. For normally distributed data, mathematical theory of the normal distribution (to be discussed in Chapter 6) suggests that the arithmetic mean is the most appropriate measure of central tendency. Finally, as we have discussed previously, if a log transformation creates normally distributed data, then the geometric mean is appropriate to the raw data.

How are the mean, median, and mode interrelated? For symmetric distributions, the mean and median are equal. If the distribution is symmetric and has only one mode, all three measures are the same, an example being the normal distribution. For skewed distributions, with a single mode, the three measures differ. (Refer to Figure 4.2.) For positively skewed distributions (where the upper, or left, tail of the distribution is longer ("fatter") than the lower, or right, tail) the measures are or-

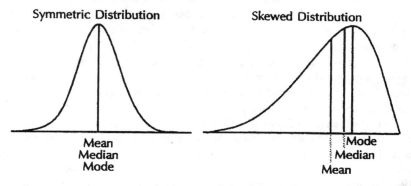

Figure 4.2. Mean, median, and mode, symmetric and skewed distributions. (Source: Centers for Disease Control and Prevention (1992). *Principles of Epidemiology,* 2nd Edition, Figure 3.11, p. 187.)

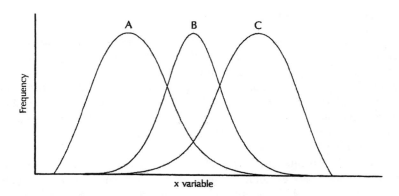

Figure 4.3. Symmetric (B) and skewed distributions: right skewed (A) and left skewed (C). (Source: Centers for Disease Control and Prevention (1992). *Principles of Epidemiology,* 2nd Edition, Figure 3.5, p. 151.)

dered as follows: mode < median < mean. For negatively skewed distributions (where the lower tail of the distribution is longer than the upper tail), the reverse ordering occurs: mean < median < mode. Figure 4.3 shows symmetric and skewed distributions. The fact that the median is closer to the mean than is the mode led Karl Pearson to observe that for moderately skewed distributions such as the gamma distribution, mode – mean ≈ 3(median – mean). See Stuart and Ord (1994) and Kotz and Johnson (1985) for more details on these relationships.

4.2 MEASURES OF DISPERSION

As you may have observed already, when we select a sample and collect measurements for one or more characteristics, these measurements tend to be different from one another. To give a simple example, height measurements taken from a sample of persons obviously will not be all identical. In fact, if we were to take measurements from a single individual at different times during the day and compare them, the measurements also would tend to be slightly different from one another; i.e., we are shorter at the end of the day than when we wake up!

How do we account for differences in biological and human characteristics? While driving through Midwestern cornfields when stationed in Michigan as a postdoctoral fellow, one of the authors (Robert Friis) observed that fields of corn stalks generally resemble a smooth green carpet, yet individual plants are taller or shorter than others. Similarly, in Southern California where oranges are grown or in the almond orchards of Tuscany, individual trees differ in height. To describe these differences in height or other biological characteristics, statisticians use the term variability.

We may group the sources of variability according to three main categories: true biological, temporal, and measurement. We will delimit our discussion of the first of the categories, variation in biological characteristics, to human beings. A range of factors cause variations in human biological characteristics, including, but not limited to, age, sex, race, genetic factors, diet and lifestyle, socioeconomic status, and past medical history.

There are many good examples of how each of the foregoing factors produces variability in human characteristics. However, let us focus on one—age, which is an important control or demographic variable in many statistical analyses. Biological characteristics tend to wax and wane with increasing age. For example, in the U.S., Europe, and other developed areas, systolic and diastolic blood pressures tend to increase with age. At the same time, age may be associated with decline in other characteristics such as immune status, bone density, and cardiac and pulmonary functioning. All of these age-related changes produce differences in measurements of characteristics of persons who differ in age. Another important example is the impact of age or maturation effects on children's performance on achievement tests and intelligence tests. Maturation effects need to be taken into account with respect to performance on these kinds of tests as children progress from lower to higher levels of education.

Temporal variation refers to changes that are time-related. Factors that are capable of producing temporal variation include current emotional state, activity level, climate and temperature, and circadian rhythm (the body's internal clock). To illustrate, we are all aware of the phenomenon of jet lag—how we feel when our normal sleep–awake rhythm is disrupted by a long flight to a distant time zone. As a consequence of jet lag, not only may our level of consciousness be impacted, but also physical parameters such as blood pressure and stress-related hormones may fluctuate. When we are forced into a cramped seat during an extended intercontinental flight, our circulatory system may produce life-threatening clots that lead to pulmonary embolism. Consequently, temporal factors may cause slight or sometimes major variations in hematologic status.

Finally, another example of a factor that induces variability in measurements is measurement error. Discrepancies between the "true" value of a variable and its measured value are called measurement errors. The topic of measurement error is an important aspect of statistics. We will deal with this type of error when we cover regression (Chapter 12) and analysis of variance (Chapter 13). Sources of measurement error include observer error, differences in measuring instruments, technical errors, variability in laboratory conditions, and even instability of chemical reagents used in experiments. Take the example of blood pressure measurement: In a multicenter clinical trial, should one or more centers use a faulty sphygmomanometer, that center would contribute measures that over- or underestimate blood pressure. Another source of error would be inaccurate measurements caused by medical personnel who have hearing loss and are unable to detect blood pressure sounds by listening with a stethoscope.

Several measures have been developed—measures of dispersion—to describe the variability of measurements in a data set. For the purposes of this text, these measures include the range, the mean absolute deviation, and the standard deviation. Percentiles and quartiles are other measures, which we will discuss in Chapter 6.

4.2.1 Range

The range is defined as the difference between the highest and lowest value in a distribution of numbers. In order to compute the range, we must first locate the highest and lowest values. With a small number of values, one is able to inspect the set of numbers in order to identify these values.

When the set of numbers is large, however, a simple way to locate these values is to sort them in ascending order and then choose the first and last values, as we did in Chapter 3. Here is an example: Let us denote the lowest or first value with the symbol X_1 and the highest value with X_n. Then the range (d) is

$$d = X_n - X_1 \tag{4.6}$$

with indices 1 and n defined after sorting the values.

Calculation is as follows:

Data set: 100, 95, 125, 45, 70
Sorted values: 45, 70, 95, 100, 125
Range = 125 − 45
Range = 80

4.2.2 Mean Absolute Deviation

A second method we use to describe variability is called the mean absolute deviation. This measure involves first calculating the mean of a set of observations or values and then determining the deviation of each observation from the mean of those values. Then we take the absolute value of each deviation, sum all of the deviations, and calculate their mean. The mean absolute deviation for a sample is

$$\text{mean absolute deviation} = \frac{\sum_{i=1}^{n} |X_i - \overline{X}|}{n} \tag{4.7a}$$

where n = number of observations in the data set.

The analogous formula for a finite population is

$$\text{mean absolute deviation} = \frac{\sum_{i=1}^{N} |X_i - \mu|}{N} \tag{4.7b}$$

where N = number of observations in the population.

Here are some additional symbols and formulae. Let

$$d_i = X_i - \overline{X}$$

where:
X_i = a particular observation, $1 \le i \le n$
$\overline{X}$ = sample mean
d_i = the deviation of a value from the mean

The individual deviations (d_i) have the mathematical property such that when we sum them

$$\sum_{i=1}^{n} d_i = 0$$

Thus, in order to calculate the mean absolute deviation of a sample, the formula must use the absolute value of d_i ($|d_i|$), as shown in Formula 4.7.

Suppose we have the following data set {80, 70, 95, 100, 125}. Table 4.5 demonstrates how to calculate a mean absolute deviation for the data set.

4.2.3 Population Variance and Standard Deviation

Historically, because of computational difficulties, the mean absolute deviation was not used very often. However, modern computers can speed up calculations of the mean absolute deviation, which has applications in statistical methods called robust procedures. Common measures of dispersion, used more frequently because of their desirable mathematical properties, are the interrelated measures variance and stan-

TABLE 4.5. Calculation of a Mean Absolute Deviation (Blood Sugar Values for a Small Finite Population)

X_i	$|X_i - \mu|$
80	14
70	24
95	1
100	6
125	31
$\Sigma 470$	76
$N = 5$	$\sum_{i=1}^{5} |X_i - \mu| = 76$

$$\mu = 470/5 = 94$$

Mean absolute deviation = 76/5 = 15.2

dard deviation. Instead of using the absolute value of the deviations about the mean, both the variance and standard deviation use squared deviations about the mean, defined for the ith observation as $(X_i - \mu)^2$. Formula 4.8, which is called the deviation score method, calculates the population variance (σ^2) for a finite population. For infinite populations we cannot calculate the population parameters such as the mean and variance. These parameters of the population distribution must be approximated through sample estimates. Based on random samples we will draw inferences about the possible values for these parameters.

$$\sigma^2 = \frac{\sum_{i=1}^{N}(X_i - \mu)^2}{N} \tag{4.8}$$

where N = the total number of elements in the population.

A related term is the population standard deviation (σ), which is the square root of the variance:

$$\sigma = \sqrt{\frac{\sum_{i=1}^{N}(X_i - \mu)^2}{N}} \tag{4.9}$$

Table 4.6 gives an example of the calculation of σ for a small finite population. The data are the same as those in Table 4.5 ($\mu = 94$).

What do the variance and standard deviation tell us? They are useful for comparing data sets that are measured in the same units. For example, a data set that has a "large" variance in comparison to one that has a "small" variance is more variable than the latter one.

TABLE 4.6. Calculation of Population Variance

Suppose we have a small finite population ($N = 5$) with the following blood sugar values:

X_i	$X_i - \mu$	$(X_i - \mu)^2$
70	−24	196
80	−14	576
95	1	1
100	6	36
125	31	961
Σ	0	1,770

$$\sigma^2 = \frac{\sum_{i=1}^{5}(X_i - \mu)^2}{5} = \frac{1770}{5} = 354 \quad \sigma = \sqrt{\sigma^2} = 18.8$$

Returning to the data set in the example (Table 4.6), the variance σ^2 is 354. If the numbers differed more from one another, e.g., if the lowest value were 60 and the highest value 180, with the other three values also differing more from one another than in the original data set, then the variance would increase substantially. We will provide several specific examples.

In the first and second examples, we will double (Table 4.6a) and triple (Table 4.6b) the individual values; we will do so for the sake of argument, forgetting momentarily that some of the blood sugar values will become unreliable. In the third

TABLE 4.6a. Effect on Mean and Variance of Doubling Each Value of a Variable

X_i	$X_i - \mu$	$(X_i - \mu)^2$
140	−48	2,304
160	−28	784
190	2	4
200	12	144
250	62	3,844
Σ	0	7,080
$\mu = 188$	$\sigma^2 = 1,416$	$\sigma = 37.6$

TABLE 4.6b. Effect on Mean and Variance of Tripling Each Value of a Variable

X_i	$X_i - \mu$	$(X_i - \mu)^2$
210	−72	5,184
240	−42	1,764
285	3	9
300	18	324
375	93	8,649
Σ	0	15,930
$\mu = 282$	$\sigma^2 = 3,186$	$\sigma = 56.4$

TABLE 4.6c. Effect on Mean and Variance of Adding a Constant (25) to Each Value of a Variable

X_i	$X_i - \mu$	$(X_i - \mu)^2$
95	−24	576
105	−14	196
120	1	1
125	6	36
150	31	961
Σ	0	1,770
$\mu = 119$	$\sigma^2 = 354$	$\sigma = 18.8$

example, we will add a constant, 25, to each individual value. The results are presented in Table 4.6c.

What may we conclude from the foregoing three examples? The individual values (X_i) differ more from one another in Table 4.6a and Table 4.6b than they did in Table 4.6. We would expect the variance to increase in the second two data sets because the numbers are more different from one another than they were in Table 4.6; in fact, σ^2 increases as the numbers become more different from one another. Note also the following additional observations. When we multiplied the original X_i by a constant (e.g., 2 or 3), the variance increased by the constant squared (e.g., 4 or 9); however, the mean was multiplied by the constant ($2 \cdot X_i \rightarrow 2\mu$, $4\sigma^2$; $3 \cdot X_i \rightarrow 3\mu$, $9\sigma^2$). When we added a constant (e.g., 25) to each X_i, there was no effect on the variance, although μ increased by the amount of the constant ($25 + X_i \rightarrow \mu + 25$; $\sigma^2 = \sigma^2$). These relationships can be summarized as follows:

Effect of multiplying X_i by a constant a or adding a constant to X_i for each i:

1. Adding a: the mean μ becomes $\mu + a$; the variance σ^2 and standard deviation σ remain unchanged.
2. Multiplying by a: the mean μ becomes μa, the variance σ^2 becomes $\sigma^2 a^2$, and the standard deviation σ becomes σa.

The standard deviation also gives us information about the shape of the distribution of the numbers. We will return to this point later, but for now distributions that have "smaller" standard deviations are narrower than those that have "larger" standard deviations. Thus, in the previous example, the second hypothetical data set also would have a larger standard deviation (obviously because the standard deviation is the square root of the variance and the variance is larger) than the original data set. Figure 4.4 illustrates distributions that have different means (i.e., different locations) but the same variances and standard deviations. In Figure 4.5, the distributions have the same mean (i.e., same locations) but different variances and standard deviations.

4.2.4 Sample Variance and Standard Deviation

Calculation of sample variance requires a slight alteration in the formula used for population variance. The symbols S^2 and S shall be used to denote sample variance and standard deviation, respectively, and are calculated by using Formulas 4.10a and 4.10b (deviation score method).

$$S^2 = \frac{\sum_{i=1}^{n}(X_i - \overline{X})^2}{n-1} \tag{4.10a}$$

$$S = \sqrt{\frac{\sum_{i=1}^{n}(X_i - \overline{X})^2}{n-1}} \tag{4.10b}$$

where n is the sample size and $\overline{X}$ is the sample mean.

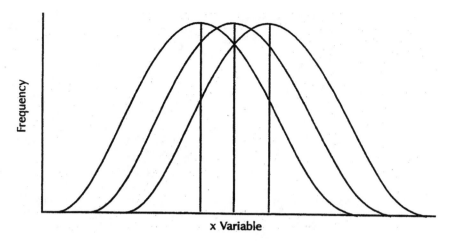

Figure 4.4. Symmetric distributions with the same variances and different means. (Source: Centers for Disease Control and Prevention (1992). *Principles of Epidemiology,* 2nd Edition, Figure 3.4, p. 150.)

Note that $n - 1$ is used in the denominator. The sample variance will be used to estimate the population variance. However, when n is used as the denominator for the estimate of variance, let us denote this estimate as $S_m^2 \cdot E(S_m^2) \neq \sigma^2$, i.e., the expected value of the estimate S_m^2 is biased; it does not equal the population variance. In order to correct for this bias, n–1 must be used in the denominator of the formula for sample variance. An example is shown in Table 4.7.

Before the age of computers, finding the difference between each score and the

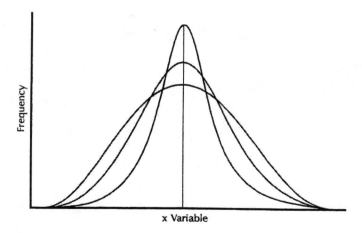

Figure 4.5. Distributions with the same mean and different variances. (Source: Centers for Disease Control and Prevention (1992). *Principles of Epidemiology,* 2nd Edition, Figure 3.4, p. 150.)

TABLE 4.7. Blood Cholesterol Measurements for a Sample of 10 Persons

Person	X	$X - \overline{X}$	$(X - \overline{X})^2$	X_2
1	276	16.3	265.69	76,176
2	304	44.3	1,962.49	92,416
3	316	56.3	3,169.69	99,856
4	188	−71.7	5,140.89	35,344
5	214	−45.7	2,088.49	45,796
6	252	−7.7	59.29	63,504
7	333	73.3	5,372.89	110,889
8	271	11.3	127.69	73,441
9	245	−14.7	216.09	60,025
10	198	−61.7	3,806.89	39,204
Sum	2,597	0	22,210.10	696,651

Mean $= \overline{X} = \Sigma X/n = 2{,}597/10 = 259.7$

Variance	2467.788
Std. Dev.	49.677

mean was a cumbersome process. Statisticians developed a shortcut formula for the sample variance that is computationally faster and numerically more stable than the difference score formula. With the speed and high precision of modern computers, the shortcut formula is no longer as important as it once was. But it is still handy for doing computations on a pocket calculator.

This alternative calculation formula of sample variance (Formula 4.11) is algebraically equivalent to the deviation score method. The formula speeds the computation by avoiding the need to find the difference between the mean and each individual value:

$$S^2 = \frac{\sum_{i=1}^{n} X_i^2 - n\overline{X}^2}{n - 1} \tag{4.11}$$

where $\overline{X} =$ sample mean and n is the sample size.

Using the data from Table 4.7, we see that:

$$S^2 = \frac{696651 - (10)(67444.09)}{9} = 2467.789$$

$$S = \sqrt{2467.789} = 49.677$$

4.2.5 Calculating the Variance and Standard Deviation from Grouped Data

For larger samples (e.g., above $n = 30$), the use of individual scores in manual calculations becomes tedious. An alternative procedure groups the data and estimates s^2 from the grouped data. The formulas for sample variance and standard deviation for grouped data using the deviation score method (shown in Formulas 4.12a and b) are analogous to those for individual scores.

Variance:
$$S^2 = \frac{\sum f(X-\bar{X})^2}{n-1}$$
(4.12a)

Standard deviation:
$$S = \frac{\sum f(X-\bar{X})^2}{n-1}$$
(4.12b)

Table 4.8 provides an example of the calculations. In Table 4.8, $\bar{X}$ is the grouped mean [$\sum fX/\sum f = 19188.50/373 \approx 51.44$ (by rounding to two decimal places)].

4.3   COEFFICIENT OF VARIATION (CV) AND COEFFICIENT OF DISPERSION (CD)

Useful and meaningful only for variables that take on positive values, the coefficient of variation is defined as the ratio of the standard deviation to the absolute value of the mean. The coefficient of variation is well defined for any variable (including a variable that can be negative) that has a nonzero mean.

Let θ and V symbolize the coefficient of variation in the population and sample, respectively. Refer to Formulas 4.13a and 4.13b for calculating θ and V.

Population:
$$\theta(\%) = 100\left(\frac{\sigma}{\mu}\right)$$
(4.13a)

Sample:
$$V(\%) = 100\left(\frac{S}{\bar{X}}\right)$$
(4.13b)

TABLE 4.8. Ages of Patients Diagnosed with Multiple Sclerosis: Sample Variance and Standard Deviation Calculations Using the Formulae for Grouped Data

Class Interval	Midpoint (X)	f	FX	$X-\bar{X}$	$(X-\bar{X})^2$	$f(X-\bar{X})^2$
20–29	24.5	4	98.00	−26.94	725.96	2,903.85
30–39	34.5	44	1,518.00	−16.94	287.09	12,631.91
40–49	44.5	124	5,518.00	−6.94	48.22	5,978.66
50–59	54.5	124	6,758.00	3.06	9.34	1,158.28
60–69	64.5	48	3,096.00	13.06	170.47	8,182.41
70–79	74.5	25	1,862.50	23.06	531.59	13,289.82
80–89	84.5	4	338.00	33.06	1,092.72	4,370.88
Σ	—	373	19,188.50	—	—	48,515.82

$$S^2 = \frac{48,515.82}{373-1} = 130.42$$

$$S = \sqrt{130.42} = 11.42$$

Usually represented as a percentage, sometimes θ is thought of as a measure of relative dispersion. A variable with a population standard deviation of σ and a mean $\mu > 0$ has a coefficient of variation $\theta = 100(\sigma/\mu)\%$.

Given a data set with a sample mean $\overline{X} > 0$ and standard deviation S, the sample coefficient of variation is $V = 100(S/\overline{X})\%$. The term V is the obvious sample analog to the population coefficient of variation.

The original purpose of the coefficient of variation was to make comparisons between different distributions. For instance, if we want to see whether the distribution of the length of the tails of mice is similar to the distribution of the length of elephants' tails, we could not meaningfully compare their actual standard deviations. In comparison to the standard deviation of the tails of mice, the standard deviation of elephants' tails would be larger simply because of the much larger measurement scale being used. However, these very differently sized animals might very well have similar coefficients of variation with respect to their tail lengths.

Another estimator, V^*, the coefficient of variation biased adjusted estimate, is often used for the sample estimate of the coefficient of variation because it has less bias in estimating θ. $V^* = V\{1 + (1/[4n])\}$, where n is the sample size. So V^* increases V by a factor of $1/(4n)$ or adds $V/(4n)$ to the estimate of V. Formula 4.14 shows the formula for V^*:

$$V^* = V\left[1 + \left(\frac{1}{4n}\right)\right] \tag{4.14}$$

This estimate and further discussion of the coefficient of variation can be found in Sokal and Rohlf (1981), pp. 58–60.

Formulas 4.15a and 4.15b present the formula for the coefficient of dispersion (CD):

Sample:
$$CD = \frac{S^2}{\overline{X}} \tag{4.15a}$$

Population:
$$CD = \frac{\sigma^2}{\mu} \tag{4.15b}$$

Similar to V, CD is the ratio of the variance to the mean. If we think of V as a ratio rather than a percentage, we see that CD is just $\overline{X}V^2$. The coefficient of dispersion is related to the Poisson distribution, which we will explain later in the text. Often, the Poisson distribution is a good model for representing the number of events (e.g., traffic accidents in Los Angeles) that occur in a given time interval. The Poisson distribution, which can take on the value zero or any positive value, has the property that its mean is always equal to its variance. So a Poisson random variable has a coefficient of dispersion equal to 1. The CD is the sample estimate of the coefficient of dispersion. Often, we are interested in count data. You will see many applications of count data when we come to the analysis of survival times in Chapter 15.

We may want to know whether the Poisson distribution is a reasonable model for our data. One way to ascertain the fit of the data to the Poisson distribution is to examine the CD. If we have sufficient data, the CD will provide a good estimate of the population coefficient of dispersion. If the Poisson model is reasonable, the estimated CD should be close to 1. If the CD is much less than 1, then the counting process is said to be underdispersed (meaning that the CD has less variance relative to the mean than a Poisson counting process). On the other hand, a counting process with a value of CD that is much greater than 1 indicates overdispersion (the opposite of underdispersion).

Overdispersion occurs commonly as a counting process that provides a mixture of two or more different Poisson counting processes. These so-called compound Poisson processes occur frequently in nature and also in some manmade events. A hypothetical example relates to the time intervals between motor vehicle accidents in a specific community during a particular year. The data for the time intervals between motor vehicle accidents might fit well to a Poisson process. However, the data aggregate information for all ages, e.g., young people (18–25 years of age), mature adults (25–65 years of age), and the elderly (above 65 years of age). The motor vehicle accident rate is likely to be higher for the inexperienced young people than for the mature adults. Also, the elderly, because of slower reflexes and poorer vision, are likely to have a higher accident rate than the mature adults. The motor vehicle accident data for the combined population of drivers represents an accumulation of three different Poisson processes (corresponding to three different age groups) and, hence, an overdispersed process.

A key assumption of linear models is that the variance of the response variable Y remains constant as predictor variables change. Miller (1986) points out that a problem with using linear models is that the variance of a response variable often does not remain constant but changes as a function of a predictor variable.

One remedy for response variables that have changing variance when predictor variables change is to use variance-stabilizing transformations. Such transformations produce a variable that has variance that does not change as the mean changes. The mean of the response variable will change in experiments in which the predictor variables are allowed to change; the mean of the response changes because it is affected by these predictors. You will appreciate these notions more fully when we cover correlation and simple linear regression in Chapter 12.

Miller (1986), p. 59, using what is known as the delta method, shows that a log transformation stabilizes the variance when the coefficient of variation for the response remains constant as its mean changes. Similarly, he shows that a square root transformation stabilizes the variance if the coefficient of dispersion for the response remains constant as the mean changes. Miller's book is advanced and requires some familiarity with calculus.

Transformations can be used as tools to achieve statistical assumptions needed for certain types of parametric analyses. The delta method is an approximation technique based on terms in a Taylor series (polynomial approximations to functions). Although understanding a Taylor series requires a first year calculus course, it is sufficient to know that the coefficient of dispersion and the coefficient of variation have statistical properties that make them useful in some analyses.

Because Poisson variables have a constant coefficient of dispersion of 1, the square root transformation will stabilize the variance for them. This fact can be very useful for some practical applications.

4.4 EXERCISES

4.1   What is meant by a measure of location? State in your own words the definitions of the following measures of location:
   a. Arithmetic mean
   b. Median
   c. Mode
   d. Uni-, bi-, and multimodal distributions
   e. Skewed distributions—positively and negatively
   f. Geometric mean
   g. Harmonic mean

4.2   How are the mean, median, and mode interrelated? What considerations lead to the choice of one of these measures of location over another?

4.3   Why do statisticians need measures of variability? State in your own words the definitions of the following measures of variability:
   a. Range
   b. Mean absolute deviation
   c. Standard deviation

4.4   How are the mean and variance of a distribution affected when:
   a. A constant is added to every value of a variable?
   b. Every value of a variable is multiplied by a constant?

4.5   Giving appropriate examples, explain what is meant by the following statement: "S_m^2 is a biased or unbiased estimator of the parameter σ^2."

4.6   Distinguish among the following formulas for variance:
   a. Finite population variance
   b. Sample variance (deviation score method)
   c. Sample variance (deviation score method for grouped data)
   d. Sample variance (calculation formula)

4.7   Define the following terms and indicate their applications:
   a. Coefficient of variation
   b. Coefficient of dispersion

4.8   The table below frequency table showing heights in inches of a sample of female clinic patients. Complete the empty cells in the table and calculate the sample variance by using the formula for grouped data.

Class Interval	Midpoint (X)	f	fX	X^2	fX^2	$X-\bar{X}$	$(\bar{X}-\bar{X})^2$	$f(\bar{X}-X)^2$
45–49		2						
50–54		3						
55–59		74						
60–64		212						
65–69		91						
70–74		18						
Total		400						

[Source: Author (Friis).]

4.9 Find the medians of the following data sets: {8, 7, 3, 5, 3}; {7, 8, 3, 6, 10, 10}.

4.10 Here is a dataset for mortality due to work-related injuries among African American women in the United States during 1997: {15–24 years (9); 25–34 years (12); 35–44 years (15); 45–54 years (7); 55–64 years (5)}.
a. Identify the modal class.
b. Calculate the estimated median.
c. Assume that the data are for a finite population and compute the variance.
d. Assume the data are for a sample and compute the variance.

4.11 A sample of data was selected from a population: {195, 179, 205, 213, 179, 216, 185, 211}.
a. Use the deviation score method and the calculation formula to calculate variance and standard deviations.
b. How do the results for the two methods compare with one another? How would you account for discrepancies between the results obtained?

4.12 Using the data from the previous exercise, repeat the calculations by applying the deviation score method; however, assume that the data are for a finite population.

4.13 Assume you have the following datasets for a sample: {3, 3, 3, 3, 3}; {5, 7, 9, 11}; {4, 7, 8}; {33, 49}
a. Compute S and S^2.
b. Describe the results you obtained.

4.14 Here again are the seasonal home run totals for the four baseball home run sluggers we compared in Chapter 3:

McGwire   49, 32, 33, 39, 22, 42, 9, 9, 39, 52, 58, 70, 65, 32
Sosa   4, 15, 10, 8, 33, 25, 36, 40, 36, 66, 63, 50
Bonds   16, 25, 24, 19, 33, 25, 34, 46, 37, 33, 42, 40, 37, 34, 49
Griffey   16, 22, 22, 27, 45, 40, 17, 49, 56, 56, 48, 40

a. Calculate the sample average number of home runs per season for each player.
b. Calculate the sample median of the home runs per season for each player.
c. Calculate the sample geometric mean for each player.
d. Calculate the sample harmonic mean for each player.

4.15 Again using the data for the four home run sluggers in Exercise 4.14, calculate the following measures of dispersion:
a. Each player's sample range
b. Each player's sample standard deviation
c. Each player's mean absolute deviation

4.16 For each baseball player in Exercise 4.14, calculate their sample coefficient of variation.

4.17 For each baseball player in Exercise 4.14, calculate their sample coefficient of dispersion.

4.18 Did any of the results in Exercise 4.17 come close to 1.0? If one of the players did have a coefficient of dispersion close to 1, what would that suggest about the distribution of his home run counts over the interval of a baseball season?

4.19 The following cholesterol levels of 10 people were measured in mg/dl: {260, 150, 165, 201, 212, 243, 219, 227, 210, 240}. For this sample:
a. Calculate the mean and median.
b. Calculate the variance and standard deviation.
c. Calculate the coefficient of variation and the coefficient of dispersion.

4.20 For the data in Exercise 4.19, add the value 931 and recalculate all the sample values above.

4.21 Which statistics varied the most from Exercise 4.19 to Exercise 4.20? Which statistics varied the least?

4.22 The eleventh observation of 931 is so different from all the others in Exercise 4.19 that it seems suspicious. Such extreme values are called outliers. Which estimate of location do you trust more when this observation is included, the mean or the median?

4.23 Answer the following questions:
a. Can a population have a zero variance?
b. Can a population have a negative variance?
c. Can a sample have a zero variance?
d. Can a sample have a negative variance?

4.5 ADDITIONAL READING

The following references provide additional information on the mean, median, and mode, and the coefficient of variation, the coefficient of dispersion, and the harmonic mean.

1. Centers for Disease Control and Prevention (1992). *Principles of Epidemiology,* 2nd Edition. USDHHS, Atlanta, Georgia.
2. Iman, R. "Harmonic Mean." In Kotz, S. and Johnson, N. L. (editors). (1983). *Encyclopedia of Statistical Sciences, Volume 3, pp.* 575–576. Wiley, New York.
3. Kotz, S. and Johnson, N. L. (editors). (1985). *Encyclopedia of Statistical Sciences, Volume 5,* pp. 364–367. Wiley, New York.
4. Kruskal, W. H. and Tanur, J. M. (editors). (1978). *International Encyclopedia of Statistics, Volume 2,* 1217. Free Press, New York.
5. Miller, R. G. (1986). *Beyond ANOVA, Basics of Applied Statistics.* Wiley, New York.
6. Stuart, A. and Ord, K. (1994). *Kendall's Advanced Theory of Statistics, Volume 1,* Sixth Edition, pp. 108–109. Edward Arnold, London.
7. Sokal, R. R. and Rohlf, F. J. (1981). *Biometry,* 2nd Edition. W. H. Freeman, New York.

CHAPTER 5

Basic Probability

As for a future life, every man must judge for himself between con-
flicting vague probabilities.
—Charles Darwin, *The Life and Letters of Charles Darwin: Religion*, p. 277

5.1   WHAT IS PROBABILITY?

Probability is a mathematical construction that determines the likelihood of occurrence of events that are subject to chance. When we say an event is subject to chance, we mean that the outcome is in doubt and there are at least two possible outcomes.

Probability has its origins in gambling. Games of chance provide good examples of what the possible events are. For example, we may want to know the chance of throwing a sum of 11 with two dice, or the probability that a ball will land on red in a roulette wheel, or the chance that the Yankees will win today's baseball game, or the chance of drawing a full house in a game of poker.

In the context of health science, we could be interested in the probability that a sick patient who receives a new medical treatment will survive for five or more years. Knowing the probability of these outcomes helps us make decisions, for example, whether or not the sick patient should undergo the treatment.

We take some probabilities for granted. Most people think that the probability that a pregnant woman will have a boy rather than a girl is 0.50. Possibly, we think this because the world's population seems to be very close to 50–50. In fact, vital statistics show that the probability of giving birth to a boy is 0.514.

Perhaps this is nature's way to maintain balance, since girls tend to live longer than boys. So although 51.4% of newborns are boys, the percentage of 50-year-old males may be in fact less than 50% of the set of 50-year-old people. Therefore, when one looks at the average sex distribution over all ages, the ratio actually may be close to 50% even though over 51% of the children starting out in the world are boys.

Another illustration of probability lies in the fact that many events in life are uncertain. We do not know whether it will rain tomorrow or when the next earthquake

Introductory Biostatistics for the Health Sciences, by Michael R. Chernick
and Robert H. Friis. ISBN 0-471-41137-X. Copyright © 2003 Wiley-Interscience.

will hit. Probability is a formal way to measure the chance of these uncertain events. Based on mathematical axioms and theorems, probability also involves a mathematical model to describe the mechanism that produces uncertain or random outcomes.

To each event, our probability model will assign a number between 0 and 1. The value 0 corresponds to events that cannot happen and the value 1 to events that are certain.

A probability value between 0 and 1, e.g., 0.6, assigned to an event has a frequency interpretation. When we assign a probability, usually we are dealing with a one-time occurrence. A probability often refers to events that may occur in the future.

Think of the occurrence of an event as the outcome of an experiment. Assume that we could replicate this experiment as often as we want. Then, if we claim a probability of 0.6 for the event, we mean that after conducting this experiment many times we would observe that the fraction of the times that the event occurred would be close to 60% of the outcomes. Consequently, in approximately 40% of the experiments the event would not occur. These frequency notions of probability are important, as they will come up again when we apply them to statistical inference.

The probability of an event A is determined by first defining the set of all possible elementary events, associating a probability with each elementary event, and then summing the probabilities of all the elementary events that imply the occurrence of A. The elementary events are distinct and are called mutually exclusive.

The term "mutually exclusive" means that for elementary events A_1 and A_2, if A_1 happens then A_2 cannot happen and vice versa. This property is necessary to sum probabilities, as we will see later. Suppose we have event A such that if A_1 occurs, A_2 cannot occur, or if A_2 occurs, A_1 cannot occur (i.e., A_1 and A_2 are mutually exclusive elementary events) and both A_1 and A_2 imply the occurrence of A. The probability of A occurring, denoted $P(A)$, satisfies the equation $P(A) = P(A_1) + P(A_2)$.

We can make this equation even simpler if all the elementary events have the same chance of occurring. In that case, we say that the events are equally likely. If there are k distinct elementary events and they are equally likely, then each elementary event has a probability of $1/k$. Suppose we denote the number of favorable outcomes as m, which is comprised of m elementary events. Suppose also that any event A will occur when any of these m favorable elementary events occur and $m < k$. The foregoing statement means that there are k equally likely, distinct, elementary events and that m of them are favorable events.

Thus, the probability that A will occur is defined as the sum of the probabilities that any one of the m elementary events associated with A will occur. This probability is just m/k. Since m represents the distinct ways that A can occur and k represents the total possible outcomes, a common description of probability in this simple model is

$$P(A) = \frac{m}{k} = \frac{\{\text{number of favorable outcomes}\}}{\{\text{number of possible outcomes}\}}$$

Example 1: Tossing a Coin Twice. Assume we have a fair coin (one that favors neither heads nor tails) and denote H for heads and T for tails. The assumption of fairness implies that on each trial the probability of heads is $P(H) = 1/2$ and the probability of tails is $P(T) = 1/2$. In addition, we assume that the trials are statistically independent—meaning that the outcome of one trial does not depend on the outcome of any other trial. Shortly, we will give a mathematical definition of statistical independence, but for now just think of it as indicating that the trials do not influence each other.

Our coin toss experiment has four equally likely elementary outcomes. These outcomes are denoted as ordered pairs, which are $\{H, H\}$, $\{H, T\}$, $\{T, H\}$, and $\{T, T\}$. For example, the pair $\{H, T\}$ denotes a head on the first trial and a tail on the second. Because of the independence assumption, all four elementary events have a probability of 1/4. You will learn how to calculate these probabilities in the next section.

Suppose we want to know the probability of the event $A = \{$one head and one tail$\}$. A occurs if $\{H, T\}$ or $\{T, H\}$ occurs. So $P(A) = 1/4 + 1/4 = 1/2$.

Now, take the event $B = \{$at least one head occurs$\}$. B can occur if any of the elementary events $\{H, H\}$, $\{H, T\}$ or $\{T, H\}$ occurs. So $P(B) = 1/4 + 1/4 + 1/4 = 3/4$.

Example 2: Role Two Dice one Time. We assume that the two dice are independent of one another. Sum the two faces; we are interested in the faces that add up to either 7, 11, or 2. Determine the probability of rolling a sum of either 7, 11, or 2.

For each die there are 6 faces numbered with 1 to 6 dots. Each face is assumed to have an equal 1/6 chance of landing up. In this case, there are 36 equally likely elementary outcomes for a pair of dice. These elementary outcomes are denoted by pairs, such as $\{3, 5\}$, which denotes a roll of 3 on one die and 5 on the other. The 36 elementary outcomes are

$\{1, 1\}$, $\{1, 2\}$, $\{1, 3\}$, $\{1, 4\}$, $\{1, 5\}$, $\{1, 6\}$, $\{2, 1\}$, $\{2, 2\}$, $\{2, 3\}$, $\{2, 4\}$, $\{2, 5\}$, $\{2, 6\}$, $\{3, 1\}$, $\{3, 2\}$, $\{3, 3\}$, $\{3, 4\}$, $\{3, 5\}$, $\{3, 6\}$, $\{4, 1\}$, $\{4, 2\}$, $\{4, 3\}$, $\{4, 4\}$, $\{4, 5\}$, $\{4, 6\}$, $\{5, 1\}$, $\{5, 2\}$, $\{5, 3\}$, $\{5, 4\}$, $\{5, 5\}$, $\{5, 6\}$, $\{6, 1\}$, $\{6, 2\}$, $\{6, 3\}$, $\{6, 4\}$, $\{6, 5\}$, and $\{6, 6\}$.

Let A denote a sum of 7, B a sum of 11, and C a sum of 2. All we have to do is identify and count all the elementary outcomes that lead to 7, 11, and 2. Dividing each sum by 36 then gives us the answers:

Seven occurs if we have $\{1, 6\}$, $\{2, 5\}$, $\{3, 4\}$, $\{4, 3\}$, $\{5, 2\}$, or $\{6, 1\}$. That is, the probability of 7 is $6/36 = 1/6 \approx 0.167$. Eleven occurs only if we have $\{5, 6\}$ or $\{6, 5\}$. So the probability of 11 is $2/36 = 1/18 \approx 0.056$. For 2 (also called snake eyes), we must roll $\{1, 1\}$. So a 2 occurs only with probability $1/36 \approx 0.028$.

The next three sections will provide the formal rules for these probability calculations in general situations.

5.2 ELEMENTARY SETS AS EVENTS AND THEIR COMPLEMENTS

The elementary events are the building blocks (or atoms) of a probability model. They are the events that cannot be decomposed further into smaller sets of events. The set of elementary events is just the collection of all the elementary events. In example 2, the event {1, 1} "snake eyes" is an elementary event. The set [{1, 1}, {1, 2}, {1, 3}, {1, 4}, {1, 5}, {1, 6}, {2, 1}, {2, 2}, {2, 3}, {2, 4}, {2, 5}, {2, 6}, {3, 1}, {3, 2}, {3, 3}, {3, 4}, {3, 5}, {3, 6}, {4, 1}, {4, 2}, {4, 3}, {4, 4}, {4, 5}, {4, 6}, {5, 1}, {5, 2}, {5, 3}, {5, 4}, {5, 5}, {5, 6}, {6, 1}, {6, 2}, {6, 3}, {6, 4}, {6, 5}, and {6, 6}] is the set of elementary events.

It is customary to use Ω, the Greek letter omega, to represent the set containing all the elementary events. This set is also called the universal set. For Ω we have $P(\Omega) = 1$. The set containing no events is denoted by $\varnothing$ and is called the null set, or empty set. For the empty set $\varnothing$ we have $P(\varnothing) = 0$.

For any set A, A^c denotes the complement of A. The complement of set A is just the set of all elementary events not contained in A. From Example 2, if $A = $ {sum of the faces on the two dice is seven}, then $A = $ [{1, 6}, {2, 5}, {3, 4}, {4, 3}, {5, 2}, {6, 1}] and the set A^c is the set [{1, 1}, {1, 2}, {1, 3}, {1, 4}, {1, 5}, {2, 1}, {2, 2}, {2, 3}, {2, 4}, {2, 6}, {3, 1}, {3, 2}, {3, 3}, {3, 5}, {3, 6}, {4, 1}, {4, 2}, {4, 4}, {4, 5}, {4, 6}, {5, 1}, {5, 3}, {5, 4}, {5, 5}, {5, 6}, {6, 2}, {6, 3}, {6, 4}, {6, 5}, and {6, 6}] .

By simply counting the elementary events in the set and dividing by the total number of elementary events in Ω, we obtain the probability for the event. In problems with a large number of elementary events, this method for finding a probability can be tedious; it also requires that the elementary events are equally likely. Formulas that we derive in later sections will allow us to compute more easily the probabilities of certain events.

Consider the probability of $A = $ {sum of the faces on the two dice is seven}. As we saw in the previous section, $P(A) = 6/36 = 1/6 \approx 0.167$. Since there are 30 elementary events in A^c, $P(A^c) = 30/36 = 5/6 \approx 0.833$. We see that $P(A^c) = 1 - P(A)$, which is always the case, as demonstrated in the next section.

5.3 INDEPENDENT AND DISJOINT EVENTS

Now we will give some formal definitions of independent events and disjoint events. But first we must explain the symbols for intersection and union of events.

Definition 5.3.1: Intersection. Let E and F be two events; then $E \cap F$ denotes the event G that is the intersection of E and F. G is the collection of elementary events that are contained in both E and F.

We often say that G occurs only if both E and F occur. Let us define the union of two events.

Definition 5.3.2: Union. Let A and B be two events; then $A \cup B$ denotes the event C that is the union of A and B. C is the collection of elementary events that are contained in both A and B or in either A or B.

In Example 2 (roll two dice independently), let $E = \{$observe the same face on each die$\}$ and let $F = \{$the first face is even$\}$. Then $E = [\{1, 1\}, \{2, 2\}, \{3, 3\}, \{4, 4\}, \{5, 5\},$ and $\{6, 6\}]$. $F = [\{2, 1\}, \{2, 2\}, \{2, 3\}, \{2, 4\}, \{2, 5\}, \{2, 6\}, \{4, 1\}, \{4, 2\}, \{4, 3\}, \{4, 4\}, \{4, 5\}, \{4, 6\}, \{6, 1\}, \{6, 2\}, \{6, 3\}, \{6, 4\}, \{6, 5\},$ and $\{6, 6\}]$. Take $G = E \cap F$. Because G consists of the common elementary events, $G = [\{2, 2\}, \{4, 4\}$ and $\{6, 6\}]$.

We see here that $P(E) = 6/36 = 1/6$, $P(F) = 18/36 = 1/2$, and $P(G) = 3/36 = 1/12$. When we intersect three or more events, for example, the events D, E, and F, we simply denote that intersection by $K = D \cap E \cap F$. This set is the same as taking the set $H = D \cap E$ and then taking $K = H \cap F$, or taking $G = E \cap F$ and then finding $K = D \cap G$.

An additional point: The order in which the successive intersections is taken and the order in which the sets are arranged do not matter.

Definition 5.3.3: Mutual Independence. Let $A_1, A_2, \ldots, A_k$ be a set of k events (k is an integer greater than or equal to 2). Then these events are said to be mutually independent if $P(A_1 \cap A_2 \cap \ldots, A_k) = P(A_1)P(A_2) \ldots P(A_k)$, and this equality of probability of intersection to product of individual probabilities must hold for any subset of these k events.

Definition 5.3.3 tells us that a set of events are mutually independent if, and only if, the probability of the intersection of any pair, or any set of three up to the set of all k events, is equal to the product of their individual probabilities. We will see shortly how this definition relates to our commonsense notion that independence means that one event does not affect the outcome of the others.

In Example 2, E and F are independent of each other. Remember that $E = \{$observe the same face on each die$\}$ and $F = \{$the first face is even$\}$. We see from the commonsense notion that whether or not the first face is even has no effect on whether or not the second face will have the same number as the first.

We verify mutual independence from the formal definition by computing $P(G)$ and comparing $P(G)$ to $P(E) P(F)$. We saw earlier that $P(G) = 1/12$, $P(E) = 1/6$, and $P(F) = 1/2$. Thus, $P(E) P(F) = (1/6) (1/2) = 1/12$. So we have verified that E and F are independent by checking the definition.

Now we will define mutually exclusive events.

Definition 5.3.4: Mutually Exclusive Events. Let A and B be two events. We say that A and B are mutually exclusive if $A \cap B = \varnothing$, or equivalently in terms of probabilites, if $P(A \cap B) = 0$. In particular, we note that A and A^c are mutually exclusive events.

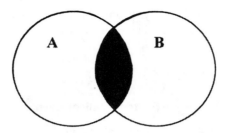

Figure 5.1. Intersection.

The distinction between the concepts of independent events and mutually exclusive events often leads to confusion. The two concepts are not related except that they both are defined in terms of probabilities of intersections.

Let us consider two nonempty events, A and B. Suppose A and B are independent. Now, $P(A) > 0$ and $P(B) > 0$, so $P(A \cap B) = P(A) P(B) > 0$. Therefore, because $P(A \cap B) \neq 0$, A and B are not mutually exclusive.

Now consider two mutually exclusive events, C and D, which are also nonempty. So $P(C) > 0$ and $P(D) > 0$, but $P(C \cap D) = 0$ because C and D are mutually exclusive. Then, since $P(C)P(D) > 0$, $P(C \cap D) \neq P(C)P(D)$; therefore, C and D are not independent.

Thus, we see that for two nonempty events, if the events are mutually exclusive, they cannot be independent. On the other hand, if they are independent, they cannot be mutually exclusive. Thus, these two concepts are in opposition.

Venn diagrams are graphics designed to portray combinations of sets such as those that represent unions and intersections. Figure 5.1 provides a Venn diagram for the intersection of events A and B.

Circles in the Venn diagram represent the individual events. In Figure 5.1, two circles, which represent events A and B, are labeled A and B. A third event, the intersection of the two events A and B, is indicated by the shaded area. Similarly, Figure 5.2 provides a Venn diagram that illustrates the union of the same two events.

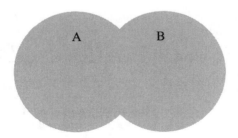

Figure 5.2. Union.

This illustration is accomplished by shading the regions covered by both of the individual sets in addition to the areas in which they overlap.

5.4   PROBABILITY RULES

Product (Multiplication) Rule for Independent Events

If A and B are independent events, their joint probability of occurrence is given by the Formula 5.1:

$$P(A \cap B) = P(A) \times P(B) \tag{5.1}$$

For a clear application of this rule, consider the experiment in which we roll two dice. What is the probability of a 1 on the first roll and a 2 or 4 on the second roll?

First of all, the outcome on the first roll is independent of the outcome on the second roll; therefore, define A = {get a 1 on one die and any outcome on the second die}, and let B = {any outcome on one die and a 2 or a 4 on the second die}. We can describe A as the following set of elementary events: A = [{1, 1}, {1, 2}, {1, 3}, {1, 4}, {1, 5}, {1, 6}] and B = [{1, 2}, {1, 4}, {2, 2}, {2, 4}, {3, 2}, {3, 4}, {4, 2}, {4, 4}, {5, 2}, {5, 4}, {6, 2}, {6, 4}].

The event $C = A \cap B$ = [{1, 2}, {1, 4}]. By the law of multiplication for independent events, $P(C) = P(A) \times P(B) = (1/6) \times (1/3) = 1/18$. You can check this by considering the elementary events associated with C. Since there are two events, each with probability 1/36, $P(C) = 2/36 = 1/18$.

Addition Rule for Mutually Exclusive Events

If A and B are mutually exclusive events, then the probability of their union (i.e., the probability that at least one of the events, A or B, occurs) is given by Formula 5.2. Mutually exclusive events are also called disjoint events. In terms of symbols, event A and event B are disjoint if $A \cap B = \varnothing$.

$$P(A \cup B) = P(A) + P(B) \tag{5.2}$$

Again, consider the example of rolling the dice; we roll two dice once. Let A be the event that both dice show the same number, which is even, and let B be the event that both dice show the same number, which is odd. Let $C = A \cup B$. Then C is the event in which the roll of the dice produces the same number, either even or odd.

For the two dice together, C occurs in six elementary ways: {1, 1}, {2, 2}, {3, 3}, {4, 4}, {5, 5}, and {6, 6}. A occurs in three elementary ways, namely, {2, 2}, {4, 4}, and {6, 6}. B also occurs in three elementary ways, namely, {1, 1}, {3, 3}, and {5, 5}.

$P(C) = 6/36 = 1/6$, whereas $P(A) = 3/36 = 1/12$ and $P(B) = 3/36 = 1/12$. By the addition law for mutually exclusive events, $P(C) = P(A) + P(B) = (1/12) + (1/12) = 2/12 = 1/6$. Thus, we see that the addition rule applies.

An application of the rule of addition is the rule for complements, shown in Formula 5.3. Since A and A^c are mutually exclusive and complementary, we have $\Omega = A \cup A^c$ and $P(\Omega) = P(A \cup A^c) = P(A) + P(A^c) = 1$.

$$P(A^c) = 1 - P(A) \tag{5.3}$$

In general, the addition rule can be modified for events A and B that are not disjoint. Let A and B be the sets identified in the Venn diagram in Figure 5.3. Call the overlap area $C = A \cap B$. Then, we can divide the set $A \cup B$ into three mutually exclusive sets as labeled in the diagram, namely, $A \cap B^c$, C, and $B \cap A^c$.

When we compute $P(A) + P(B)$, we obtain $P(A) = P(A \cap B) + P(A \cap B^c)$ and $P(B) = P(B \cap A) + P(B \cap A^c)$. Now $A \cap B = B \cap A$. So $P(A) + P(B) = P(A \cap B) + P(A \cap B^c) + P(B \cap A) + P(B \cap A^c) = P(A \cap B^c) + P(B \cap A^c) + 2P(C)$. But $P(A \cup B) = P(A \cap B^c) + P(B \cap A^c) + P(C)$ because it is the union of these three mutually exclusive events.

The problem with the summation formula is that $P(C)$ is counted twice. We remedy this error by subtracting $P(C)$ once. This subtraction yields the generalized addition formula for union of arbitrary events, shown as Formula 5.4:

$$P(A \cup B) = P(A) + P(B) - P(A \cap B) \tag{5.3}$$

Note that Formula 5.4 applies to mutually exclusive events A and B as well, since for mutually exclusive events, $P(A \cap B) = 0$. Next we will generalize the multiplication rule, but first we need to define conditional probabilities.

Suppose we have two events, A and B, and we want to define the probability of A occurring given that B will occur. We call this outcome the conditional probability of A given B and denote it by $P(A|B)$. Definition 5.4.1 presents the formal mathematical definition of $P(A|B)$.

Definition 5.4.1: Conditonal Probability of A Given B. Let A and B be arbitrary events. Then $P(A|B) = P(A \cap B)/P(B)$.

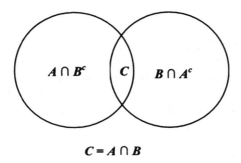

$$C = A \cap B$$

Figure 5.3. Decomposition of $A \cup B$ into disjoint sets.

Consider rolling one die. Let $A = \{$a 2 occurs$\}$ and let $B = \{$an even number occurs$\}$. Then $A = \{2\}$ and $B = [\{2\}, \{4\}, \{6\}]$. $P(A \cap B) = 1/6$ because $A \cap B = A = \{2\}$ and there is 1 chance out of 6 for 2 to come up. $P(B) = 1/2$ since there are 3 ways out of 6 for an even number to occur. So by definition, $P(A|B) = P(A \cap B)/P(B) = (1/6)/(1/2) = 2/6 = 1/3$.

Another way to understand conditional probabilities is to consider the restricted outcomes given that B occurs. If we know that B occurs, then the outcomes $\{2\}$, $\{4\}$, and $\{6\}$ are the only possible ones and they are equally likely to occur. So each outcome has the probability 1/3; hence, the probability of a 2 is 1/3. That is just what we mean by $P(A|B)$. Directly from Definition 5.4.1, we derive Formula 5.5 for the general law of conditional probabilities:

$$P(A|B) = P(A \cap B)/P(B) \tag{5.5}$$

Multiplying both sides of the equation by $P(B)$, we have $P(A|B) P(B) = P(A \cap B)$. This equation, shown as Formula 5.6, is the generalized multiplication law for the intersection of arbitrary events:

$$P(A \cap B) = P(A|B)P(B) \tag{5.6}$$

The generalized multiplication formula holds for arbitrary events A and B. Consequently, it also holds for independent events.

Suppose now that A and B are independent; then, from Formula 5.1, $P(A \cap B) = P(A) P(B)$. On the other hand, from Formula 5.6, $P(A \cap B) = P(A|B) P(B)$. So $P(A|B) P(B) = P(A) P(B)$.

Dividing both sides of $P(A|B) P(B) = P(A) P(B)$ by $P(B)$ (since $P(B) > 0$), we have $P(A|B) = P(A)$. That is, if A and B are independent, then the probability of A given B is the same as the unconditional probability of A.

This result agrees with our intuitive notion of independence, namely, conditioning on B does affect the chances of A's occurrence. Similarly, one can show that if A and B are independent, then $P(B|A) = P(B)$.

5.5 PERMUTATIONS AND COMBINATIONS

In this section, we will derive some results from combinatorial mathematics. These results will be useful in obtaining shortcut calculations of probabilities of events linked to specific probability distributions to be discussed in Sections 5.6 and 5.7.

In the previous sections, we presented a common method for calculating probabilities: We calculated the probability of an event by counting the number of possible ways that the event can occur and dividing the resulting number by the total number of equally likely elementary outcomes. Because we used simple examples, with 36 possibilities at most, we had no difficulty applying this formula.

However, in many applied situations the number of ways that an event can occur is so large that complete enumeration is tedious or impractical. The combinatorial methods discussed in this section will facilitate the computation of the numerator and denominator for the probability of interest.

Let us again consider the experiment where we toss dice. On any roll of a die, there are six elementary outcomes. Suppose we roll the die three times so that each roll is independent of the other rolls. We want to know how many ways we can roll a 4 or less on all three rolls of the die without repeating a number.

We could do direct enumeration, but there are a total of $6 \times 6 \times 6 = 216$ possible outcomes. In addition, the number of successful outcomes may not be obvious. There is a shortcut solution that becomes even more important as the space of possible outcomes, and possible successful outcomes, becomes even larger than in this example.

Thus far, our problem is not well defined. First we must specify whether or not the order of the distinct numbers matters. When order matters we are dealing with permutations. When order does not matter we are dealing with combinations.

Let us consider first the case in which order is important; therefore, we will be determining the number of permutations. If order matters, then the triple {4, 3, 2} is a successful outcome but differs from the triple {4, 2, 3} because order matters. In fact, the triples {4, 3, 2}, {4, 2, 3}, {3, 4, 2}, {3, 2, 4}, {2, 4, 3}, and {2, 3, 4} are six distinct outcomes when order matters but count only as one outcome when order does not matter, because they all correspond to an outcome in which the three numbers 2, 3, and 4 each occur once.

Suppose the numbers 4 or lower comprise a successful outcome. In this case we have four objects—the numbers 1, 2, 3, and 4—to choose from because a choice of 5 or 6 on any trial leads to a failed outcome. Since there are only three rolls of the die, and a successful roll requires a different number on each trial, we are interested in the number of ways of selecting three objects out of four when order matters. This type of selection is called the number of possible permutations for selecting three objects out of four.

Let us think of the problem of selecting the objects as filling slots. We will count the number of ways we can fill the first slot and then, given that the first slot is filled, we consider how many ways are left to fill the second slot. Finally, given that we have filled the first two slots, we consider how many ways remain to fill the third slot. We then multiply these three numbers together to get the number of permutations of three objects taken out of a set of four objects.

Why do we multiply these numbers together? This procedure is based on a simple rule of counting. To illustrate, let us consider a slightly different case that involves two trials. We want to observe an even number on the first trial (call that event A) and an even number on the second trial. However, the number on the second trial must differ from the one chosen on the first (call that event B).

On the first trial, we could get a 2, 4, or 6. So there are three possible ways for A to occur. On the second trial, we also can get a 2, 4, or 6, but we can't repeat the result of the first trial. So if 2 occurred for A, then 4 and 6 are the only possible outcomes for B. Similarly, if 4 occurred for A, then 2 and 6 are the only possible outcomes for B.

Finally, if the third possible outcome for A occurred, namely 6, then only 2 and 4 are possible outcomes for B. Note that regardless of what number occurs for A, there are always two ways for B to occur. Since A does not depend on B, there are always three ways for A to occur.

According to the multiplication rule, the number of ways A and B can occur together is the product of the individual number of ways that they can occur. In this example, $3 \times 2 = 6$ ways. Let us enumerate these pairs to see that 6 is in fact the right number.

We have $\{2, 4\}, \{2, 6\}, \{4, 2\}, \{4, 6\}, \{6, 2\}$, and $\{6, 4\}$. This set consists of the number of permutations of two objects taken out of three, as we have two slots to fill with three distinct even numbers: 2, 4, and 6.

Now let us go back to our original, more complicated, problem of selecting three (since we are filling three slots) from four objects: 1, 2, 3, and 4. By using mathematical induction, we can show that the multiplication law extends to any number of slots. Let us accept this assertion as a fact. We see that our solution to the problem involves taking the number of permutations for selecting three objects out of four; the multiplication rule tells us that this solution is $4 \times 3 \times 2 = 24$.

The following list enumerates these 24 cases: $\{4, 3, 2\}, \{4, 3, 1\}, \{4, 2, 3\}$, $\{4, 2, 1\}, \{4, 1, 3\}, \{4, 1, 2\}, \{3, 4, 2\}, \{3, 4, 1\}, \{3, 2, 4\}, \{3, 1, 4\}, \{2, 4, 3\}$, $\{2, 4, 1\}, \{2, 3, 4\}, \{2, 1, 4\}, \{1, 4, 3\}, \{1, 4, 2\}, \{1, 3, 4\}, \{1, 2, 4\}, \{3, 2, 1\}$ $\{3, 1, 2\}, \{2, 3, 1\}, \{2, 1, 3\}, \{1, 3, 2\}$, and $\{1, 2, 3\}$. Note that a systematic method of enumeration is important; otherwise, it is easy to miss some cases or to accidentally count cases twice.

Our system is to start with the highest available number in the first slot; once the first slot is chosen, we select the next highest available number for the second slot, and then the remaining highest available number for the third slot. This process is repeated until all cases with 4 in the first slot are exhausted. Then we consider the cases with 3 in the first slot, the highest available remaining number for the second slot, and then the highest available remaining number for the third slot. After the 3s are exhausted, we repeat the procedure with 2 in the first slot, and finally with 1 in the first slot.

In general, let r be the number of objects to choose and n the number of objects available. We then denote by $P(n, r)$ the number of permutations of r objects chosen out of n. As an example of permutations, we denote the quantity $3 \times 2 = 3 \times 2 \times 1$ as $3!$, where the symbol "!" represents the function called the factorial. In our notation and formulae, $0!$ exists and is equal to 1. Formula 5.7 shows the permutations of r objects taken from n objects:

$$P(n, r) = n!/(n - r)! \qquad (5.7)$$

From Formula 5.7, we see that when $n = 3$ and $r = 2$, $P(3, 2) = 3!/(3 - 2)! = 3!/1!$ $= 3! = 6$. This result agrees with our enumeration of distinct even numbers on two rolls of the die. Also, $P(4, 3) = 4!/(4 - 3)! = 4!/1! = 4! = 24$. This number agrees with the result we obtained for three independent rolls less than 5.

Now we will examine combinations. For combinations, we consider only distinct subsets but not their order. In the example of distinct outcomes of three rolls of the die where success means three distinct numbers less than 5 without regard to order, the triplets {2, 3, 4}, {2, 4, 3}, {3, 2, 4}, {3, 4, 2}, {4, 3, 2}, and {4, 2, 3} differ only in order and not in the objects included.

Notice that for each different set of three distinct numbers, the common number of permutations is always 6. For example, the set 1, 2, and 3 contains the six triplets {1, 2, 3}, {1, 3, 2}, {2, 1, 3}, {2, 3, 1}, {3, 1, 2}, and {3, 2, 1}. Notice that the number six occurs because it is equal to $P(3, 3) = 3!/0! = 3! = 6$.

Because for every distinct combination of r objects selected out of n there are $P(r, r)$ orders for these objects, we have $P(n, r) = C(n, r)P(r, r)$ where $C(n, r)$ denotes the number of combinations for choosing r objects out of n. Therefore, we arrive at the following equation for combinations, with the far-right-hand side of the chain of equalities obtained by substitution, since $P(r, r) = r!$ $C(n, r) = P(n, r)/P(r, r) = n!/[(n - r)! \, P(r, r)] = n!/[(n - r)! \, r!]$. Formula 5.8 shows the formula for combinations of r objects taken out of n:

$$C(n, r) = n!/[(n - r)! \, r!] \qquad (5.8)$$

In our example of three rolls of the die leading to three distinct numbers less than 5, we obtain the number of combinations for choosing 3 objects out of 4 as $C(4, 3) = 4!/[1! \, 3!] = 4$. These four distinct combinations are enumerated as follows: (1) 1, 2 and 3; (2) 1, 2 and 4; (3) 1, 3 and 4; and (4) 2, 3 and 4.

5.6   PROBABILITY DISTRIBUTIONS

Probability distributions describe the probability of events. Parameters are characteristics of probability distributions. The statistics that we have used to estimate parameters are also called random variables. We are interested in the distributions of these statistics and will use them to make inferences about population parameters.

We will be able to draw inferences by constructing confidence intervals or testing hypotheses about the parameters. The methods for doing this will be developed in Chapters 8 and 9, but first you must learn the basic probability distributions and the underlying bases for the ones we will use later.

We denote the statistic, or random variable, with a capital letter—often "X." We distinguish the random variable X from the value it takes on in a particular experiment by using a lower case x for the latter value. Let $A = [X = x]$. Assume that $A = [X = x]$ is an event that is similar to the events described earlier in this chapter. If X is a discrete variable that takes on only a finite set of values, the events of the form $A = [X = x]$ have positive probabilities associated with some finite set of values for x and zero probability for all other values of x.

A discrete variable is one that can take on distinct values for each individual measurement. We can assign a positive probability to each number. The probabilities associated with each value of a discrete variable can form an infinite set of values, known as an infinite discrete set. The discrete set also could be finite. The most common example of an infinite discrete set is a Poisson random variable, which assigns a positive probability to all the non-negative integers, including zero. The

Poisson distribution is a type of distribution used to portray events that are infrequent (such as the number of light bulb failures). The degree of occurrence of events is determined by the rate parameter. By infrequent we mean that in a short interval of time there cannot be two events occurring. An example of a distribution that is discrete and finite is the binomial distribution, to be discussed in detail later. For the binomial distribution, the random variable is the number of successes in n trials; it can take on the $n + 1$ discrete values $0, 1, 2, 3, \ldots, n$.

Frequently, we will deal with another type of random variable, the absolutely continuous random variable. This variable can take on values over a continuous range of numbers. The range could be an interval such as [0, 1], or it could be the entire set of real numbers. A random variable with a uniform distribution illustrates a distribution that uses a range of numbers in an interval such as [0, 1]. A uniform distribution is made from a dataset in which all of the values have the same chance of occurrence. The normal, or Gaussian, distribution is an example of an absolutely continuous distribution that takes on values over the entire set of real numbers.

Absolutely continuous random variables have probability densities associated with them. You will see that these densities are the analogs to probability mass functions that we will define for discrete random variables.

For absolutely continuous random variables, we will see that events such as $A = P(X = x)$ are meaningless because for any value x, $P(X = x) = 0$. To obtain meaningful probabilities for absolutely continuous random variables, we will need to talk about the probability that X falls into an interval of values such as $P(0 < X < 1)$. On such intervals, we can compute positive probabilities for these random variables.

Probability distributions have certain characteristics that can apply to both absolutely continuous and discrete distributions. One such property is symmetry. A probability distribution is symmetric if it has a central point at which we can construct a vertical line so that the shape of the distribution to the right of the line is the mirror image of the shape to the left.

We will encounter a number of continuous and discrete distributions that are symmetric. Examples of absolutely continuous distributions that are symmetric are the normal distribution, Student's t distribution, the Cauchy distribution, the uniform distribution, and the particular beta distribution that we discuss at the end of this chapter.

The binomial distribution previously mentioned (covered in detail in the next section) is a discrete distribution. The binomial distribution is symmetric if, and only if, the success probability $p = 1/2$. To review, the toss of a fair coin has two possible outcomes, heads or tails. If we want to obtain a head when we toss a coin, the head is called a "success." The probability of a head is $1/2$.

Probability distributions that are not symmetric are called skewed distributions. There are two kinds of skewed distributions: positively skewed and negatively skewed. Positively skewed distributions have a higher concentration of probability mass or density to the left and a long, declining tail to the right, whereas negatively skewed distributions have probability mass or density concentrated to the right with a long, declining tail to the left.

Figure 5.4 shows continuous probability densities corresponding to: (1) a sym-

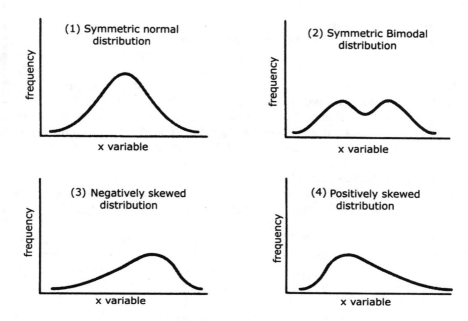

Figure 5.4. Continuous probability densities.

metric normal distribution, (2) a symmetric bimodal distribution, (3) a negatively skewed distribution, and (4) a positively skewed distribution. The negative exponential distribution and the chi-square distribution are examples of positively skewed distributions.

Beta distributions and binomial distributions (both to be described in detail later) can be symmetric, positively skewed, or negatively skewed depending on the values of certain parameters. For instance, the binomial distribution is positively skewed if $p < 1/2$, is symmetric if $p = 1/2$, and is negatively skewed if $p > 1/2$.

Now let us look at a familiar experiment and define a discrete random variable associated with that experiment. Then, using what we already know about probability, we will be able to construct the probability distribution for this random variable.

For the experiment, suppose that we are tossing a fair coin three times in independent trials. We can enumerate the elementary outcomes: a total of eight. With H denoting heads and T tails, the triplets are: $\{H, H, H\}$, $\{H, H, T\}$, $\{H, T, H\}$, $\{H, T, T\}$, $\{T, H, H\}$, $\{T, H, T\}$, $\{T, T, H\}$, and $\{T, T, T\}$. We can classify these eight elementary events as follows: $E_1 = \{H, H, H\}$, $E_2 = \{H, H, T\}$, $E_3 = \{H, T, H\}$, $E_4 = \{H, T, T\}$, $E_5 = \{T, H, H\}$, $E_6 = \{T, H, T\}$, $E_7 = \{T, T, H\}$, and $E_8 = \{T, T, T\}$.

We want Z to denote the random variable that counts the number of heads in the experiment. By looking at the outcomes above, you can see that Z can take on the values 0, 1, 2, and 3. You also know that the 8 elementary outcomes above are equally likely because the coin is fair and the trials are independent. So each triplet has a probability of 1/8. You have learned that elementary events are mutually exclusive (also called disjoint). Consequently, the probability of the union of elementary events is just the sum of their individual probabilities.

You are now ready to compute the probability distribution for Z. Since Z can be only 0, 1, 2, or 3, we know its distribution once we compute $P(Z = 0)$, $P(Z = 1)$, $P(Z = 2)$, and $P(Z = 3)$. Each of these events $\{Z = 0\}$, $\{Z = 1\}$, $\{Z = 2\}$, and $\{Z = 3\}$ can be described as the union of a certain set of these elementary events.

For example, $Z = 0$ only if all three tosses are tails. E_8 denotes the elementary event $\{T, T, T\}$. We see that $P(Z = 0) = P(E_8) = 1/8$. Similarly, $Z = 3$ only if all three tosses are heads. E_1 denotes the event $\{H, H, H\}$; therefore, $P(Z = 3) = P(E_1) = 1/8$.

Consider the event $Z = 1$. For $Z = 1$, we have exactly one head and two tails. The elementary events that lead to this outcome are $E_4 = \{H, T, T\}$, $E_6 = \{T, H, T\}$, and $E_7 = \{T, T, H\}$. So $P(Z = 1) = P(E_4 \cup E_6 \cup E_7)$. By the addition law for mutually exclusive events, we have $P(Z = 1) = P(E_4 \cup E_6 \cup E_7) = P(E_4) + P(E_6) + P(E_7) = 1/8 + 1/8 + 1/8 = 3/8$.

Next, consider the event $Z = 2$. For $Z = 2$ we have exactly one tail and two heads. Again there are three elementary events that give this outcome. They are $E_2 = \{H, H, T\}$, $E_3 = \{H, T, H\}$, and $E_5 = \{T, H, H\}$. So $P(Z = 2) = P(E_2 \cup E_3 \cup E_5)$. By the addition law for mutually exclusive events, we have $P(Z = 2) = P(E_2 \cup E_3 \cup E_5) = P(E_2) + P(E_3) + P(E_5) = 1/8 + 1/8 + 1/8 = 3/8$.

Table 5.1 gives the distribution for Z. The second column of the table is called the probability mass function for Z. The third column is the cumulative probability function. The value shown in the first cell of the third column is carried over from the first cell of the second column. The value shown in the second cell of the third column is the sum of the values shown in cell one and in all of the cells above cell two of the second column. Each of the remaining values shown in the third column can be found in a similar manner, e.g., the third cell in column 3 (0.875) = (0.125 + 0.375 + 0.375). We will find analogs for the absolutely continuous distribution functions.

Recall another way to perform the calculation. In the previous section, we learned how to use permutations and combinations as a shortcut to calculating such probabilities. Let us see if we can determine the distribution of Z using combinations.

To obtain $Z = 0$, we need three tails for three objects. There are $C(3, 3)$ ways to do this. $C(3, 3) = 3!/[(3 - 3)! \, 3!] = 3!/[0! \, 3!] = 1$. So $P(Z = 0) = C(3, 3)/8 = 1/8 = 0.125$.

TABLE 5.1. Probability Distribution for Number of Heads in Three Coin Tosses

Value for Z	$P(Z = \text{Value})$	$P(Z \leq \text{Value})$
0	1/8 = 0.125	1/8 = 0.125
1	3/8 = 0.375	4/8 = 0.500
2	3/8 = 0.375	7/8 = 0.875
3	1/8 = 0.125	8/8 = 1.000

To find $Z = 1$, we need two tails and one head. Order does not matter, so the number of ways of choosing exactly two tails out of three is $C(3, 2) = 3!/[(3 - 2)! \, 2!] = 3!/[1! \, 2!] = 3 \times 2/2 = 3$. So $P(Z = 1) = C(3, 2)/8 = 3/8 = 0.375$.

Now for $Z = 2$, we need one tail and two heads. Thus, we must select exactly one tail out of three choices; order does not matter. So $P(Z = 2) = C(3, 1)/8$ and $C(3, 1) = 3!/[(3 - 1)! \, 1!] = 3!/[2! \, 1!] = 3 \times 2/2 = 3$. Therefore, $P(Z = 2) = C(3, 1)/8 = 3/8 = 0.375$.

For $P(Z = 3)$, we must have no tails out of three selections. Again, order does not matter, so $P(Z = 3) = C(3, 0)/8$ and $C(3, 0) = 3!/[(3 - 0)! \, 0!] = 3!/[3! \, 0!] = 3!/3! = 1$. Therefore, $P(Z = 3) = C(3, 0)/8 = 1/8 = 0.125$.

Once one becomes familiar with this method for computing permutations, it is simpler than having to enumerate all of the elementary outcomes. The saving in time and effort becomes much more apparent as the space of possible outcomes increases markedly. Consider how tedious it would be to compute the distribution of the number of heads when we toss a coin 10 times!

The distribution we have just seen is a special case of the binomial distribution that we will discuss in Section 5.7. We will denote the binomial distribution as $Bi(n, p)$. The two parameters n and p determine the distribution. We will see that n is the number of trials and p is the probability of success on any one trial. The binomial random variable is just the count of the number of successes.

In our example above, if we call a head on a trial a success and a tail a failure, then we see that because we have a fair coin, $p = 1/2 = 0.50$. Since we did three independent tosses of the coin, $n = 3$. Therefore, our exercise derived the distribution $Bi(3, 0.50)$.

In previous chapters we talked about means and variances as parameters that measure location and scale for population variables. We saw how to estimate means and variances from sample data. Also, we can define and compute these population parameters for random variables if we can specify the distribution of these variables.

Consider a discrete random variable such as the binomial, which has a positive probability associated with a finite set of discrete values $x_1, x_2, x_3, \ldots, x_n$. To each value we associate the probability mass p_i for $i = 1, 2, 3, \ldots, n$. The mean μ for this random variable is defined as $\mu = \Sigma_{i=1}^{n} p_i x_i$. The variance σ^2 is defined as $\sigma^2 = \Sigma_{i=1}^{n} p_i (x_i - \mu)^2$. For the $Bi(n, p)$ distribution it is easy to verify that $\mu = np$ and $\sigma^2 = npq$, where $q = 1 - p$. For an example, refer to Exercise 5.21 at the end of this chapter.

Up to this point, we have discussed only discrete distributions. Now we want to consider random variables that have absolutely continuous distributions. The simplest example of an absolutely continuous distribution is the uniform distribution on the interval [0, 1]. The uniform distribution represents the distribution we would like to have for random number generation. It is the distribution that gives every real number in the interval [0, 1] an "equal" chance of being selected, in the sense that any subinterval of length L has the same probability of selection as any other subinterval of length L.

Let U be a uniform random variable on [0, 1]; then $P\{0 \leq U \leq x) = x$ for any x

satisfying $0 \leq x \leq 1$. With this definition and using calculus, we see that the function $F(x) = P\{0 \leq U \leq x\} = x$ is differentiable on $[0, 1]$. We denote its derivative by $f(x)$. In this case, $f(x) = 1$ for $0 \leq x \leq 1$, and $f(x) = 0$ otherwise.

Knowing that $f(x) = 1$ for $0 \leq x \leq 1$, and $f(x) = 0$ otherwise, we find that for any a and b satisfying $0 \leq a \leq b \leq 1$, $P(a \leq U \leq b) = b - a$. So the probability that U falls in any particular interval is just the length of the interval and does not depend on a. For example, $P(0 \leq U \leq 0.2) = P(0.1 \leq U \leq 0.3) = P(0.3 \leq U \leq 0.5) = P(0.4 \leq U \leq 0.6) = P(0.7 \leq U \leq 0.9) = P(0.8 \leq U \leq 1.0) = 0.2$.

Many other absolutely continuous distributions occur naturally. Later in the text, we will discuss the normal distribution and the negative exponential distribution, both of which are important absolutely continuous distributions.

The material described in the next few paragraphs uses results from elementary calculus. You are not expected to know calculus. However, if you read this material and just accept the results from calculus as facts, you will get a better appreciation for continuous distributions than you would if you skip this section.

It is easy to define absolutely continuous distributions. All you need to do is define a continuous function, g, on an interval or on the entire line such that g has a finite integral.

Suppose the value of the integral is c. One then obtains a density function $f(x)$ by defining $f(x) = g(x)/c$. Then, integrating f over the region where g is not zero gives the value 1. The integral of f we will call F, which when integrated from the smallest value with a nonzero density to a specified point x is the cumulative distribution function. It has the property that it starts out at zero at the first real value for which $f > 0$ and increases to 1 as we approach the largest value of x for which $f > 0$.

Let us consider a special case of a family of continuous distributions on $[0, 1]$ called the beta family. The beta family depends on two parameters α and β. We will look at a special case where $\alpha = 2$ and $\beta = 2$. In general, the beta density is $f(x) = B(\alpha, \beta)x^{\alpha-1}(1-x)^{\beta-1}$. The term $B(\alpha, \beta)$ is a constant that is chosen so that the integral of the function g from 0 to 1 is equal to 1. This function is known as the beta function. In the special case we simply define $g(x) = x(1-x)$ for $0 \leq x \leq 1$ and $g(x) = 0$ for all other values of x. Call the integral of g, G.

By integral calculus, $G(x) = x^2/2 - x^3/3$ for all $0 \leq x \leq 1$, $G(x) = 0$ for $x > 0$, and $G(x) = 1/6$ for all $x > 1$. Now $G(1) = 1/6$ is the integral of g over the interval $[0, 1]$. Therefore, $G(1)$ is the constant c that we want.

Let $f(x) = g(x)/c = x(1-x)/(1/6) = 6x(1-x)$ for $0 \leq x \leq 1$ and $f(x) = 0$ for all other x. The quantity $1/G(1)$ is the constant for the beta density f. In our general formula it was $B(\alpha, \beta)$. In this case, since $\alpha = 2$ and $\beta = 2$ we have $B(2, 2) = 1/G(1) = 6$. This function f is a probability density function (the analog for absolutely continuous random variables to the probability mass function for discrete random variables). The cumulative probability distribution function is $F(x) = x^2(3 - 2x) = 6G(x)$ for $0 \leq x \leq 1$, $F(x) = 0$ for $x < 0$, and $F(x) = 1$ for $x > 1$. We see that $F(x) = 6G(x)$ for all x.

We can define, by analogy to the definitions for discrete random variables, the mean μ and the variance σ^2 for a continuous random variable. We simply use the integration symbol in place of the summation sign, with the density function f taking the place of the probability mass function. Therefore, for an absolutely continuous random variable X, we have $\mu = \int x f(x) dx$ and $\sigma^2 = \int (x - \mu)^2 f(x) dx$.

For the uniform distribution on $[0, 1]$, you can verify that $\mu = 1/2$ and $\sigma^2 = 1/12$ if you know some basic integral calculus.

5.7   THE BINOMIAL DISTRIBUTION

As introduced in the previous section, the binomial random variable is the count of the number of successes in n independent trials when the probability of success on any given trial is p. The binomial distribution applies in situations where there are only two possible outcomes, denoted as S for success and F for failure.

Each such trial is called a Bernoulli trial. For convenience, we let X_i be a Bernoulli random variable for trial i. Such a random variable is assigned the value 1 if the trial is a success and the value 0 if the trial is a failure.

For Z (the number of successes in n trials) to be $Bi(n, p)$, we must have n independent Bernoulli trials with each trial having the same probability of success p. Z then can be represented as the sum of the n independent Bernoulli random variables X_i for $i = 1, 2, 3, \ldots, n$. This representation is convenient and conceptually important when we are considering the Central Limit Theorem (discussed in Chapter 7) and the normal distribution approximation to the binomial.

The binomial distribution arises naturally in many problems. It may represent appropriately the distribution of the number of boys in families of size 3, 4, or 5, for example, or the number of heads when a coin is flipped n times. It could represent the number of successful ablation procedures in a clinical trial. It might represent the number of wins that your favorite baseball team achieves this season or the number of hits your favorite batter gets in his first 100 at bats.

Now we will derive the general binomial distribution, $Bi(n, p)$. We simply generalize the combinatorial arguments we used in the previous section for $Bi(3, 0.50)$. We consider $P(Z = r)$ where $0 \leq r \leq n$. The number of elementary events that lead to r successes out of n trials (i.e., getting exactly r successes and $n - r$ failures) is $C(n, r) = n! / [(n - r)! \, r!]$.

Recall our earlier example of filling slots. Applying that example to the present situation, we note that one such outcome that leads to r successes and $n - r$ failures would be to have the r successes in the first r slots and the $n - r$ failures in the remaining $n - r$ slots. For each slot, the probability of a success is p, and the probability of a failure is $1 - p$. Given that the events are independent from trial to trial, the multiplication rule for independent events applies, i.e., products of terms which are either p or $1 - p$. We see that for this particular arrangement, p is multiplied r times and $1 - p$ is multiplied $n - r$ times.

The probability for a success on each of the first r trials and a failure on each of the remaining trials is $p^r(1 - p)^{n-r}$. The same argument could be made for any other arrangement. The quantity p will appear r times in the product and $1 - p$ will appear $n - r$ times. The product of multiplication does not change when the order of the

TABLE 5.2. Binomial Distributions for $n = 8$ and p ranging from 0.05 to 0.95

No. of successes	$p = 0.05$	$p = 0.10$	$p = 0.20$	$p = 0.40$	$p = 0.50$	$p = 0.60$	$p = 0.80$	$p = 0.90$	$p = 0.95$
0	0.66342	0.43047	0.16777	0.01680	0.00391	0.00066	0.00000	0.00000	0.00000
1	0.27933	0.38264	0.33554	0.08958	0.03125	0.00785	0.00008	0.00000	0.00000
2	0.05146	0.14880	0.29360	0.20902	0.10938	0.04129	0.00115	0.00002	0.00000
3	0.00542	0.03307	0.14680	0.27869	0.21875	0.12386	0.00918	0.00041	0.00002
4	0.00036	0.00459	0.04588	0.23224	0.27344	0.23224	0.04588	0.00459	0.00036
5	0.00002	0.00041	0.00918	0.12386	0.21875	0.27869	0.14680	0.03307	0.00542
6	0.00000	0.00002	0.00115	0.04129	0.10938	0.20902	0.29360	0.14880	0.05146
7	0.00000	0.00000	0.00008	0.00785	0.03125	0.08958	0.33554	0.38264	0.27933
8	0.00000	0.00000	0.00000	0.00066	0.00391	0.01680	0.16777	0.43047	0.66342

terms is changed. Therefore, each arrangement of the r successes and $n - r$ failures has the same probability of occurrence as the one that we just computed.

The number of such arrangements is just the number of ways to select exactly r out of the n slots for success. This number denotes combinations for selecting r objects out of n, namely, $C(n, r)$. Therefore, $P(Z = r) = C(n, r)(1 - p)^{n-r} = \{n!/[r!(n - r)!]\}p^r(1 - p)^{n-r}$. Because the formula for $P(Z = r)$ applies for any value of r between 0 and n (including both 0 and n), we have the general binomial distribution.

Table 5.2 shows for $n = 8$ how the binomial distribution changes as p ranges from small values such as 0.05 to large values such as 0.95. From the table, we can see the relationship between the probability distribution for $Bi(n, p)$ and the one for $Bi(n, 1 - p)$. We will derive this relationship algebraically using the formula for $P(Z = r)$.

Suppose Z has the distribution $Bi(n, p)$; then $P(Z = r) = n!/[(n - r)!r!]p^r(1 - p)^{n-r}$. Now suppose W has the distribution $Bi(n, 1 - p)$. Let us consider $P(W = n - r)$. $P(W = n - r) = n!/[\{n - (n - r)\}!(n - r)!](1 - p)^{n-r}p^r = n!/[r!\ (n - r)!](1 - p)^{n-r}p^r$. Without changing the product, we can switch terms around in the numerator and switch terms around in the denominator: $P(W = n - r) = n!/[r!\ (n - r)!](1 - p)^{n-r}\ p^r = n!/[(n - r)!\ r!]p^r(1 - p)^{n-r}$. But we recognize that the term on the far-right-hand side of the chain of equalities equals $P(Z = r)$. So $P(W = n - r) = P(Z = r)$. Consequently, for $0 \leq r \leq n$, the probability that a $Bi(n, p)$ random variable equals r is the same as the probability that a $Bi(n, 1 - p)$ random variable is equal to $n - r$.

Earlier in this chapter, we noted that $Bi(n, p)$ has a mean of $\mu = np$ and a variance of $\sigma^2 = npq$, where $q = 1 - p$. Now that you know the probability mass function for the $Bi(n, p)$, you should be able to verify these results in Exercise 5.21.

5.8 THE MONTY HALL PROBLEM

Although probability theory may seem simple and very intuitive, it can be very subtle and deceptive. Many results found in the field of probability are counterintuitive;

some examples are the St. Petersburg Paradox, Benford's Law of Lead Digits, the Birthday Problem, Simpson's Paradox, and the Monty Hall Problem.

References for further reading on the foregoing problems include Feller (1971), which provides a good treatment of Benford's Law, the Waiting Time Paradox, and the Birthday Problem. We also recommend the delightful account (Bruce, 2000), written in the style of Arthur Conan Doyle, wherein Sherlock Holmes teaches Watson about many probability misconceptions. Simpson's Paradox, which is important in the analysis of categorical data in medical studies, will be addressed in Chapter 11.

The Monty Hall Problem achieved fame and notoriety many years ago. Marilyn Vos Savant, in her *Parade* magazine column, presented a solution to the problem in response to a reader's question. There was a big uproar; many readers responded in writing (some in a very insulting manner), challenging her answer. Many of those who offered the strongest challenges were mathematicians and statisticians. Nevertheless, Vos Savant's solution, which was essentially correct, can be demonstrated easily through computer simulation.

In the introduction to her book (1997), Vos Savant summarizes this problem, which she refers to as the Monty Hall Dilemma, as well as her original answer. She repeats this answer on page 5 of the text, where she discusses the problem in more detail and provides many of the readers' written arguments against her solution.

On pages 5–17, she presents the succession of responses and counterresponses. Also included in Vos Savant (Appendix, pages 169–196) is Donald Granberg's well-formulated and objective treatment of the mathematical problem. Granberg provides insight into the psychological mechanisms that cause people to cling to incorrect answers and not consider opposing arguments. Vos Savant (1997) is also a good source for other statistical fallacies and misunderstandings of probability.

The Monty Hall Problem may be stated as follows: At the end of each "Let's Make a Deal" television program, Monty Hall would let one of the contestants from that episode have a shot at the big prize. There were three showcase doors to choose from. One of the doors concealed the prize, and the other two concealed "clunkers" (worthless prizes sometimes referred to as "goats").

In fact, a real goat actually might be standing on the stage behind one of the doors! Monty would ask a contestant to choose a door; then he would expose one of the other doors that was hiding a clunker. Then the contestant would be offered a bribe ($500, $1000, or more) to give up the door. Generally, the contestants chose to keep the door, especially if Monty offered a lot of cash for the bribe; the grand prize was always worth a lot more than the bribe. The more Monty offered, the more the contestants suspected that they had the right door. Since Monty knew which door held the grand prize, contestants suspected that he was tempting them to give up the grand prize.

The famous problem that Vos Savant addressed in her column was a slight variation, which Monty may or may not have actually used. Again, after one of the three doors is removed, the contestant selects one of the two remaining doors. Instead of offering money, the host (for example, Monty Hall) allows the contestant to keep the selected door or switch to the remaining door. Marilyn said that the contestant should switch because his chance of winning if he switches is 2/3, while the door he originally chose has only a 1/3 chance of being the right door.

Those who disagreed said that it would make no difference whether or not the contestant switches, as the removal of one of the empty doors leaves two doors, each with an equal 1/2 chance of being the right door. To some, this seemed to be a simple exercise in conditional probabilities. But they were mistake*n*!

One correct argument would be that initially one has a 1/3 chance of selecting the correct door. Once a door is selected, Monty will reveal a door that hides a clunker. He can do this only because he knows which door has the prize. If the first door selected is the winner, Monty is free to select either of the two remaining doors. However, if the contestant does not have the correct door, Monty must show the contestant the one remaining door that conceals a clunker.

But the correct door will be found two-thirds of the time using a switching strategy. So in two-thirds of the cases, switching is going to lead one to the winning door; only in one-third of the cases will switching backfire. Consequently, a strategy of always switching will win about 67% of the time, and a strategy of remaining with the selected door will win only 33% of the time.

Some of the mathematicians erred because they ignored the fact that the contestant picked a door first, thus affecting Monty's strategy. Had Monty picked one of the two "clunker" doors first at random, the problem would be different. The contestant then would know that each of the two remaining doors has an equal (50%) chance of being the right door. Then, regardless of which door the contestant chose, the opportunity to switch would not affect the chance of winning: 50% if he stays, and 50% if he switches. The subtlety here is that the difference in the order of the decisions completely changes the game and the probability of the final outcome.

If you still do not believe that switching doubles your chances of winning, construct the game on a computer. Use a uniform random number generator to pick the winning door and let the computer follow Monty's rule for showing a clunker door. That is the best way to see that after playing the game many times (e.g., at least 100 times employing the switching strategy and 100 times employing the staying strategy), you will win nearly 67% of the time when you switch and only about 33% of the time when you keep the same door.

If you are not adept at computer programming, you can go to the Susan Holmes Web site at the Stanford University Statistics Department (www.stat. stanford.edu/~susan). She has a computerized version of the game that you can play; she will keep a tally of the number of wins out of the number of times you switch and also a tally of the number of wins out of the number of times you remain with your first choice.

The game works as follows: Susan shows you a cartoon with three doors. First, you click on the door you want. Next, her computer program uncovers a door showing a cartoon picture of a donkey. Again, you click on your door if you want to keep it or click on the remaining door if you want to switch. In response, the program shows you what is behind your door: either you win or find another donkey.

Then you are asked if you want to play again. You can play the game as many times as you like using whatever strategy you like. Finally, when you decide to stop, the program shows you how many times you won when you switched and the total number of times you switched. The program also tallies the number of times you won when you used the staying strategy, along with the total number of times you chose this strategy.

5.9   A QUALITY ASSURANCE PROBLEM*

One of the present authors provided consultation services to a medical device company that was shipping a product into the field. Before shipping, the company routinely subjected the product to a sequence of quality control checks. In the field, it was discovered that one item had been shipped with a mismatched label. After checking the specifics, the company identified a lot of 100 items that included the mislabeled item at the time of shipment. These 100 items were sampled in order to test for label mismatches (failures).

The company tested a random sample of 13 out of 100 and found no failures. Although the company believed that this one mismatch was an isolated case, they could not be certain. They were faced with the prospect of recalling the remaining items in the lot in order to inspect them all for mismatches. This operation would be costly and time-consuming. On the other hand, if they could demonstrate with high enough assurance that the chances of having one or more mismatched labels in the field is very small, they would not need to conduct the recall.

The lot went through the following sequence of tests:

1. Thirteen out of 100 items were randomly selected for label mismatch checking.
2. No mismatches were found and the 13 were returned to the lot; two items were pulled and destroyed for other reasons.
3. Of the remaining 98 items, 13 were chosen at random and used for a destructive test (one that causes the item to be no longer usable in the field).
4. The remaining 85 items were then released.

In the field, it was discovered that one of these 85 had a mismatched label. A statistician (Chernick) was asked to determine the probability that at least one more of the remaining 84 items in the field could have a mismatch, assuming:

a) Exactly two are known to have had mismatches.
b) The mismatch inspection works perfectly and would have caught any mismatches.
c) In the absence of any information to the contrary, the two items pulled at the second stage could equally likely have been any of the 100 items.

*This section is the source of Exercise 5.22.

The statistician also was asked to determine the probability that at least one more of the remaining 84 items in the field could have a mismatch, assuming that exactly three are known to have had mismatches. This problem entails calculating two probabilities and adding them together: (1) the probability that all three mislabeled items passed the inspection, and (2) the probability that one was destroyed among the two pulled while the other two passed. The first of these two probabilities was of primary interest.

In addition, for baseline comparison purposes, the statistician was to consider what the probability was of the outcome that if only one item out of the 100 in the lot were mismatched, it would be among the 85 that passed the sequence of tests. This probability, being the easiest to calculate, will be derived first.

For the one mismatched label to pass with the 85 that survived the series of inspections, it must not have been selected from the first 13 for label mismatch check; otherwise, it would not have survived (assuming mismatch checking is perfectly accurate). Selecting 13 items at random from 100 is the same as drawing 13 one at a time at random without replacement. The probability that the item is not in these 13 is the product of 13 probabilities.

Each of these 13 probabilities represents the probability that among the 13 draws, the item is not drawn. On the first draw, this probability is 99/100. On the second draw, there are now only 99 items to select, resulting in the probability of 98/99 of the items not being selected. Continuing in this way and multiplying these probabilities together, we see that the probability of the item not being drawn in any one of the 13 draws is

$$(99/100)(98/99)(97/98)(96/97)(95/96)(94/95)(93/94)$$

$$(92/93)(91/92)(90/91)(89/90)(88/89)(87/88)$$

This calculation can be simplified greatly by canceling common numerators and denominators to 87/100, which gives us the probability that the item survives the first inspection.

The second and third inspections occur independently of the first. The probability we calculate for the third inspection is conditional on the result of the second inspection. So we calculate the probability of surviving those inspections and then multiply the three probabilities together to get our final result.

In the second stage, the 13 items that passed the initial inspection are replaced with others. So we again have 100 items to select from. Now, for the item with the mismatched label to escape destruction, it must not be one of the two items that were originally drawn. As we assumed that each item is equally likely to be drawn, the probability that the item with the mismatched label is not drawn is the probability that it is not the first one drawn multiplied by the probability that it is not the second one drawn, given that it was not the first one drawn. That probability is (98/100)(97/99).

At the third stage, there are only 98 items left and 13 are chosen at random for destructive testing. Consequently, the method to compute the probability is the same as the method used for the first stage, except that the first term in the product is 97/98 instead of 99/100. After multiplication and cancellation, we obtain 85/98.

The final result is then the product of these three probabilities, namely [(87/100)][(98/100)(97/99)][(85/98)]. This simplifies to (87/100)(97/100)(85/99) after cancellation. The result equals 0.72456 or 72.46%. (Note that a proportion also may be expressed as a percentage.)

Next we calculate the probability that there are two items with mismatched labels out of the 100 items in the lot. We want to determine the probability that both are missed during the three stages of inspection. Probability calculations that are similar to the foregoing calculations apply. Accordingly, we multiply the three probabilities obtained in the first three stages together.

To repeat, the probabilities obtained in the first three stages (the probability that both mismatched items are missed during inspection) are as follows:

- The first stage—(87/100)(86/99)
- The second stage, given that they survive the first stage—(98/100)(97/99)
- The third stage, given that they are among the remaining 98—(85/98)(84/97)

The final result is (87/100)(86/99)(98/100)(97/99)(85/98)(84/97). This result simplifies to (87/100)(86/99)(85/100)(84/99) = 0.54506 or 54.51%.

In the case of three items with mismatched labels out of the 100 total items in the lot, we must add the probability that all three pass inspection to the probability that two out of three pass. To determine the latter probability, we must have exactly one of the three thrown out at stage two. This differs from the previous calculation in that we are adding the possibility of two passing and one failing.

The first term follows the same logic as the previous two calculations. We compute at each stage the probability that all the items with mismatched labels pass inspection and multiply these probabilities together. The arguments are similar to those presented in the foregoing paragraphs. We present this problem as Exercise 5.22.

5.10 EXERCISES

5.1 By using a computer algorithm, an investigator can assign members of twin pairs at random to an intervention condition in a clinical trial. Assume that each twin pair consists of dizygotic twins (one male and one female). The probability of assigning one member of the pair to the intervention condition is 50%. Among the first four pairs, what is the probability of assigning to the intervention condition: 1) zero females, 2) one female, 3) two females, 4) three females, 4) four females?

5.2 In this exercise, we would like you to toss four coins at the same time into the air and record and observe the results obtained for various numbers of coin tosses. Count the frequencies of the following outcomes: 1) zero heads, 2) one head, 3) two heads, 4) three heads, 5) four heads.

a. Toss the coins one time (and compare to the results obtained in Exercise 5.1).

b. Toss the coins five times.

c. Toss the coins 15 times.

d. Toss the coins 30 times.

e. Toss the coins 60 times.

5.3   In the science exhibit of a museum of natural history, a coin-flipping machine tosses a silver dollar into the air and tallies the outcome on a counting device. What are all of the respective possible outcomes in any three consecutive coin tosses? In any three consecutive coin tosses, what is the probability of: a) at least one head, *b*) not more than one head, c) at least two heads, d) not more than two heads, e) exactly two heads, f) exactly three heads.

5.4   A certain laboratory animal used in preclinical evaluations of experimental catheters gives birth to only one offspring at a time. The probability of giving birth to a male or a female offspring is equally likely. In three consecutive pregnancies of a single animal, what is the probability of giving birth to: (a) two males and one female, (b) no females, (c) two males first and then a female, and (d) at least one female. State how the four probabilities are different from one another. For the foregoing scenario, note all of the possible birth outcomes in addition to (a) through (d).

5.5   What is the expected distribution—numbers and proportions—of each of the six faces (i.e., 1 through 6) of a die when it is rolled 1000 times?

5.6   A pharmacist has filled a box with six different kinds of antibiotic capsules. There are a total of 300 capsules, which are distributed as follows: tetracycline (15), penicillin (30), minocycline (45), Bactrim (60), streptomycin (70), and Zithromax (80). She asks her assistant to mix the pills thoroughly and to withdraw a single capsule from the box. What is the probability that the capsule selected is: a) either penicillin or streptomycin, *b*) neither Zithromax nor tetracycline, c) Bactrim, d) not penicillin, e) either minocycline, Bactrim, or tetracycline?

5.7   In an ablation procedure, the probability of acute success (determined at completion of the procedure) is 0.95 when an image mapping system is used. Without the image mapping system, the probably of acute success is only 0.80. Suppose that Patient A is given the treatment with the mapping system and Patient *B* is given the treatment without the mapping system. Determine the following probabilities:

a. Both patients *A* and *B* had acute successes.

b. *A* had an acute success but *B* had an acute failure.

   c. B had an acute success but A had an acute failure.
   d. Both *A* and *B* had acute failures.
   e. At least one of the patients had an acute success.
   f. Describe two ways that the result in (e) can be calculated based on the re-
      sults from (a), (b), (c), and (d).

5.8   Repeat Exercise 5.4 but this time assume that the probability of having a male
          offspring is 0.514 and the probability of having a female offspring is 0.486. In
          this case, the elementary outcomes are not equally likely. However, the trials
          are Bernoulli and the binomial distribution applies. Use your knowledge of
          the binomial distribution to compute the probabilities [(a) through (e) from
          Exercise 5.5].

5.9   Refer to Formula 5.7, permutations of *r* objects taken from *n* objects. Com-
          pute the following permutations:
          a. $P(8, 3)$
          b. $P(7, 5)$
          c. $P(4, 2)$
          d. $P(6, 4)$
          e. $P(5, 2)$

5.10 Nine volunteers wish to participate in a clinical trial to test a new medication
          for depression. In how many ways can we select five of these individuals for
          assignment to the intervention trial?

5.11 Use Formula 5.8, combinations of *r* objects taken out of *n*, to determine the
          following combinations:
          a. $C(7, 4)$
          b. $C(6, 4)$
          c. $C(6, 2)$
          d. $C(5, 2)$
          e. What is the relationship between 5.11 (d) and 5.9 (e)?
          f. What is the relationship between 5.11 (b) and 5.9 (d)?

5.12 In how many ways can four different colored marbles be arranged in a row?

5.13 Provide definitions for each of these terms:
          a. Elementary events
          b. Mutually exclusive events
          c. Equally likely events
          d. Independent events
          e. Random variable

5.14 Give a definition or description of the following:
          a. $C(4, 2)$
          b. $P(5, 3)$

c. The addition rule for mutually exclusive events
d. The multiplication rule for independent events

5.15 Based on the following table of hemoglobin levels for miners, compute the probabilities described below. Assume that the proportion in each category for this set of 90 miners is the true proportion for the population of miners.

Class Interval for Hemoglobin (g/cc)	Number of Miners
12.0–17.9	24
18.0–21.9	53
22.0–27.9	13
Total	90

Source: Adapted from Dunn, O. J. (1977). *Basic Statistics: A Primer for the Biomedical Sciences,* 2nd Edition. Wiley, New York, p. 17.

a. Compute the probability that a miner selected at random from the population has a hemoglobin level in the 12.0–17.9 range.
b. Compute the probability that a miner selected at random from the population has a hemoglobin level in the 18.0–21.9 range.
c. Compute the probability that a miner selected at random from the population has a hemoglobin level in the 22.0–27.9 range.
d. What is the probability that a miner selected at random will have a hemoglobin count at or above 18.0?
e. What is the probability that a miner selected at random will have a hemoglobin count at or below 21.9?
f. If two miners are selected at random from the "infinite population" of miners with the distribution for the miners in the table, what is the probability that one miner will fall in the lowest class and the other in the highest (i.e., one has a hemoglobin count in the 12.0 to 17.9 range and the other has a hemoglobin count in the 22.0 to 27.9 range)?

5.16 Consider the following 2 × 2 table that shows incidence of myocardial infarction (denoted MI) for women who had used oral contraceptives and women who had never used oral contraceptives. The data in the table are fictitious and are used just for illustrative purposes.

	MI Yes	MI No	Totals
Used oral contraceptives	55	65	120
Never used oral contraceptives	25	125	150
Totals	80	190	270

Assume that the proportions in the table represent the "infinite population" of adult women. Let A = {woman used oral contraceptives} and let B = {woman had an MI episode}

a. Find $P(A)$, $P(B)$, $P(A^c)$, and $P(B^c)$.
b. What is $P(A \cap B)$?
c. What is $P(A \cup B)$?
d. Are A and B mutually exclusive?
e. What are $P(A|B)$ and $P(B|A)$?
f. Are A and B independent?

5.17 For the binomial distribution, do the following:
a. Give the conditions necessary for the binomial distribution to apply to a random variable.
b. Give the general formula for the probability of r successes in n trials.
c. Give the probability mass function for $Bi(10, 0.40)$.
d. For the distribution in c, determine the probability of no more than four successes.

5.18 Sickle cell anemia is a genetic disease that occurs only if a child inherits two recessive genes. Each child receives one gene from the father and one from the mother. A person can be characterized as follows: The person can have: (a) two dominant genes (cannot transmit the disease to a child), (b) one dominant and one recessive gene (has the trait and is therefore a carrier who can pass on the disease to a child, but does not have the disease), or (c) has both recessive genes (in which case the person has the disease and is a carrier of the disease). For each parent there is a 50–50 chance that the child will inherit either the dominant or the recessive gene. Calculate the probability of the child having the disease if:
a. Both parents are carriers
b. One parent is a carrier and the other has two dominant genes
c. One parent is a carrier and the other has the disease
Calculate the probability that the child will be a carrier if:
d. Both parents are carriers
e. One parent is a carrier and the other has the disease
f. One parent is a carrier and the other has two dominant genes

5.19 Under the conditions given for Exercise 5.18, calculate the probability that the child will have two dominant genes if:
a. One of the parents is a carrier and the other parent has two dominant genes
b. Both of the parents are carriers

5.20 Compute the mean and variance of the binomial distribution $Bi(n, p)$. Find the arithmetic values for the special case in which both $n = 10$ and $p = 1/2$.

5.21 a. Define the probability density and cumulative probability function for an absolutely continuous random variable.
b. Which of these functions is analogous to the probability mass function of a discrete random variable?

c. Determine the probability density function and the cumulative distribution function for a uniform random variable on the interval [0, 1].

5.22 In the example in Section 5.9, consider the probability that three items have mismatched labels and one of these items is found.

a. Calculate the probability that all three items would pass inspection and, therefore, there would be two additional ones out of the 84 remaining in the field.

b. Calculate the probability that exactly one of the two remaining items with mismatched labels is among the 84 items still in the field. (Hint: Add together two probabilities, namely the probability that exactly one item is removed at the second stage but none at the third, added to the probability that exactly one item is removed at the third stage but none at the second).

c. Use the results from (a) and (b) above to calculate the probability that at least one of the two additional items with mismatched labels is among the 84 remaining in the field.

d. Based on the result in (c), do you think the probability is small enough not to recall the 84 items for inspection?

5.11   ADDITIONAL READING

As references 1 and 3 are written for general audiences, students should be comfortable with the writing style and level of presentation. A different approach is represented by reference 2, which is an advanced text on probability intended for graduate students in mathematics and statistics. However, Feller (reference 2) has an interesting writing style and explains the paradoxes very well. Students should be able to follow his arguments but should stay away from any mathematical derivations. We recommend it because it is one of those rare books that gives the reader insight into probability results and demonstrates the subtle problems, in particular, that can arise.

1. Bruce, C. (2000). *Conned again, Watson!* Cautionary Tales of Logic, Math, and Probability. Perseus Publishing, Cambridge, Massachusetts.
2. Dunn, O. J. (1977). *Basic Statistics: A Primer for the Biomedical Sciences* 2nd Edition. Wiley, New York.
3. Feller, W. (1971). *An Introduction to Probability Theory and Its Applications: Volume II.* 2nd Edition, Wiley, New York.
4. Vos Savant, M. (1997). *The Power of Logical Thinking: Easy Lessons in the Art of Reasoning . . . and Hard Facts about Its Absence in Our Lives.* St Martin's Griffin, New York.

CHAPTER 6

The Normal Distribution

We know not to what are due the accidental errors, and precisely because we do not know, we are aware they obey the law of Gauss. Such is the paradox.
—Henri Poincare, *The Foundation of Science: Science and Method,* p. 406.

6.1   THE IMPORTANCE OF THE NORMAL DISTRIBUTION IN STATISTICS

The normal distribution is an absolutely continuous distribution (defined in Chapter 5) that plays a major role in statistics. Unlike the examples we have seen thus far, the normal distribution has a nonzero density function over the entire real number line. You will discover that because of the central limit theorem, many random variables, particularly those obtained by averaging others, will have distributions that are approximately normal.

The normal distribution is determined by two parameters: the mean and the variance. The fact that the mean and the variance of the normal distribution are the natural parameters for the normal distribution explains why they are sometimes preferred as measures of location and scale.

For a normal distribution, there is no need to make the distinction among the mean, median, and mode. They are all equal to one another. The normal distribution is a unimodal (i.e., has one mode) symmetric distribution. We will describe its density function and discuss its important properties in Section 6.2. For now, let us gain a better appreciation of its importance in statistics and statistical applications.

The normal distribution was discovered first by the French mathematician Albert DeMoivre in the 1730s. Two other famous mathematicians, Pierre Simon de Laplace (also from France) and Karl Friedrich Gauss from Germany, motivated by applications to social and natural sciences, independently rediscovered the normal distribution.

Gauss found that the normal distribution with a mean of zero was often a useful model for characterizing measurement errors. He was very much involved in astronomical measurements of the planetary orbits and used this theory of errors to help fit elliptic curves to these planetary orbits.

Introductory Biostatistics for the Health Sciences, by Michael R. Chernick and Robert H. Friis. ISBN 0-471-41137-X. Copyright © 2003 Wiley-Interscience.

DeMoivre and Laplace both found that the normal distribution provided an increasingly better approximation to the binomial distribution as the number of trials became large. This discovery was a special form of the Central Limit Theorem that later was to be generalized by 20th century mathematicians including Liapunov, Lindeberg, and Feller.

In the 1890s in England, Sir Francis Galton found applications for the normal distribution in medicine; he also generalized it to two dimensions as an aid in explaining his theory of regression and correlation. In the 20th century, Pearson, Fisher, Snedecor, and Gosset, among others, further developed applications and other distributions including the chi-square, F distribution, and Student's t distribution, all of which are related to the normal distribution. Some of the most important early applications of the normal distribution were in the fields of agriculture, medicine, and genetics. Today, statistics and the normal distribution have a place in almost every scientific endeavor.

Although the normal distribution provides a good probability model for many phenomena in the real world, it does not apply universally. Other parametric and nonparametric statistical models also play an important role in medicine and the health sciences.

A common joke is that theoreticians say the normal distribution is important because practicing statisticians have discovered it to be so empirically. But the practicing statisticians say it is important because the theoreticians have proven it so mathematically.

6.2   PROPERTIES OF NORMAL DISTRIBUTIONS

The normal distribution has three main characteristics. First, its probability density is bell-shaped, with a single mode at the center. As the tails of the normal distribution extend to $\pm\infty$, the distribution decreases in height and remains positive. It is symmetric in shape about μ, which is both its mean and mode. As detailed as this description may sound, it does not completely characterize the normal distribution. There are other probability distributions that are symmetric and bell-shaped as well. The normal density function is distinguished by the rate at which it drops to zero. Another parameter, σ, along with the mean, completes the characterization of the normal distribution.

The relationship between σ and the area under the normal curve provides the second main characteristic of the normal distribution. The parameter σ is the standard deviation of the distribution. Its square is the variance of the distribution.

For a normal distribution, 68.26% of the probability distribution falls in the interval from $\mu - \sigma$ to $\mu + \sigma$. The wider interval from $\mu - 2\sigma$ to $\mu + 2\sigma$ contains 95.45% of the distribution. Finally, the interval from $\mu - 3\sigma$ to $\mu + 3\sigma$ contains 99.73% of the distribution, nearly 100% of the distribution. The fact that nearly all observations from a normal distribution fall within $\pm 3\sigma$ of the mean explains why the three-sigma limits are used so often in practice.

Third, a complete mathematical description of the normal distribution can be found in the equation for its density. The probability density function $f(x)$ for a normal distribution is given by

$$f(x) = \frac{1}{\sigma\sqrt{2\pi}} e^{\frac{-(x-\mu)^2}{2\sigma^2}}$$

One awkward fact about the normal distribution is that its cumulative distribution does not have a closed form. That means that we cannot write down an explicit formula for it. So to calculate probabilities, the density must be integrated numerically. That is why for many years statisticians and other practitioners of statistical methods relied heavily on tables that were generated for the normal distribution.

One important feature was very helpful in making those tables. Although to specify a particular normal distribution one has to provide the two parameters, the mean and the variance, a simple equation relates the general normal distribution to one particular normal distribution called the standard normal distribution.

For the general normal distribution, we will use the notation $N(\mu, \sigma^2)$. This expression denotes a normal distribution with mean μ and variance σ^2. The standard normal distribution has mean 0 and variance 1. So $N(0, 1)$ denotes the standard normal distribution. Figure 6.1 presents a standard normal distribution with standard deviation units shown on the x-axis.

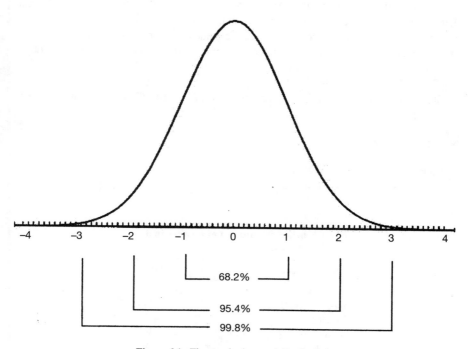

Figure 6.1. The standard normal distribution.

Suppose X is $N(\mu, \sigma^2)$; if we let $Z = (X - \mu)/\sigma$, then Z is $N(0, 1)$. The values for Z, an important distribution for statistical inference, are available in a table. From the table, we can find the probability P for any values $a < b$, such that $P(a \le Z \le b)$. But, since $Z = (X - \mu)/\sigma$, this is just $P(a \le (X - \mu)/\sigma \le b) = P(a\sigma \le (X - \mu) \le b\sigma) = P(a\sigma + \mu \le X \le b\sigma + \mu)$. Thus, to make inferences about X, all we need to do is to convert X to Z, a process known as standardization.

So, probability statements about Z can be translated into probability statements about X through this relationship. Therefore, a single table for Z suffices to tell us everything we need to know about X (assuming both μ and σ are specified).

6.3 TABULATING AREAS UNDER THE STANDARD NORMAL DISTRIBUTION

Let us suppose that in a biostatistics course, students are given a test that has 100 total possible points. Assume that the students who take this course have a normal distribution of scores with a mean of 75 and a standard deviation of 7. The instructor uses the grading system presented in Table 6.1. Given this grading system and the assumed normal distribution, let us determine the percentage of students that will receive A, B, C, D, and F. This calculation will involve exercises with tables of the standard normal distribution.

First, let us repeat this table with the raw scores replaced by the Z scores. This process will make it easier for us to go directly to the standard normal tables. Recall that we arrive at Z by the linear transformation $Z = (X - \mu)/\sigma$. In this case $\mu = 75$, $\sigma = 7$, and the X values we are interested in are the grade boundaries 60, 70, 80, and 90. Let us go through these calculations step by step for $X = 90$, $X = 80$, $X = 70$, and $X = 60$.

Step 1: Subtract μ from X: $90 - 75 = 15$.

Step 2: Divide the result of step one by σ: $15/7 = 2.143$ (The resulting Z score = 2.143)

Now take $X = 80$.

Step 1: Subtract μ from X: $80 - 75 = 5$.

Step 2: Divide the result of step one by σ: $5/7 = 0.714$ ($Z = 0.714$)

TABLE 6.1. Distribution of Grades in a Biostatistics Course

Range of Scores	Grade
Below 60	F
60–69	D
70–79	C
80–89	B
90–100	A

Now take $X = 70$.

> Step 1: Subtract μ from X: $70-75 = -5$.
> Step 2: Divide the result of step one by σ: $-5/7 = -0.714$ ($Z = -0.714$)

Now take $X = 60$.

> Step 1: Subtract μ from X: $60 - 75 = -15$.
> Step 2: Divide the result of step one by σ: $-15/7 = -2.143$ ($Z = -2.143$)

The distribution of percentiles and corresponding grades are shown in Table 6.2.

To determine the probability of an F we need to compute $P(Z < -2.143)$ and find its value in a table of Z scores. The tables in our book (see Appendix D) give us $P(0 < Z < b)$, where b is a positive number. Other probabilities are obtained using properties of the standard normal distribution. These properties are given in Table 6.3. The areas associated with these properties are given in Figure 6.2.

Using the properties shown in the equations in Figure 6.2, Parts (a) through (g), we can calculate any desired probability. We are seeking probabilities on the left-hand side of each equation. The terms farthest to the right in these equations are the probabilities that can be obtained directly from the Z Table. (Refer to Appendix E.)

For $P(Z < -2.143)$ we use the property in Part (d) and see that the result is $0.50-P(0 < Z < 2.143)$. The table of Z values is carried to only two decimal places. For greater accuracy we could interpolate between 2.14 and 2.15 to get the answer. But for simplicity, let us round 2.143 to 2.14 and use the probability that we obtain for $Z = 2.14$.

TABLE 6.2. Distribution of Z Scores and Grades

Range of Z Scores	Grade
Below -2.143	F
Between -2.143 and -0.714	D
Between -0.714 and 0.714	C
Between 0.714 and 2.143	B
Above 2.143	A

TABLE 6.3. Properties of the Table of Standard Scores (Used for Finding Z Scores)

a. $P(Z > b) = 0.50 - P(0 < Z < b)$
b. $P(-b < Z < b) = 2P(0 < Z < b)$
c. $P(-b < Z < b) = P(0 < Z < b)$
d. $P(Z < -b) = P(Z > b) = 0.50 - P(0 < Z < b)$
e. $P(-a < Z < b) = P(0 < Z < a) + P(0 < Z < b)$, where $a > 0$
f. $P(a < Z < b) = P(0 < Z < b) - P(0 < Z < a)$, where $0 < a < b$
g. $P(-a < Z < -b) = P(b < Z < a) = P(0 < Z < a) - P(0 < Z < b)$, where $-a < -b < 0$ and hence $a > b > 0$

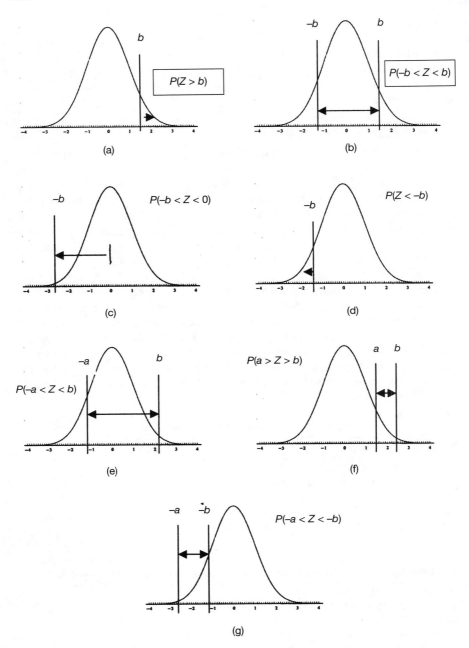

Figure 6.2. The properties of Z Scores illustrated. Parts (a) through (g) illustrate the properties shown in Table 6.3. Note that b is symmetric. A negative letter (−a or −b) indicates that the Z score falls to the left of the mean, which is 0.

The Z table shows us that $P(0 < Z < 2.14) = 0.4838$. So the probability of getting an F is just $0.5000 - 0.4838 = 0.0162$.

The probability of a D is $P(-2.14 < Z < -0.71)$ by rounding to two decimal places. For this probability we must use the property in Part (g). So we have $P(-2.14 < Z < -0.71) = P(0 < Z < 2.14) - P(0 < Z < 0.71) = 0.4838 - 0.2611 = 0.2227$.

The probability of a C is $P(-0.71 < Z < 0.71)$. Here we use property in Part (b). We have $P(-0.71 < Z < 0.71) = 2P(0 < Z < 0.71) = 2(0.2611) = 0.5222$.

The probability of a B is $P(0.71 < Z < 2.14)$. We could calculate this probability directly by using the property in Part (f). However, looking closely at Part (g), we see that it is the same as $P(-2.14 < Z < -0.71)$, a probability that we have already calculated for a D. So we save some work and notice that the probability of a B is 0.2227.

The probability of an A is $P(Z > 2.14)$. We can obtain this value directly from the property in Part (a). Again, if we look carefully at the property in Part (d), we see that $P(Z > 2.14) = P(Z < -2.14)$, which equals the right-hand side that we calculated previously for an F. So again, careful use of the properties can save us some work! The probability of an A is 0.0162.

We might feel that we are giving out too many Ds and Bs, possibly because the test is a little harder than the usual test for this class. If the instructor wants to adjust the test based on what the standard deviation should be (i.e., curve the test), the instructor can make the following adjustments. The mean of 75 is where it should be, so only an adjustment is needed to take account of the spread of the score. If the observed mean were 70, an adjustment for this bias also could be made.

We will not go through the exercise of curving the tests, but let us see what would happen if we in fact did have a lower standard deviation of 5, for example, with an average of 75. In that case, what would we find for the distribution of grades?

We will repeat all the steps we went through before. The only difference will be in the final Z scores that we obtain, because we divide by 5 instead of 7.

Step 1: Subtract μ from X: $90 - 75 = 15$

Step 2: Divide the result of step one by σ: $15/5 = 3.00$. (The resulting Z score = 3.00.)

Now take $X = 80$.

Step 1: Subtract μ from X: $80 - 75 = 5$

Step 2: Divide the result of step one by σ: $5/5 = 1.00$ $(Z = 1.00)$

Now take $X = 70$.

Step 1: Subtract μ from X: $70 - 75 = -5$

Step 2: Divide the result of step one by σ: $-5/5 = -1.00$ $(Z = -1.00)$

Now take $X = 60$.

  Step 1: Subtract μ from X: $60 - 75 = -15$
  Step 2: Divide the result of step one by σ: $-15/5 = -3.00$ ($Z = -3.00$)

These results are summarized in Table 6.4. In this case we obtained whole integers that are easy to work with. Since we already know how to interpret 1σ and 3σ in terms of normal probabilities, we do not even need the tables but we will use them anyway.

  We will use shorthand notation: $P(F)$ = probability of receiving an F = $P(Z < -3)$. Recall that by symmetry, $P(F) = P(A)$ and $P(D) = P(B)$. First compute $P(A)$: $P(A) = P(Z > 3) = 0.50\text{-}P(0 < Z < 3) = 0.50\text{-}0.4987 = 0.0013 = P(F)$.

  Only about 1 in 1000 students will receive an F. Although the low number of Fs will please the students, an A will be nearly impossible! By symmetry, $P(B) = P(1 < Z < 3) = P(0 < Z < 3) - P(0 < Z < 1) = 0.4987 - 0.3413 = 0.1574 = P(D)$. As a result, approximately 16% of the class will receive a B and 16% a D. These proportions of Bs and Ds represent fairly reasonable outcomes. Now $P(C) = P(-1 < Z < 1) = 2\,P(0 < Z < 1) = 2\,(0.3413) = 0.6826$. As expected, more than two-thirds of the class will receive the average grade of C.

  Until now, you have learned how to use the Z table (Appendix E) by applying the seven properties shown in Table 6.3 to find grade distributions. In these examples, we always started with specific endpoints or intervals for Z and looked up the probabilities associated with them. In other situations, we may know the specified probability for the normal distribution and want to look up the corresponding Z values for an endpoint or interval.

  Consider that we want to find a symmetric interval for a C grade on a test but we do not have specific cutoffs in mind. Rather, we specify that the interval should be centered at the mean of 75, be symmetric, and contain 62% of the population. Then $P(C)$ should have the form: $P(-a < Z < a) = 2P(0 < Z < a)$. We want $P(C) = 0.62$, so $P(0 < Z < a) = 0.31$. We now look for a value a that satisfies $P(0 < Z < a) = 0.31$. Scanning the Z table, we see that a value of $a = 0.88$ gives $P(0 < Z < a) = 0.3106$. That is good enough. So $a = 0.88$.

TABLE 6.4. Distribution of Z Scores When σ Changes from 7 to 5

Range of Z Scores	Grade
Below -3.00	F
Between -3.00 and -1.00	D
Between -1.00 and 1.00	C
Between 1.00 and 3.00	B
Above 3.00	A

6.4   EXERCISES

6.1   Define the following terms in your own words:
    Continuous distribution
    Normal distribution
    Standard normal distribution
    Probability density function
    Standardization
    Standard score
    Z score
    Percentile

6.2   The following questions pertain to some important facts to know about a normal distribution:
    a. What are three important properties of a normal distribution?
    b. What percentage of the values are:
        i. within 1 standard deviation of the mean?
        ii. 2 standard deviations or more above the mean?
        iii. 1.96 standard deviations or more below the mean?
        iv. between the mean and ±2.58 standard deviations?
        v. 1.28 standard deviations above the mean?

6.3   The following questions pertain to the standard normal distribution:
    a. How is the standard normal distribution defined?
    b. How does a standard normal distribution compare to a normal distribution?
    c. What is the procedure for finding an area under the standard normal curve?
    d. How would the typical normal distribution of scores on a test administered to a freshman survey class in physics differ from a standard normal distribution?
    e. What characteristics of the standard normal distribution make it desirable for use with some problems in biostatistics?

6.4   If you were a clinical laboratory technician in a hospital, how would you apply the principles of the standard normal distribution to define normal and abnormal blood test results (e.g., for low-density lipoprotein)?

To solve Exercises 6.5 through 6.9, you will need to refer to the standard normal table.

6.5   Referring to the properties shown in Table 6.3, find the standard normal score (Z score) associated with the following percentiles: (a) 5th, (b) 10th, (c) 20th, (d) 25th, (e) 50th, (f) 75th, (g) 80th, (h) 90th, and (i) 95th.

6.6 Determine the areas under the standard normal curve that fall between the following values of Z:
  a. 0 and 1.00
  b. 0 and 1.28
  c. 0 and –1.65
  d. 1.00 and 2.33
  e. –1.00 and –2.58

6.7 The areas under a standard normal curve also may be considered to be probabilities. Find probabilities associated with the area:
  a. Above $Z = 2.33$
  b. Below $Z = -2.58$
  c. Above $Z = 1.65$ and below $Z = -1.65$
  d. Above $Z = 1.96$ and below $Z = -1.96$
  e. Above $Z = 2.33$ and below $Z = -2.33$

6.8 Another way to express probabilities associated with Z scores (assuming a standard normal distribution) is to use parentheses according to the format: $P(Z > 0) = 0.5000$, for the case when $Z = 0$. Calculate the following probabilities:
  a. $P(Z < -2.90) =$
  b. $P(Z > -1.11) =$
  c. $P(Z < 0.66) =$
  d. $P(Z > 3.00) =$
  e. $P(Z < -1.50) =$

6.9 The inverse of Exercise 6.8 is to be able to find a Z score when you know a probability. Assuming a standard normal distribution, identify the Z score indicated by a # sign that is associated with each of the following probabilities:
  a. $P(Z < \#) = 0.9920$
  b. $P(Z > \#) = 0.0005$
  c. $P(Z < \#) = 0.0250$
  d. $P(Z < \#) = 0.6554$
  e. $P(Z > \#) = 0.0049$

6.10 A first year medical school class ($n = 200$) took a first midterm examination in human physiology. The results were as follows ($\overline{X} = 65$, $S = 7$). Explain how you would standardize any particular score from this distribution, and then solve the following problems:
  a. What Z score corresponds to a test score of 40?
  b. What Z score corresponds to a test score of 50?
  c. What Z score corresponds to a test score of 60?
  d. What Z score corresponds to a test score of 70?
  e. How many students received a score of 75 or higher?

6.11 The mean height of a population of girls aged 15 to 19 years in a northern province in Sweden was found to be 165 cm with a standard deviation of 15 cm. Assuming that the heights are normally distributed, find the heights in centimeters that correspond to the following percentiles:
  a. Between the 20th and 50th percentiles.
  b. Between the 40th and 60th percentiles.
  c. Between the 10th and 90th percentiles.
  d. Above the 80th percentile.
  e. Below the 10th percentile.
  f. Above the 5th percentile.

6.12 In a health examination survey of a prefecture in Japan, the population was found to have an average fasting blood glucose level of 99.0 with a standard deviation of 12. Determine the probability that an individual selected at random will have a blood sugar reading:
  a. Greater than 120 (let the random variable for this be denoted as X; then we can write the probability of this event as $P(X > 120)$
  b. Between 70 and 100, $P(70 < X < 100)$
  c. Less than 83, $P(X < 83)$
  d. Less than 70 or greater than 110, $P(X > 110) + P(X < 70)$
  e. That deviates by more than 2 standard deviations (24 units) from the mean

6.13 Repeat Exercise 6.12 but with a standard deviation of 9 instead of 12.

6.14 Repeat Exercise 6.12 again, but this time with a mean of 110 and a standard deviation of 15.

6.15 A community epidemiology study conducted fasting blood tests on a large community and obtained the following results for triglyceride levels (which were normally distributed): males—$\mu = 100$, $\sigma = 30$; females—$\mu = 85$, $\sigma = 25$. If we decide that persons who fall within two standard deviations of the mean shall not be referred for medical workup, what triglyceride values would fall within this range for males and females, respectively? If we decide to refer persons who have readings in the top 5% for medical workup, what would these triglyceride readings be for males and females, respectively?

6.16 Assume the weights of women between 16 and 30 years of age are normally distributed with a mean of 120 pounds and a standard deviation of 18 pounds. If 100 women are selected at random from this population, how many would you expect to have the following weights (round off to the nearest integer):
  a. Between 90 and 145 pounds
  b. Less than 85 pounds
  c. More than 150 pounds
  d. Between 84 and 156 pounds

6.17 Suppose that the population of 25-year-old American males has an average remaining life expectancy of 50 years with a standard deviation of 5 years and that life expectancy is normally distributed.
   a. What proportion of these 25-year-old males will live past 75?
   b. What proportion of these 25-year-old males will live past 85?
   c. What proportion of these 25-year-old males will live past 90?
   d. What proportion will not live past 65?

6.18 The population of 25-year-old American women has a remaining life expectancy that is also normally distributed and differs from that of the males in Exercise 6.17 only in that the women's average remaining life expectancy is 5 years longer than for the males.
   a. What proportion of these 25-year-old females will live past 75?
   b. What proportion of these 25-year-old females will live past 85?
   c. What proportion of these 25-year-old females will live past 95?
   d. What proportion will not live past 65?

6.19 It is suspected that a random variable has a normal distribution with a mean of 6 and a standard deviation of 0.5. After observing several hundred values, we find that the mean is approximately equal to 6 and the standard deviation is close to 0.5. However, we find that 53% percent of the observations are between 5.5 and 6.5 and 83% are between 5.0 and 6.0. Does this evidence increase or decrease your confidence that the data are normally distributed? Explain your answer.

6.5 ADDITIONAL READING

The following is a list of a few references that can provide more detailed information about the properties of the normal distribution. Reference #1 (Johnson and Kotz, 1970) covers the normal distribution. Reference #2 (Kotz and Johnson, 1985) cites I. W. Molenaar's article on normal approximations to other distributions. Reference #3 (also Kotz and Johnson, 1985) cites C. B. Read's article on the normal distribution.

1. Johnson, N. L. and Kotz, S. (1970). *Distributions in Statistics: Continuous Univariate Distributions, Volume 1* (Chapter 13). Wiley, New York.
2. Kotz, S. and Johnson, N. L. (editors). (1985). *Encyclopedia of Statistical Sciences, Volume 6,* pp. 340–347, Wiley, New York.
3. Kotz, S. and Johnson, N. L. (editors). (1985). *Encyclopedia of Statistical Sciences, Volume 6,* pp. 347–359, Wiley, New York.
4. Patel, J. K. and Read, C. B. (1982). *Handbook of the Normal Distribution.* Marcel Dekker, New York.
5. Stuart, A. and Ord, K. (1994). *Kendall's Advanced Theory of Statistics, Volume 1: Distribution Theory,* Sixth Edition, pp. 191–197. Edward Arnold, London.

CHAPTER 7

Sampling Distributions for Means

[T]o quote a statement of Poincare who said (partly in jest no doubt) that there must be something mysterious about the normal law since mathematicians think it is a law of nature, whereas physicists are convinced that it is a mathematical theorem.
—Mark Kac, *Statistical Independence in Probability, Analysis and Number Theory,*
Chapter 3: The Normal Law, p. 52

7.1 POPULATION DISTRIBUTIONS AND THE DISTRIBUTION OF SAMPLE AVERAGES FROM THE POPULATION

What is the strategy of statistical inference? Statistical inference refers to reaching conclusions about population parameters based on sample data. Statisticians make inferences based on samples from finite populations (even large ones such as the U.S. population) or conceptually infinite populations (a probability model of a distribution for which our sample can be thought of as a set of independent observations drawn from this distribution). Other examples of finite populations include all of the patients seen in a hospital clinic, all patients known to a tumor registry who have been diagnosed with cancers, or all residents of a nursing home.

As an example of a rationale for sampling, we note that it would be prohibitively expensive for a research organization to conduct a health survey of the U.S. population by administering a health status questionnaire to everyone in the United States. On the other hand, a random sample of this population, say 2000 Americans, may be feasible. From the sample, we would estimate health parameters for the population based on responses from the random sample. These estimates are random because they depend on the particular sample that was chosen.

Suppose that we calculate a sample mean $(\bar{X})$ as an estimate of the population mean (μ). It is possible to select many samples of size n from a population. The value of this sample estimate of the parameter would differ from one random sample to the next. By determining the distribution of these estimates, a statistician is then able to draw an inference (e.g., confidence interval statement or conclusion of a hypothesis test) based on the distribution of sample statistics. This distribution that is so important to us is called the sampling distribution for the estimate.

Similarly, we will observe for many different parameters of populations the sampling distribution of their estimates. First, we will start out with the simplest, namely, the sample estimate of a population mean.

Let us be clear on the difference between the sample distribution of an observation and the sampling distribution of the mean of the observations. We will note that the parent populations for some data may have highly skewed distributions (either left or right), multimodal distributions, or a wide variety of other possible shapes. However, the central limit theorem, which we will discuss in this chapter, will show us that regardless of the shape of the distribution of the observations for the parent population, the sample average will have a distribution that is approximately a normal distribution. This important result partially explains the importance in statistics of the normal or Gaussian distribution that we studied in the previous chapter.

We will see examples of data with distributions very different from the normal distribution (both theoretical and actual) and will see that the distribution of the average of several samples, even for sample sizes as small as 5 or 10, will become symmetric and approximately normal—an amazing result! This result can be proved by using tools from probability theory, but that involves advanced probability tools that are beyond the scope of the course. Instead, we hope to convince you of the result by observing what the exact sampling distribution is for small sample sizes. You will see how the distribution changes as the sample size increases.

Recall from a previous exercise the seasonal home run totals of four current major league sluggers—Ken Griffey Jr, Mark McGwire, Sammy Sosa, and Barry Bonds. The home run totals for their careers, starting with their "rookie" season (i.e., first season with enough at bats to qualify as a rookie) is given as follows:

McGwire	49, 32, 33, 39, 22, 42, 9, 9, 39, 52, 58, 70, 65, 32
Sosa	4, 15, 10, 8, 33, 25, 36, 40, 36, 66, 63, 50
Bonds	16, 25, 24, 19, 33, 25, 34, 46, 37, 33, 42, 40, 37, 34, 49
Griffey	16, 22, 22, 27, 45, 40, 17, 49, 56, 56, 48, 40

This gives us a total of 53 seasonal home run totals for top major league home run hitters. Let us consider this distribution (combining the totals for these four players) to be a population distribution for home run hitters. Now let us first look at a histogram of this distribution taking the intervals 0–9, 10–19, 20–29, 30–39, 40–49, 50–59, and 60–70 as the class intervals. Table 7.1 shows the histogram for these data.

The mean for this population is 35.26 and the population variance is 252.95. The population standard deviation is 15.90. These three parameters have been computed by rounding to two decimal places. Figure 7.1 is a bar graph of the histogram for this population.

We notice that although the distribution is not a normal distribution, it is not highly skewed either. Now let us look at the means for random samples of size 5.

TABLE 7.1. Histogram for Home run Hitters "Population" Distribution

Class Interval	Frequency
0–9	4
10–19	6
20–29	8
30–39	14
40–49	12
50–59	5
60–70	4
Total	53

We shall use a random number table to generate 25 random samples each of size 5. For each sample we will compute the average and the sample estimate of standard deviation and variance. The indices for the 53 seasonal home run totals will be selected randomly from the table of uniform numbers. The indices correspond to the home run totals as shown in Table 7.2.

We sample across the table of random numbers until we have generated 25 samples of size 5. For each sample, we are sampling without replacement. So if a particular index is repeated, we will use the rejection sampling method that we learned in Chapter 2.

We refer to Table 2.1 for the random numbers. Starting in column row one and going across the columns and down we get the following numbers: 69158, 38683, 41374, 17028, and 09304. Interpreting these numbers as decimals 0.69158, 0.38683, 0.41374, 0.17028, and 0.09304 we then must determine the indices and decide whether we must reject any numbers because of repeats. To determine the indices, we divide the interval [0, 1] into 53 equal parts so that the indices correspond to random numbers in intervals as shown in Table 7.3.

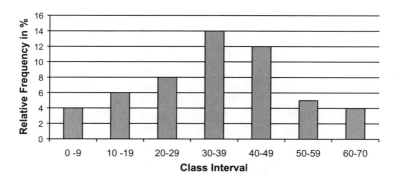

Figure 7.1. Relative frequency histogram for home run sluggers population distribution.

TABLE 7.2. Home Runs: Correspondence to Indices

Index	Home Run Total
1	49
2	32
3	33
4	39
5	22
6	42
7	9
8	9
9	39
10	52
11	58
12	70
13	65
14	32
15	4
16	15
17	10
18	8
19	33
20	25
21	36
22	40
23	36
24	66
25	63
26	50
27	16
28	25
29	24
30	19
31	33
32	25
33	34
34	46
35	37
36	33
37	42
38	40
39	37
40	34
41	49
42	16
43	22
44	22
45	27
46	45

TABLE 7.2. *Continued*

Index	Home Run Total
47	40
48	17
49	49
50	56
51	56
52	48
53	40

Scanning Table 7.3 we find the following correspondences: $0.69158 \rightarrow 37$, $0.38683 \rightarrow 21$, $0.41374 \rightarrow 22$, $0.17028 \rightarrow 10$, and $0.09304 \rightarrow 5$. Since none of the indices repeated, we do not have to reject any random numbers and the first sample is obtained by matching the indices to home runs in Table 7.2.

We see that the correspondence is $37 \rightarrow 42$, $21 \rightarrow 36$, $22 \rightarrow 40$, $10 \rightarrow 52$, and $5 \rightarrow 22$. So the random sample is 42, 36, 40, 52, and 22. The sample mean, sample variance, and sample standard deviation rounded to two decimal places for this sample are 38.40, 118.80, and 10.90, respectively.

Although these numbers will vary from sample to sample, they should be comparable to the population parameters. However, thus far we have computed only one sample estimate of the mean, namely, 38.40. We will focus attention on the distribution of the 25 sample means that we generate and the standard deviation and variance for that distribution.

Picking up where we left off in Table 2.1, we obtain for the next sequence of 5 random numbers 10834, 10332, 07534, 79067, and 27126. These correspond to the indices 6, 6, 4, 42, and 15 respectively. Because 10332 led to a repeat of the index 6, we have to reject it and we complete the sample by adding the next number 00858 which corresponds to the index 1.

The second sample now consists of the indices 6, 4, 42, 15, and 1, and these indices correspond to the following homerun totals: 42, 39, 16, 4, and 49. The mean,

TABLE 7.3. Random Number Correspondence to Indices

Index	Interval of Uniform Random Numbers
1	0.00000–0.01886
2	0.01887–0.03773
3	0.03774–0.05659
4	0.05660–0.07545
5	0.07546–0.09431
6	0.09432–0.11317
7	0.11318–0.13203
8	0.13204–0.15089

(continues)

TABLE 7.3. *Continued*

Index	Interval of Uniform Random Numbers
9	0.15090–0.16975
10	0.16976–0.18861
11	0.18861–0.20747
12	0.20748–0.22633
13	0.22634–0.24519
14	0.24520–0.26405
15	0.26406–0.28291
16	0.28292–0.30177
17	0.30178–0.32063
18	0.32064–0.33949
19	0.33950–0.35835
20	0.35836–0.37721
21	0.37722–0.39607
22	0.39608–0.41493
23	0.41494–0.43379
24	0.43380–0.45265
25	0.45266–0.47151
26	0.47152–0.49037
27	0.49038–0.50923
28	0.50924–0.52809
29	0.52810–0.54695
30	0.54696– 0.56581
31	0.56582–0.58467
32	0.58468–0.60353
33	0.60354–0.62239
34	0.62240–0.64125
35	0.64126–0.66011
36	0.66012–0.67897
37	0.67898–0.69783
38	0.69784–0.71669
39	0.71670–0.73555
40	0.73556–0.75441
41	0.75442–0.77327
42	0.77328–0.79213
43	0.79214–0.81099
44	0.81100–0.82985
45	0.82986–0.84871
46	0.84872–0.86757
47	0.86758–0.88643
48	0.88644–0.90529
49	0.90530–0.92415
50	0.92416–0.94301
51	0.94302–0.96187
52	0.96188–0.98073
53	0.98074–0.99999

standard deviation, and variance for this sample are 30.0, 19.09, and 364.50, respectively.

We leave it to the reader to go through the rest of the steps to verify the remaining 23 samples. We will merely list the 25 samples along with their mean values:

1. 42 36 40 52 22   38.40
2. 42 39 16 4 49   30.00
3. 33 52 40 63 17   41.00
4. 8 37 49 40 28   31.80
5. 33 39 56 27 24   35.80
6. 45 48 49 10 66   43.60
7. 15 22 32 22 34   25.00
8. 37 46 56 16 33   37.60
9. 36 9 40 39 4   25.60
10. 42 39 34 17 33   33.00
11. 33 34 49 15 40   34.20
12. 34 52 56 42 24   41.60
13. 22 22 33 34 48   31.80
14. 15 39 22 16 50   28.40
15. 33 40 52 42 40   41.40
16. 40 42 45 49 16   38.40
17. 65 40 42 50 33   46.00
18. 25 37 33 49 8   30.40
19. 32 52 65 39 70   51.60
20. 49 50 39 40 25   40.60
21. 52 48 42 40 49   46.20
22. 42 40 66 33 25   41.20
23. 40 42 10 16 50   31.60
24. 9 46 19 17 34   25.00
25. 9 25 58 33 46   34.20

The average of the 25 estimates of the mean is 36.18, its sample standard deviation is 7.06, and the sample variance is 49.90.

Figure 7.2 shows the histogram for the sample means. We should compare it to the histogram for the original observations. The new histogram that we have drawn appears to be centered at approximately the same point but has a much smaller standard deviation and is more symmetric, just like the histogram for a normal distribution might look.

We note that the range of the averages is from 25 to 51.60, whereas the range of the original observations went from 4 to 70. The observations have a mean of 35.26, a standard deviation of 15.90, and a variance of 252.94, whereas the averages have a mean of 36.18, a standard deviation of 7.06, and a variance of 49.90.

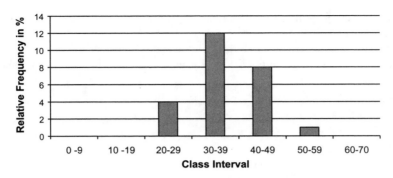

Figure 7.2. Relative frequency histogram for home run sluggers sample distribution for the mean of 25 samples.

We note that the means are close, differing only by 0.92 in absolute magnitude. The standard deviation is reduced by a factor of $15.90/7.06 \approx 2.25$ and the variance is reduced by a factor of $252.94/49.90 \approx 5.07$. This agrees very well with the theory you will learn in the next two sections. Based on that theory, the average has the same mean as the original samples (i.e., it is an unbiased estimate of the population mean), the standard deviation for the mean of 5 samples is the population standard deviation divided by $\sqrt{5} \approx 2.24$, and the variance therefore by the population variance divided by 5.

We compare these values based on comparing the population parameters to the observed samples with the theoretical values 0.92 to 0.00, 2.25 to 2.24, and 5.07 to 5.00. The reason that the results differ slightly from the theory is because we only took 25 random samples and therefore only got 25 averages for the distribution. Had we done 100 or 1000 random samples, the observed results would have been closer to the theoretical results for the distribution of an average of 5 samples.

The histogram in Figure 7.2 does not look as symmetric as a normal distribution because we have a few empty class intervals and the filled ones are too wide. For the original data, we set up 7 class intervals for 53 observations that ranged from 4 to 70. For the means, we only have 25 values but their range is narrower—from 25 to 51.6. So we may as well take 7 class intervals of width 4 going from 24 to 52 as follows (see Figure 7.3):

Greater than or equal to 24 and less than or equal to 28
Greater than 28 and less than or equal to 32
Greater than 32 and less than or equal to 36
Greater than 36 and less than or equal to 40
Greater than 40 and less than or equal to 44
Greater than 44 and less than or equal to 48
Greater than 48 and less than or equal to 52.

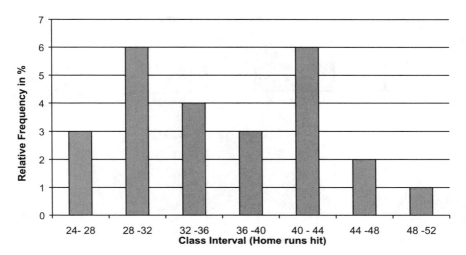

Figure 7.3. Relative frequency histogram for home run sluggers sample distribution for the mean of 25 samples (new class intervals).

This picture is not as close to a normal distribution as the theory suggests. First of all, because we are only averaging 5 samples, the normal approximation will not be as good as if we averaged 20 or 50. Also, the histogram is only based on 25 samples. A much larger number of random samples might be necessary for the histogram to closely approximate the sampling distribution of the mean of 5 sample seasonal home run totals.

7.2   THE CENTRAL LIMIT THEOREM

Section 7.1 illustrated that as we average sample values (regardless of the shape of the distribution for the observations for the parent population), the sample average has a distribution that becomes more and more like the shape of a normal distribution (i.e., symmetric and unimodal) as the sample size increases. Figure 7.4, taken from Kuzma (1998), shows how the distribution of the sample mean changes as the sample size n increases from 1 to 2 to 5 and finally to 30 for a uniform distribution, a bimodal distribution, a skewed distribution, and a symmetric distribution.

In all cases, by the time $n = 30$, the distribution in very symmetric and the variance continually decreases as we noticed for the home run data in the previous section. So, the figure gives you an idea of how the convergence depends on both the sample size n and the shape of the population distribution function.

What we see from the figure is remarkable. Regardless of the shape of the population distribution, the sample averages will have a nearly symmetric distribution approximating the normal distribution in shape as the sample size gets large! This is

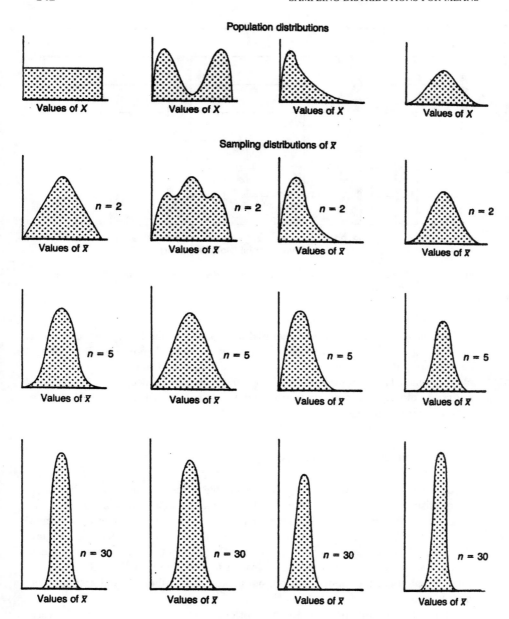

Figure 7.4. The effect of shape of population distribution and sample size on the distribution of means of random samples. (Source: Kuzma, J. W. *Basic Statistics for the Health Sciences.* Mountain View, California: Mayfield Publishing Company, 1984, Figure 7.3, p. 82.)

a surprising result from probability that is called the central limit theorem. Let us now state the results of the central limit theorem formally.

Suppose we have taken a random sample of size n from a population (generally, n needs to be at least 25 for the approximation to be accurate, but sometimes larger samples sizes are needed and occasionally, for symmetric populations, you can do fine with only 5 to 10 samples). We assume the population has a mean μ and a standard deviation σ. We then can assert the following:

1. The distribution of sample means $\overline{X}$ is approximately a normal distribution regardless of the population distribution. If the population distribution is normal, then the distribution for $\overline{X}$ is exactly normal.
2. The mean for the distribution of sample means is equal to the mean of the population distribution (i.e., $\mu_{\overline{X}} = \mu$ where $\mu_{\overline{X}}$ denotes the mean of the distribution of the sample means). This statement signifies that the sample mean is an unbiased estimate of the population mean.
3. The standard deviation of the distribution of sample means is equal to the standard deviation of the population divided by the square root of the sample size [i.e., $\sigma_{\overline{X}} = (\sigma/n)$, where $\sigma_{\overline{X}}$ is the standard deviation of the distribution of sample means based on n observations]. We call $\sigma_{\overline{X}}$ the standard error of the mean.

Property 1 is actually the central limit theorem. Properties 2 and 3 hold for any sample size n when the population has a finite mean and variance.

7.3   STANDARD ERROR OF THE MEAN

The measure of variability of sample means, the standard deviation of the distribution of the sample mean, is called the standard error of the mean (s.e.m.). The s.e.m. is to the distribution of the sample means what the standard deviation is to the population distribution. It has the nice property that it decreases in magnitude as the sample size increases, showing that the sample mean becomes a better and better approximation to the population mean as the sample size increases.

Because of the central limit theorem, we can use the normal distribution approximation to assert that the population mean μ will be within plus or minus two standard errors of the sample mean with a probability of approximately 95%. This is because slightly over 95% of a standard normal distribution lies between ± 2 and the sampling distribution for the mean is centered at μ with a standard deviation equal to one standard error of the mean.

A proof of the central limit theorem is beyond the scope of the course. However, the sampling experiment of Section 7.1 should be convincing to you. If you generate random samples of larger sizes on the computer using an assumed population distribution, you should be able to generate histograms that will have the changing shape illustrated in Figure 7.4 as you increase the sample size.

Suppose we know the population standard deviation σ. Then we can transform the sample mean so that it has an approximate standard normal distribution, as we will show you in the next section.

7.4   *Z* DISTRIBUTION OBTAINED WHEN STANDARD DEVIATION IS KNOWN

Recall that if X has a normal distribution with mean μ and standard deviation σ, then the transformation $Z = (X - \mu)/\sigma$ leads to a random variable Z with a standard normal distribution. We can do the same for the sample mean $\overline{X}$. Assume n is large so that the sample mean has an approximate normal distribution. Now, let us pretend for the moment that the distribution of the sample mean is exactly normal. This is reasonable since it is approximately so. Then define the standard or normal Z score as follows:

$$Z = \frac{\overline{X} - \mu}{\sigma/\sqrt{n}} \tag{7.1}$$

Then Z would have a standard normal distribution because $\overline{X}$ has a normal distribution with mean $\mu_{\overline{X}} = \mu$ and standard deviation $\sigma/\sqrt{n}$.

Because in practice we rarely know σ, we can approximate σ by the sample estimate,

$$S = \sqrt{\frac{\sum_{i=1}^{n}(X_i - \overline{X})^2}{n-1}}$$

For large sample sizes, it is acceptable to use S in place of σ; under these conditions, the standard normal approximation still works. So we use the following formula for the approximate Z score for large sample sizes:

$$Z = \frac{\overline{X} - \mu}{S/\sqrt{n}} \tag{7.2}$$

However, in small samples such as $n < 20$, even if the observations are normally distributed, using Formula 7.2 does not give a good approximation to the normal distribution. In a famous paper under the pen name Student, William S. Gosset found the distribution for the statistic in Formula 7.2 and it is now called the Student's t statistic; the distribution is called the Student's t distribution with $n - 1$ degrees of freedom. This is the subject of the next section.

7.5   STUDENT'S *t* DISTRIBUTION OBTAINED WHEN STANDARD DEVIATION IS UNKNOWN

The Guinness Brewery in Dublin employed an English chemist, William Sealy Gosset, in the early 1900s. Gosset's research involved methods for growing hops in order to improve the taste of beer. His experiments, which generally involved small samples, used statistics to compare hops developed by different procedures.

In his experiments, Gosset used Z statistics similar to the ones we have seen thus far (as in Formula 7.2). However, he found that the distribution of the Z statistic tended to have more extreme negative and positive values than one would expect to see from a standard normal distribution. This excess variation in the sampling distribution was due to the presence of s instead of σ in the denominator. The variability of s, which depended on the sample size n, needed to be accounted for in small samples.

Eventually, Gosset was able to fit a Pearson distribution to observed values of his standardized statistic. The Pearson distributions were a large family of distributions that could have symmetric or asymmetric shapes and have short or long tails. They were developed by Karl Pearson and were known to Gosset and other researchers. Instead of Z, we now use the notation t for the statistic that Gosset developed. It turned out that Gosset had derived empirically the exact distribution for t when the sample observations have exactly a normal distribution. His t distribution provides the appropriate correction to Z in small samples where the normal distribution does not provide an accurate enough approximation to the distribution of the sample mean because the effect of s on the statistic matters.

Ultimately, tables similar to those used for the standard normal distribution were created for the t distribution. Unfortunately, unlike the standard normal, the distribution of t changes as n changes (either increases or decreases).

Figure 7.5 shows how the shape of the t distribution changes as n increases. Three distributions are plotted on the graph, the t with 2 degrees of freedom, the t with 20 degrees of freedom, and the standard normal distribution. The term "degrees of freedom" for a t distribution is a parameter denoted by "*df*" that is equal to $n - 1$ where n is the sample size.

We can see from Figure 7.5 that the t is symmetric about zero but is more spread out than the standard normal distribution. Tables for the t distribution as a function

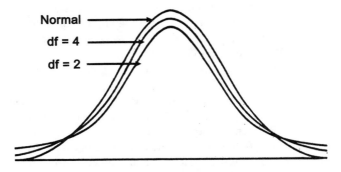

Figure 7.5. Comparison of normal distribution with t distributions of degrees of freedom (*df*) 4 and 2. (Source: Adapted from Kuzma, J. W. *Basic Statistics for the Health Sciences.* Mountain View, California: Mayfield Publishing Company, 1984, Figure 7.4, p. 84.)

of the percentile point of interest and the degrees of freedom are given in Appendix F. Formula 7.3 presents the t statistic.

$$t = \frac{\overline{X} - \mu}{S/\sqrt{n}} \tag{7.3}$$

For $n \leq 30$, use the table of the t distribution with $n - 1$ degrees of freedom. When $n > 30$, there is very little difference between the standard normal distribution and the t distribution.

Let us illustrate the difference between Z and t with a medical example. We consider the blood glucose data from the Honolulu Heart Study (Kuzma, 1998, p. 93, Figure 7.1). The population distribution in this example, a finite population of $N = 7683$ patients, was highly skewed. The population mean and standard deviation were $\mu = 161.52$ and $\sigma = 58.15$, respectively. Suppose we select a random sample of 25 patients from this population; what proportion of the sample would fall below 164.5?

First, let us use Z with μ and σ as given above (assumed to be known). Then $Z = (164.5 - 161.52)/(58.15/\sqrt{25}) = 2.98/11.63 = 0.2562$. Looking in Appendix E at the table for the standard normal distribution, we will use 0.26, since the table carries only two decimal places: $P(Z > 0.26) = 0.5 - P(0 \leq Z \leq 0.26) = 0.5 - 0.1026 = 0.3974$.

Suppose that (1) the mean μ is known to be 161.52, (2) the standard deviation σ is unknown, and (3) we use our sample of 25 to estimate σ. Although the sample estimate is not likely to equal the population value of 58.15, let us assume (for the sake of argument) that it does. When $S = 58.15$, $t = 0.2562$.

Now we must refer to Appendix E to determine the probability for a t with 24 degrees of freedom—$P(t > 0.2562)$. As the table provides $P(t \leq a)$, in order to find $P(t > a)$ we use the relationship that $P(t > a) = 1 - P(t \leq a)$; in our case, $a = 0.2562$. The table tells us that $P(t \leq 0.2562) = 0.60$. So $P(t > 0.2562) = 0.40$. Note that there is not much difference between 0.40 for the t and the value 0.3974 that we obtained using the standard normal distribution. The reason for the similar results obtained for the t and Z distributions is that the degrees of freedom ($df = 24$) are close to 30.

Let us assume that $n = 9$ and repeat the foregoing calculations, this time for the probability of observing an average blood glucose level below 178.75. First, for Z we have $Z = (178.75 - 161.52)/(58.15/\sqrt{9}) = 17.23/(58.15/3) = 17.23/19.383 = 0.889$. Rounding 0.889 to two decimal places, $P(Z < 0.89) = 0.50 + P(0 < Z < 0.89) = 0.50 + 0.3133 = 0.8133$.

If we assume correctly that the standard deviation is estimated from the sample, we should apply the t distribution with 8 degrees of freedom. The calculated t statistic is again 0.889. Referencing Appendix F, we see for a t distribution with 8 degrees of freedom $P(t < 0.889) = 0.80$. The difference between the probabilities obtained by the Z test and t test ($0.8133 - 0.8000$) equals 0.0133, or 1.33%. We see that because the t ($df = 8$) has more area in the upper tail than does the Z distribution, the proportion of the distribution below 0.889 will be smaller than the proportion we obtained for a standard normal distribution.

7.6 ASSUMPTIONS REQUIRED FOR *t* DISTRIBUTION

For the *t* distribution to apply strictly we need the following two assumptions:

1. The observations are selected at random from the population.
2. The population distribution is normal.

Sometimes these assumptions may not be met (particularly the second one). The *t* test is robust for departures from the normal distribution. That means that even when assumption 2 is not satisfied because the population differs from the normal distribution, the probabilities calculated from the *t* table are still approximately correct. This outcome is due to the central limit theorem, which implies that the sample mean will still be approximately normal even if the observations themselves are not.

7.7 EXERCISES

7.1 Define in your own words the following terms:
  a. Central limit theorem
  b. Standard error of the mean
  d. Student's *t* statistic

7.2 Calculate the standard error of the mean for the following sample sizes ($\mu = 100$, $\sigma = 10$). Describe how the standard error of the mean changes as n increases.
  a. $n = 4$
  b. $n = 9$
  c. $n = 16$
  d. $n = 25$
  e. $n = 36$

7.3 The average fasting cholesterol level of an entire community in Michigan is $\mu = 200$ ($\sigma = 20$). A sample ($n = 25$) is selected from this population. Based on the information provided, sketch the sampling distribution of μ.

7.4 The population mean (μ) blood levels of lead of children who live in a city is 11.93 with a standard deviation of 3. For a sample size of 9, what is the probability that a mean blood level will be:
  a. Between 8.93 and 14.93
  b. Below 7.53
  c. Above 16.43

7.5 Repeat Exercise 7.4 with a sample size of 36.

7.6   Based on the findings obtained from Exercises 7.4 and 7.5, what general statement can be made regarding the effect of sample size on the probabilities for the sample means?

7.7   The average height of male physicians employed by a Veterans Affairs medical center is 180.18 cm with a standard deviation of 4.75 cm. Find the probability of obtaining a mean height of 184.93 cm or greater for a sample size of:
   a. 5
   b. 10
   c. 20

7.8   A health researcher collected blood samples from a population of female medical students. The following cholesterol measurements were obtained: $\mu = 211$, $\sigma = 44$. If we select any student at random, what is the probability that her cholesterol value (X) will be:
   a. $P(150 < X < 250)$
   b. $P(X < 140)$
   c. $P(X > 300)$
   What do you need to assume in order to solve this problem?

7.9   Using the data from Exercise 7.8, for a sample of 25 female students, calculate the standard error of the mean, draw the sampling distribution about μ, and find:
   a. $P(200 < \overline{X} < 220)$
   b. $P(\overline{X} < 196)$
   c. $P(\overline{X} > 224)$

7.10 The following questions pertain to the central limit theorem:
   a. Describe the three main consequences of the central limit theorem for the relationship between a sampling distribution and a parent population.
   b. What conditions must be met for the central limit theorem to apply?
   c. Why is the central limit theorem so important to statistical inference?

7.11 Here are some questions about sampling distributions in comparison to the parent populations from which samples are selected:
   a. Describe the difference between the distribution of the observed sample values from a population and the distribution of means calculated from samples of size n.
   b. What is the difference between the population standard deviation and the standard error of the mean?
   c. When would you use the standard error of the mean?
   d. When would you use the population standard deviation?

7.12 The following questions relate to comparisons between the standard normal distribution and the t distribution:

     a. What is the difference between the standard normal distribution (used to determine Z scores) and the t distribution?

     b. When are the values for t and Z almost identical?

     c. Assume that a distribution of data is normally distributed. For a sample size $n = 7$, by using a sample mean, which distribution would you employ (t or Z) to make an inference about a population?

7.13 Based on a sample of six cases, the mean incubation period for a gastrointestinal disease is 26.0 days with a standard deviation of 2.83 days. The population standard deviation (σ) is unknown, but $\mu = 28.0$ days. Assume the data are normally distributed and normalize the sample mean. What is the probability that a sample mean would fall below 24 days based on this normalized statistic t where the actual standard deviation is unknown and the sample estimate must be used.

7.14 Assume that we have normally distributed data. From the standard normal table, find the probability area bounded by ±1 standard deviation units about a population mean and by ±1 standard errors about the mean for any distribution of sample means of a fixed size. How do the areas compare?

7.8   ADDITIONAL READING

1. Kuzma, J. W. (1998). *Basic Statistics for the Health Sciences,* 3rd Edition. Mayfield Publishing Company, Mountain View, California.

2. Kuzma, J. W. and Bohnenblust, S. E. (2001). *Basic Statistics for the Health Sciences,* 4th Edition. Mayfield Publishing Company, Mountain View, California.

3. Salsburg, D. (2001). *The Lady Tasting Tea: How Statistics Revolutionized Science in the Twentieth Century.* W. H. Freeman, New York.

CHAPTER 8

Estimating Population Means

*[Q]uantities which are called errors in one case, may really be
most important and interesting phenomena in another
investigation. When we speak of eliminating error we really
mean disentangling the complicated phenomena of nature.*
—W. J. Jevons, *The Principles of Science,* Chapter 15, p. 339

8.1 ESTIMATION VERSUS HYPOTHESIS TESTING

In this section, we move from descriptive statistics to inferential statistics. In descriptive statistics, we simply summarize information available in the data we are given. In inferential statistics, we draw conclusions about a population based on a sample and a known or assumed sampling distribution. Implicit in statistical inference is the assumption that the data were gathered as a random sample from a population.

Examples of the types of inferences that can be made are estimation, conclusions from hypothesis tests, and predictions of future observations. In estimation, we are interested in choosing the "best" estimate of a population parameter based on the sample and statistical theory.

For example, as we saw in Chapter 7, when data are sampled from a normal distribution, the sample mean has a normal distribution that is on average equal to the population mean with a variance equal to the population variance divided by the sample size n. Recall that the distribution of a statistic such as a sample mean is called a sampling distribution. The Gauss–Markov theory goes on to determine that the sample mean is the best estimate of the population mean. That means that for a sample of size n it gives us the most accurate answer (e.g., has properties such as smallest mean square error and minimum variance among unbiased estimators).

The sample mean is a point estimate, but we know it has a sampling distribution. Hence, the sample mean will not be exactly equal to the population mean. However, the theory we have tells us about its sampling distribution; thus, statistical theory can aid us in describing our uncertainty about the population mean based on our knowledge of the sampling distribution for the sample mean.

In Section 8.2, we will further discuss point estimates and in Section 8.3 we will

Introductory Biostatistics for the Health Sciences, by Michael R. Chernick
and Robert H. Friis. ISBN 0-471-41137-X. Copyright © 2003 Wiley-Interscience.

discuss confidence intervals. Confidence intervals are merely interval estimates (based on the observed data) of population parameters that express a range of values that are likely to contain the parameter. We will describe how the sampling distribution of the point estimate is used to get confidence intervals in Section 8.3.

In hypothesis testing, we construct a null and an alternative hypothesis. Usually, the null hypothesis is an uninteresting hypothesis that we would like to reject. You will see examples in Chapter 9. The alternative hypothesis is generally the interesting scientific hypothesis that we would like to "prove." However, we do not actually "prove" the alternative hypothesis; we merely reject the null hypothesis and retain a degree of uncertainty about its status.

Due to statistical uncertainty, one can never absolutely prove a hypothesis based on a sample. We will draw conclusions based on our sample data and associate an error probability with our possible conclusion. When our conclusion favors the null hypothesis, we prefer to say that we fail to reject the null hypothesis rather than that we accept the null hypothesis.

In setting up the hypothesis test, we will determine a critical value in advance of looking at the data. This critical value is selected to control the type I error (i.e., the probability of falsely rejecting the null hypothesis). This is the so-called Neyman–Pearson formulation that we will describe in Section 9.2.

In Section 9.9, we will describe a relationship between confidence intervals and hypothesis tests that enables one to construct a hypothesis test from a confidence interval or a confidence interval from a hypothesis test. Usually, hypothesis tests are constructed based directly on the sampling distribution of the point estimate. However, in Chapter 9 we will introduce the simplest form of bootstrap hypothesis testing. This test is based on a bootstrap percentile method confidence interval that we will introduce in Section 8.8.

8.2   POINT ESTIMATES

In Chapter 4, you learned about summary statistics. We discussed population parameters for central tendency (e.g., the mean, median and the mode) and for dispersion (e.g., the range, variance, mean absolute deviation, and standard deviation). We also presented formulas for sample analogs based on data from random samples taken from the population. These sample analogs are often also used as point estimates of the population parameters. A point estimate is a single value that is chosen as an estimate for a population parameter.

Often the estimates are obvious, such as with the use of the sample mean to estimate the population mean. However, sometimes we can select from two or more possible estimates. Then the question becomes which point estimate should you use?

Statistical theory offers us properties to compare point estimates. One important property is consistency. The property of consistency requires that as the sample size becomes large, the estimate will tend to approximate more closely the population parameter.

For example, we saw that the sampling distribution of the sample mean was centered at the true population mean; its distribution approached the normal distribution as the sample size grew large. Also, its variance tended to decrease by a factor of $1/\sqrt{n}$ as the sample size n increased. The sampling distribution was concentrated closer and closer to the population mean as n increased.

The facts stated in the foregoing paragraph are sufficient to demonstrate consistency of the sample mean. Other point estimates, such as the sample standard deviation, the sample variance, and the sample median, are also consistent estimates of their respective population parameters.

In addition to consistency, another property of point estimates is unbiasedness. This property requires the sample estimate to have a sampling distribution whose mean is equal to the population parameter (regardless of the sample size n). The sample mean has this property and, therefore, is unbiased. The sample variance (the estimate obtained by dividing by $n - 1$) is also unbiased, but the sample standard deviation is not.

To review:

$E\overline{X} = \mu$ (The sample mean is an unbiased estimate of the population mean.)

$E(S^2) = \sigma^2$ where $S^2 = \Sigma_{i=1}^{n} (X_i - \overline{X})^2/(n - 1)$ (The sample variance is an unbiased estimate of the population variance.)

$E(S) \neq \sigma$ (The sample standard deviation is a biased estimate of the population standard deviation.)

Similarly $S/\sqrt{n}$ is the usual estimate of the standard error of the mean, namely, $\sigma/\sqrt{n}$. However, since $E(S) \neq \sigma$ it also follows that $E(S/\sqrt{n}) \neq \sigma/\sqrt{n}$. So our estimate of the standard error of the mean is also biased. These results are summarized in Display 8.1.

If we have several estimates that are unbiased, then the best estimate to choose is the one with the smallest variance for its sampling distribution. That estimate would be the most accurate. Biased estimates are not necessarily bad in all circumstances. Sometimes, the bias is small and decreases as the sample size increases. This situation is the case for the sample standard deviation.

An estimate with a small bias and a small variance can be better than an estimate with no bias (i.e., an unbiased estimate) that has a large variance. When comparing

---

Display 8.1.   Bias Properties of Some Common Estimates

$E(X) = \mu$—The sample mean is an unbiased estimator of the population mean.

$E(S^2) = \sigma^2$—The sample variance is an unbiased estimator of the population variance.

$E(S) \neq \sigma$—The sample standard deviation is a biased estimator of the population standard deviation.

a biased estimator to an unbiased estimator, we should consider the accuracy that can be measured by the mean-square error.

The mean-square error is defined as $MSE = \beta^2 + \sigma^2$, where β is the bias of the estimator and σ^2 is the variance of the estimator. An unbiased estimator has $MSE = \sigma^2$.

Here we will show an example in which a biased estimator is better than an unbiased estimator because the former has a smaller mean square error than the latter. Suppose that A and B are two estimates of a population parameter. A is unbiased and has $MSE = \sigma_A^2$. We use the subscript A to denote that σ_A^2 is the variance for estimator A. B is a biased estimate and has $MSE = \beta_B^2 + \sigma_B^2$. Here we use B as the subscript for the bias and β_B^2 to denote the variance for estimator B. Now if $\beta_B^2 + \sigma_B^2 < \sigma_A^2$, then B is a better estimate of the population parameter than A. This situation happens if $\sigma_B^2 < \sigma_A^2 - \beta_B^2$. To illustrate this numerically, suppose A is an unbiased estimator for a parameter θ and A has a variance of 50. Now B is a biased estimate of θ with a bias of 4 and a variance of 25. Then A has a mean square error of 50 but B has a mean square error of $16 + 25 = 41$. (B's variance is 25 and the square of the bias is 16.) Because 41 is less than 50, B is a better estimate of θ (i.e., it has a lower mean square error).

As another example, suppose A is an unbiased estimate for θ with variance 36 and B is a biased estimate with variance 30 but bias 4. Which is the better estimate? Surprisingly, it is A. Even though B has a smaller variance than A, B tends to be farther away from θ than A. In this case, B is more precise but misses the target, whereas A is a little less precise but is centered at the target. Numerically, the mean square error for A is 36 and for B it is $30 + (4)^2 = 30 + 16 = 46$. Here, a biased estimate with a lower variance than an unbiased estimate was less accurate than the unbiased estimator because it had a higher mean square error. So we need the mean square error and not just the variance to determine the better estimate when comparing unbiased and biased estimates. (See Figure 8.1.)

In conclusion, precise estimates with large bias are never desirable, but precise estimates with small bias can be good. Unbiased estimates that are precise are good, but imprecise unbiased estimates are bad. The trade-off between accuracy and precision is well expressed in one quantity: the mean square error.

8.3 CONFIDENCE INTERVALS

Point estimates can be used to obtain our best determination of a single value that operates as a parameter. However, point estimates by themselves do not express the uncertainty in the estimate (i.e., the variability in its sampling distribution). However, under certain statistical assumptions the sampling distribution of the estimate can be determined (e.g., for the sample mean when the population distribution is normal with known variance). In other circumstances, the sampling distribution can be approximated (e.g., for the sample mean under the assumptions needed for the central limit theorem to hold along with the standard deviation estimated from a sample). This information enables us to quantify the uncertainty in a confidence in-

Unbiased and Accurate

Unbiased and Inaccurate

Biased and Accurate

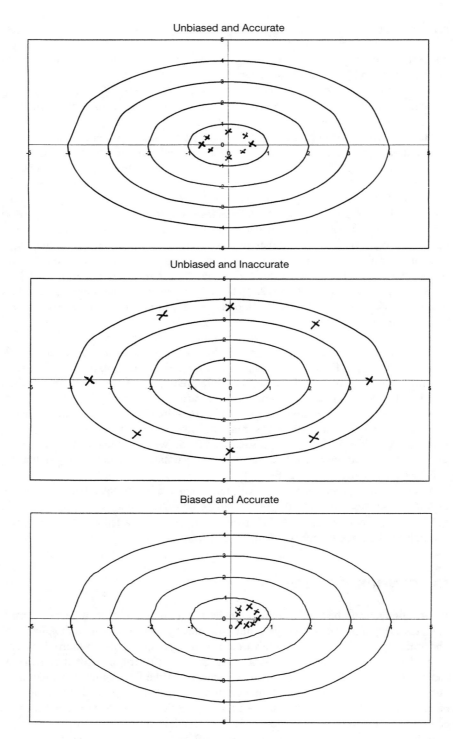

Figure 8.1.

terval. Confidence intervals express the probability that a prescribed interval will contain the true parameter.

8.4 CONFIDENCE INTERVALS FOR A SINGLE POPULATION MEAN

To understand how confidence intervals work, we will first illustrate them by the simplest case, in which the observations have a normal distribution with a known variance σ^2 and we want to estimate the population mean, μ. Then we know that the sample mean is $\overline{X}$ and its sampling distribution has mean equal to the population mean μ and a variance σ^2/n, where n is the number of samples. Thus, $Z = (\overline{X} - \mu)/(\sigma/\sqrt{n})$ has a standard normal distribution. We can therefore state that $P(-1.96 \leq Z \leq 1.96) = 0.95$ based on the standard normal distribution. Substituting $(\overline{X} - \mu)/(\sigma/\sqrt{n})$ for Z we obtain $P(-1.96 \leq (\overline{X} - \mu)/(\sigma/\sqrt{n}) \leq 1.96) = 0.95$ or $P(-1.96\sigma/\sqrt{n} \leq (\overline{X} - \mu) \leq 1.96\sigma/\sqrt{n}) = 0.95$ or $P(-1.96(\sigma/\sqrt{n}) - \overline{X} \leq -\mu \leq 1.96(\sigma/\sqrt{n}) - \overline{X}) = 0.95$. Multiplying throughout by -1 and reversing the inequality, we find that $P(1.96(\sigma/\sqrt{n}) + \overline{X} \geq \mu \geq -1.96(\sigma/\sqrt{n}) + \overline{X}) = 0.95$. Rearranging the foregoing formula, we have $P(\overline{X} - 1.96\sigma/\sqrt{n} \leq \mu \leq \overline{X} + 1.96\sigma/\sqrt{n}) = 0.95$. The confidence interval is an interpretation of this probability statement. The confidence interval $[\overline{X} - 1.96\sigma/\sqrt{n}, \overline{X} + 1.96\sigma/\sqrt{n}]$ is a random interval determined by the sample value of $\overline{X}$, σ, n, and the confidence level (e.g., 95%). $\overline{X}$ is the component to this interval that makes it random. (See Display 8.2.)

The probability statement $P[\overline{X} - 1.96(\sigma/\sqrt{n}) \leq \mu \leq \overline{X} + 1.96(\sigma/\sqrt{n})] = 0.95$ says only that the probability that this random interval includes the population mean is 0.95. This probability pertains to the procedure for generating random confidence intervals. It does not say what will happen to the parameter on any particular outcome. If, for example, σ is 5 and $n = 25$ and we obtain from a sample a sample mean of 5.96, then the outcome for the random interval is $[5.96 - 1.96, 5.96 + 1.96] = [4.00, 7.92]$. The population mean will either be inside or outside the interval. If the mean $\mu = 7$, then it is contained in the interval. On the other hand, if $\mu = 8$, μ is not contained in the interval.

We *cannot* say that the probability is 0.95 that the single fixed interval [4.00, 7.92] contains μ. It either does or it does not. Instead, we say that we have 95% confidence that such an interval would include (or cover) μ. This means that the process will tend to include the true value of the parameter 95% of the time if we

---

**Display 8.2. A 95% Confidence Interval for a Population
Mean μ When the Population Variance σ^2 is Known**

The confidence interval is formed by the following equation:

$$[\overline{X} - 1.96\sigma/\sqrt{n}, \overline{X} + 1.96\sigma/\sqrt{n}]$$

where n is the sample size.

were to repeat the process many times. That is to say, if we generated 100 samples
of size 25 and for each sample we generated the confidence interval as described
above, approximately 95 of the intervals would include μ and the remaining ones
would not. (See Figure 8.2.)

Why did we choose 95%? There is no strong reason. The probability 0.95 is high
and indicates we have high confidence that the interval will include the true parameter. However, in some situations we may feel comfortable only with a higher
confidence level such as 99%. Let "C" denote the Z value associated with a particular level of confidence that corresponds to a particular section of the normal curve.
To obtain a 99% confidence interval, we just go to the table of the standard normal
distribution to find the value C such that $P(-C \leq Z \leq C) = 0.99$. We find that $C =$
2.576. This leads to the interval $[\overline{X} - 2.576\sigma/\sqrt{n}, \overline{X} + 2.576\sigma/\sqrt{n}]$. In the example

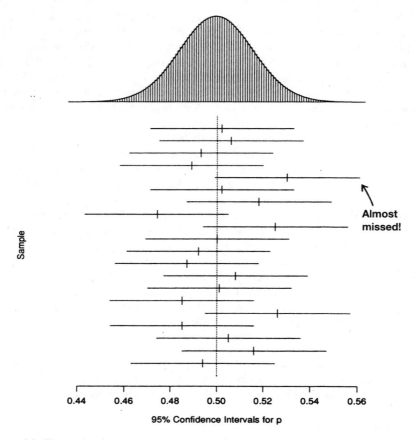

Figure 8.2. The results of a computer simulation of 20 samples of size $n = 1000$. We assumed that the
true value of $p = 0.5$. At the top is the sampling distribution of $\hat{p}$ [normal, with mean p and $\sigma =$
$\sqrt{p(1-p)/n}$]. Below are the 95% confidence intervals from each sample. On average, one out of 20 (or
5%) of these intervals will not cover the point $p = 0.5$.

above where the sample mean is 5.96, σ is 5, and $n = 25$, the resulting interval would be [5.96 − 2.576(5)/$\sqrt{25}$, 5.96 + 2.576(5)/$\sqrt{25}$] = [3.384, 8.536]. Compare this to the 95% interval [4.00, 7.92].

Notice that for the same standard deviation and sample size, increasing the confidence level increases the length of the interval and also increases the chance that such intervals generated by this prescription would contain the parameter μ. Note that in this case, if $\mu = 8$, the 95% interval would not have contained μ but the 99% interval would. This example could have been one of the 5% of cases where a 95% confidence interval does not contain the mean but the 99% interval does. The 99% interval has to be wider because it has to capture the true mean in 4/5ths of the cases where the 99% confidence interval does not. That is why the 95% interval is contained within the 99% interval.

We pay a price for the higher confidence in a much wider interval. For example, by establishing an extremely wide confidence interval, we are increasingly certain that it contains μ. Thus, for example, we could say with extremely high confidence that the confidence interval for the mean age of the U.S. population is between 0 and 120 years. However, this interval would not be helpful, as we would like to have a more precise estimate of μ.

If we were willing to accept a lower confidence level such as 90%, we would obtain a value of 1.645 for C, where $P(-C \le Z \le C) = 0.90$. In that case, for the example we are considering the interval would be [5.96 − 1.645, 5.96 + 1.645] = [4.315, 7.505]. This is a much tighter interval that is contained within the 95% interval. Here we gain a tighter interval at the price of lower confidence.

Another important point to note is the gain in precision of the estimate with increase in sample size. This point can be illustrated by the narrowing of the width of the confidence interval. Let us consider the 95% confidence interval for the mean that we obtained with a sample of size 25 and an estimated mean of 5.96. Suppose we increase the sample size to 100 (a factor of 4 increase) and assume that we still get a sample mean of 5.96. The 95% interval (assuming the population standard deviation is known to be 5) is then [5.96 − 1.96 (5/$\sqrt{100}$), 5.96 + 1.96 (5/$\sqrt{100}$)] = [5.96 − 0.98, 5.96 + 0.98] = [4.98, 6.94].

This interval is much narrower and is contained inside the previous one. The interval width is 6.94 − 4.98 = 1.96 as compared to 7.92 − 4.00 = 3.92. Notice this interval is exactly half the width of the other interval. That is, if the confidence level is left unchanged and the sample size n is increased by a factor of 4, $\sqrt{n}$ is increased by a factor of 2; because the interval width is 2(1.96)/$\sqrt{n}$, the interval width is reduced by a factor of 2. Exhibit 8.1 summarizes the critical values of the standard normal distribution for calculating confidence intervals at various levels of confidence.

If the population standard deviation is unknown and we want to estimate the mean, we must use the t distribution instead of the normal distribution. So we calculate the sample standard deviation S and construct the t score $(\overline{X} - \mu)/(S/\sqrt{n})$. Recall that this quantity has Student's t distribution with $n - 1$ degrees of freedom. Note that this distribution does not depend on the unknown parameters μ and σ, but it does depend on the sample size n through the degrees of freedom. This dif-

---

**Exhibit 8.1.   Two-Sided Critical Values of the
Standard Normal Distribution**

For standard normal distributions, we have the following critical points for two-sided confidence intervals:

$$C_{0.90} = 1.645 \qquad C_{0.95} = 1.960 \qquad C_{0.99} = 2.576$$

---

fers from the standard normal distribution that does not depend on the sample size n.

For a 95% confidence interval, we need to determine C so that $P(-C \le t \le C) = 0.95$. For $n = 25$, again assume that the sample mean is 5.96, the sample standard deviation is 5, and $n = 25$. Then the degrees of freedom are 24, and from the table for the t distribution we see that $C = 2.064$. The statement $P(-C \le t \le C) = 0.95$ is equivalent to $P[\overline{X} - C(S/\sqrt{n}) \le \mu \le \overline{X} + C(S/\sqrt{n})] = 0.95$. So the interval is $[\overline{X} - C(S/\sqrt{n}), \overline{X} + C(S/\sqrt{n})]$. Using $C = 2.064$, $S = 5$, $n = 25$, and a sample mean of 5.96, we find [5.96 − 2.064, 5.96 + 2.064] or [3.896, 8.024]. Display 8.3 summarizes the procedure for calculating a 95% confidence interval for a population mean when the population variance is unknown.

You should note that the interval is wider than in the case in which we knew the variance and used the normal distribution. This result occurs because there is extra variability in the t statistic due to the fact that the random quantity s is used in place of a fixed quantity σ. Remember that the t with 24 degrees of freedom has heavier tails than the standard normal distribution; this fact is reflected in the quantity $C = 2.064$ in place of $C = 1.96$ for the standard normal distribution.

Suppose we obtained the same estimates for the sample mean $\overline{X}$ and the sample standard deviation S but the sample size was increased to 100; the interval width again would decrease by a factor of 2, because the width of the interval is $2C(S/\sqrt{n})$ and only n is changing.

**Display 8.3.   A 95% Confidence Interval for a Population
Mean μ When the Population Variance is Unknown**

The confidence interval is given by the formula

$$\left[\overline{X} - C\frac{S}{\sqrt{n}} \le \mu \le \overline{X} + C\frac{S}{\sqrt{n}} \right]$$

where n is the sample size, C is the 97.5 percentile of Student's t distribution with $n - 1$ degrees of freedom, and s is the sample standard deviation.

8.5   *Z* AND *t* STATISTICS FOR TWO INDEPENDENT SAMPLES

Now consider a situation in which we compare the difference between means of samples selected from two populations. In a clinical trial, we could be comparing the mean of a variable (commonly referred to as an endpoint) for a control group to the corresponding mean for a treatment group.

First assume that both groups have normally distributed observations with known and possibly different variances σ_t and σ_c for the treatment and control groups, respectively. Assume that the sample size for the treatment group is n_t and for the control group is n_c. Also assume that the means are μ_t and μ_c for the treatment and control groups, respectively.

Let us select two samples independently from the two groups (treatment and control) and compute the means of the samples. We denote the means of the samples from the control and treatment groups, $\overline{X}_t$ and $\overline{X}_c$, respectively. The difference between the sample means $\overline{X}_t - \overline{X}_c$ comes from a normal distribution with mean $\mu_t - \mu_c$, variance $(\sigma_t^2/n_t) + (\sigma_c^2/n_c)$, and standard error for $\overline{X}_t - \overline{X}_c$ equal to $\sqrt{(\sigma_t^2/n_t) + (\sigma_c^2/n_c)}$. The *Z* transformation of $\overline{X}_t - \overline{X}_c$ is defined as

$$Z = \frac{(\overline{X}_t - \overline{X}_c) - (\mu_t - \mu_c)}{\sqrt{\left(\dfrac{\sigma_t^2}{n_t} + \dfrac{\sigma_c^2}{n_c} \right)}}$$

which has a standard normal distribution. Here is an interesting statistical observation: Even though we are finding the difference between two sample means, the variance of the distribution of their differences is equal to the sum of the two squared standard errors associated with each of the individual sample means. The standard errors of the treatment and control groups are calculated by dividing the population variance of each group by the respective sample size of each independently selected sample.

As demonstrated in Section 8.6, the *Z* transformation, which employs the addition of the error variances of the two means, enables us to obtain confidence intervals for the difference between the means. In the special case where we can assume that $\sigma_t^2 = \sigma_c^2 = \sigma^2$, the *Z* formula reduces to

$$Z = \frac{(\overline{X}_t - \overline{X}_c) - (\mu_t - \mu_c)}{\sigma\sqrt{(1/n_t) + (1/n_c)}}$$

The term σ^2 is referred to as the common variance. Since $P\{[-1.96 \leq Z \leq 1.96] = 0.95$, we find after algebraic manipulation that $[(\overline{X}_t - \overline{X}_c) - 1.96\{\sigma\sqrt{\{(1/n_t) + (1/n_c)\}}, (\overline{X}_t - \overline{X}_c)\} + 1.96\{\sigma\sqrt{\{(1/n_t) + (1/n_c)\}}\}]$ is a 95% confidence interval for $\mu_t - \mu_c$.

In practice, the population variances of the treatment and control groups are unknown; if the two variances can be assumed to be equal, we can calculate an estimate of the common variance σ^2, called the pooled estimate. Let S_t^2 and S_c^2 be the sample estimates of the variance for the treatment and control groups, respectively. The pooled variance estimate S_p^2 is then given by the formula

$$S_p^2 = \frac{S_t^2(n_t - 1) + S_c^2(n_c - 1)}{[n_t + n_c - 2]}$$

The corresponding t statistic is

$$t = \frac{(\overline{X}_t - \overline{X}_c) - (\mu_t - \mu_c)}{S_p \sqrt{(1/n_t) + (1/n_c)}}$$

This formula is obtained by replacing the common σ in the formula above for Z with the pooled estimate S_p. The resulting statistic has Student's t distribution with $n_t + n_c - 2$ degrees of freedom. We will use this formula in Section 8.7 to obtain a confidence interval for the mean difference based on this t statistic when the population variances can be assumed to be equal.

Although not covered in this text, the hypothesis of equal variances can be tested by an F test similar to the F tests that are used in the analysis of variance (discussed in Chapter 13). If the F test indicates that the variances are different, then one should use a statistic based on the assumption of unequal variances.

This problem with unequal and unknown variances is called the Behrens–Fisher problem. Let "k" denote the test statistic that is commonly used in the Behrens–Fisher problem. The test statistic k does not have a t distribution, but it can be approximated by a t distribution with a degrees of freedom parameter that is not necessarily an integer. The statistic k is obtained by replacing the Z statistic in the unequal variance case as given below:

$$Z = \frac{(\overline{X}_t - \overline{X}_c) - (\mu_t - \mu_c)}{\sqrt{(\sigma_t^2/n_t) + (\sigma_c^2/n_c)}}$$

with

$$k = \frac{(\overline{X}_t - \overline{X}_c) - (\mu_t - \mu_c)}{\sqrt{(S_t^2/n_t) + (S_c^2/n_c)}}$$

where S_t^2 and S_c^2 are the sample estimates of variance for the treatment and control groups, respectively.

We use a t distribution with ν degrees of freedom to approximate the distribution of k. The degrees of freedom ν are

$$\nu = \frac{\{(S_t^2/n_t) + (S_c^2/n_c)\}^2}{[1/(n_c - 1)](S_c^2/n_c)^2 + [1/(n_t - 1)](S_t^2/n_t)^2}$$

This is the formula we use for confidence intervals in Section 8.7 when the variances are assumed to be unequal and also for hypothesis testing under the same assumptions (not covered in the text).

8.6 CONFIDENCE INTERVALS FOR THE DIFFERENCE BETWEEN MEANS FROM TWO INDEPENDENT SAMPLES (VARIANCES KNOWN)

When the population variances are known, we use the Z statistic defined in the previous section, namely

$$Z = \frac{(\overline{X}_t - \overline{X}_c) - (\mu_t - \mu_c)}{\sqrt{(\sigma_t^2/n_t) + (\sigma_c^2/n_c)}}$$

Z has exactly a standard normal distribution when the observations in both samples are normally distributed. Also, based on the central limit theorem, Z is approximately normal if conditions for the central limit theorem are satisfied for each population being sampled. For a 95% confidence interval we know that $P(-C \le Z \le C) = 0.95$ if $C = 1.96$. So $P(-1.96 \le \{(\overline{X}_t - \overline{X}_c) - (\mu_t - \mu_c)\}/\sqrt{(\sigma_t^2/n_t) + (\sigma_c^2/n_c)} \le 1.96)$. After some algebra we find that $P[(\overline{X}_t - \overline{X}_c) - 1.96\sqrt{(\sigma_t^2/n_t) + (\sigma_c^2/n_c)} \le (\mu_t - \mu_c) \le (\overline{X}_t - \overline{X}_c) + 1.96\sqrt{(\sigma_t^2/n_t) + (\sigma_c^2/n_c)}]$. The 95% confidence interval is $[(\overline{X}_t - \overline{X}_c) - 1.96\sqrt{(\sigma_t^2/n_t) + (\sigma_c^2/n_c)}, (\overline{X}_t - \overline{X}_c) + 1.96\sqrt{(\sigma_t^2/n_t) + (\sigma_c^2/n_c)}]$. If $\sigma^2 = \sigma_t^2 = \sigma_c^2$, then the formula for the interval reduces to $[(\overline{X}_t - \overline{X}_c) - 1.96\,\sigma\sqrt{(1/n_t) + (1/n_c)}, (\overline{X}_t - \overline{X}_c) + 1.96\,\sigma\sqrt{(1/n_t) + (1/n_c)}]$. If, in addition, $n = n_t = n_c$, then the formula becomes $[(\overline{X}_t - \overline{X}_c) - 1.96\,\sigma\sqrt{(2/n)}, (\overline{X}_t - \overline{X}_c) + 1.96\,\sigma\sqrt{(2/n)}]$. For other confidence levels, we just change the constant C to 1.645 for 90% or 2.575 for 99%. Display 8.4 provides the formula for the 95% confidence interval for the difference between two population means, assuming common known population variance.

8.7 CONFIDENCE INTERVALS FOR THE DIFFERENCE BETWEEN MEANS FROM TWO INDEPENDENT SAMPLES (POPULATION VARIANCE UNKNOWN)

In the case when the variances of the parent populations from which the samples are selected are unknown, we use the t statistic with the pooled variance formula from Section 8.5 assuming normal distributions and equal variances. When the variances are assumed to be unequal and the distributions normal, we use the k statistic from Section 8.5 with the individual sample variances. When using k, we apply the Welch–Aspin t approximation with ν degrees of freedom where ν is defined as in Section 8.5.

In the first case the 95% confidence interval is $[(\overline{X}_t - \overline{X}_c) - CS_p\sqrt{(1/n_t) + (1/n_c)}, (\overline{X}_t - \overline{X}_c) + CS_p\sqrt{(1/n_t) + (1/n_c)}]$, where S_p is the pooled estimate of the standard deviation and C is the appropriate constant such that $P(-C \le t \le C) = 0.95$ when t has a Student's t distribution with $n_t + n_c - 2$ degrees of freedom. The formula for the 95% confidence interval for the difference between two population means assuming unknown and common population variances is given in Display 8.5.

Now recall that $S_p^2 = \{S_t^2(n_t - 1) + S_c^2(n_c - 1)/[n_t + n_c - 2]\}$; $S_p^2 = \{(115)^2(8) + (125)^2(15)\}/(9 + 16{-}2) = \{13225(8) + 15625\,(15)\}/23 = \{105800 + 2343750/23\} = 340175/23 = 14790.22$. S_p is the square root of $14790.22 = 121.62$. So the interval is

Display 8.4. 95% Confidence Interval For the Difference Between Two Population Means (Common Population Variance Known)

$$[(\overline{X}_t - \overline{X}_c) - 1.96\sigma\sqrt{(1/n_t) + (1/n_c)}, (\overline{X}_t - \overline{X}_c) + 1.96\sigma\sqrt{(1/n_t) + (1/n_c)}]$$

where:

n_t is the sample size for the treatment group

n_c is the sample size for the control group

σ is the common variance for the two populations

Example:

$\overline{X}_t$	$\overline{X}_c$
311.9	212.4
n_t	n_c
9	16

$\sigma = 120$ for both populations.

$$311.9 - 212.4 \pm 1.96(120)\sqrt{\frac{1}{9} + \frac{1}{16}} = 99.5 \pm 1.96(120)\sqrt{0.111 + 0.0625}$$

$$= 99.5 \pm 1.96(120)\sqrt{0.1736}$$

$$= 99.5 \pm 1.96(120)(0.4167)$$

$$99.5 \pm 1.96(50.00): \text{limits } 1.5 \leftrightarrow 197.5$$

as follows: $[(\overline{X}_t - \overline{X}_c) - C\{S_p\sqrt{(1/n_t) + (1/n_c)}\}. (\overline{X}_t - \overline{X}_c) + C\{S_p\sqrt{(1/n_t) + (1/n_c)}\}] = [99.5 - C\{121.62\sqrt{(1/9) + (1/16)}\}, 99.5 + C\{121.62\sqrt{(1/9) + (1/16)}\}]$. From the t table we see that $C = 2.0687$ since the degrees of freedom are 23. Using this value for C we get the following:

$$[99.5 - 2.0687\{121.62\sqrt{(1/9) + (1/16)}\}, 99.5 + 2.0687\{121.62\sqrt{(1/9) + (1/16)}\}]$$

$$= [99.5 - 249.53(0.1736, 99.5 + 249.53(0.1736] =$$

$$= [99.5 - 249.53(0.4167), 99.5 + 249.53(0.4167)] =$$

$$= [99.5 - 103.98, 99.5 + 103.98] = [-4.48, 203.48]$$

In the second case, the 95% confidence interval is $[(\overline{X}_t - \overline{X}_c) - C\sqrt{(S_t^2/n_t) + (S_c^2/n_c)}, (\overline{X}_t - \overline{X}_c) + C\sqrt{(S_t^2/n_t) + (S_c^2/n_c)}]$, where S_t^2 is the sample estimate of variance for the treatment group and S_c^2 is the sample estimate of variance for the control group. The quantity C is calculated such that $P(-C \leq k \leq C) = 0.95$ when k has Student's t distribution with ν degrees of freedom. Refer to Display 8.6 for the formula for a 95% confidence interval for a difference between two population means, assuming different unknown population variances.

Display 8.5.   95% Confidence Interval For the Difference Between Two Population Means (Common Population Variance Unknown)

$$[(\overline{X}_t - \overline{X}_c) - C\{S_p\sqrt{(1/n_t) + (1/n_c)}\}, (\overline{X}_t - \overline{X}_c) + C\{S_p\sqrt{(1/n_t) + (1/n_c)}\}]$$

where:
n_t is the sample size for the treatment group
n_c is the sample size for the control group
C is the 97.5 percentile of the t distribution with $n_t + n_c - 2$ degrees of freedom
S_p is the pooled estimate of the common variance for the two populations

Example:

$\overline{X}_t$	$\overline{X}_c$
311.9	212.4
n_t	n_c
9	16
s_t	s_c
115	125

Let us consider an example from the pharmaceutical industry. A company is interested in marketing a clotting agent that reduces blood loss when an accident causes an internal injury such as liver trauma. To study possible doses of the agent and obtain some indication of safety and efficacy, the company conducts an experiment in which a controlled liver injury is induced in pigs and blood loss is measured. Pigs are randomized as to whether they receive the drug after the injury or do not receive drug therapy—the treatment and control groups, respectively.

The following data were taken from a study in which there were 10 pigs in the treatment group and 10 in the control group. The blood loss was measured in milliliters and is given in Table 8.1.

When the variances are known, we use the Z statistic defined in the previous section, namely

$$Z = \frac{\{(\overline{X}_t - \overline{X}_c) - (\mu_t - \mu_c)\}}{\sqrt{(\sigma_t^2/n_t) + (\sigma_c^2/n_c)}}$$

Z has exactly the standard normal distribution when the observations in both samples are normally distributed. Also, based on the central limit theorem, Z is approximately normal if conditions for the central limit theorem are satisfied for each population being sampled. So for a 95% confidence interval we know that $P(-C \le Z \le C) = 0.95$ if $C = 1.96$. So $P(-1.96 \le \{(\overline{X}_t - \overline{X}_c) - (\mu_t - \mu_c)\}/\sqrt{(\sigma_t^2/n_t) + (\sigma_c^2/n_c)} \le 1.96)$. After some algebra we find that $P[(\overline{X}_t - \overline{X}_c) - 1.96\sqrt{(\sigma_t^2/n_t) + (\sigma_c^2/n_c)} \le (\mu_t - \mu_c) \le (\overline{X}_t - \overline{X}_c) + 1.96\sqrt{(\sigma_t^2/n_t) + (\sigma_c^2/n_c)}]$. So the 95% confidence interval is

TABLE 8.1. Pig Blood Loss Data (ml)

Control Group Pigs	Treatment Group Pigs
786	543
375	666
4446	455
2886	823
478	1716
587	797
434	2828
4764	1251
3281	702
3837	1078
Sample mean = 2187.40	Sample mean = 1085.90
Sample standard deviation = 1824.27	Sample standard deviation = 717.12

$[(\overline{X}_t - \overline{X}_c) - 1.96\sqrt{(\sigma_t^2/n_t) + (\sigma_c^2/n_c)}, (\overline{X}_t - \overline{X}_c) + 1.96\sqrt{(\sigma_t^2/n_t) + (\sigma_c^2/n_c)}]$. If $\sigma^2 = \sigma_t^2$ $= \sigma_c^2$, then the formula for the interval reduces to $[(\overline{X}_t - \overline{X}_c) - 1.96\,\sigma\sqrt{(1/n_t) + (1/n_c)}$, $(\overline{X}_t - \overline{X}_c) + 1.96\,\sigma\sqrt{(1/n_t) + (1/n_c)}]$. If, in addition, $n = n_t = n_c$, then the formula becomes $[(\overline{X}_t - \overline{X}_c) - 1.96\,\sigma(2/n), (\overline{X}_t - \overline{X}_c) + 1.96\,\sigma\sqrt{(2/n)}]$. For other confidence levels we just change the constant C to 1.645 for 90% or 2.575 for 99%.

For these data, we note a large difference between the sample standard deviations: 717.12 for the treatment group versus 1824.27 for the control group. This result is not compatible with the assumption of equal variance. We will make the assumption anyway to illustrate the calculation. We will then revisit this example and calculate the confidence interval obtained, dropping the equal variance assumption and using the t approximation with the k statistic. In Section 8.9, we will look at the result we would obtain from a bootstrap percentile method confidence interval where the questionable normality assumption can be dropped. In Chapter 9, we will look at the conclusions of various hypothesis tests based on these pig blood loss data and various assumptions about the population variances. We will revisit the example one more time in Section 14.3, where we will apply a nonparametric technique called the Wilcoxon rank–sum test to these data.

Using the formula for the estimated common variance (Display 8.5), we must calculate the pooled variance S_p^2. The term $S_p^2 = \{S_t^2(n_t - 1) + S_c^2(n_c - 1)\}/[n_t + n_c - 2] = \{(717.12)^2\,9 + (1824.27)^2\,9\}/18$, where $n_t = n_c = 10$, $S_t = 717.12$, and $S_c = 1824.27$. So $S_p^2 = 2178241.61$; taking the square root we obtain $S_p = 1475.89$. Since the degrees of freedom are $n_t + n_c - 2 = 18$, we find that the constant C from the table of the Student's t distribution is 2.101. The interval is then $[(\overline{X}_t - \overline{X}_c) - CS_p\sqrt{(1/n_t) + (1/n_c)}, (\overline{X}_t - \overline{X}_c) + CS_p\sqrt{(1/n_t) + (1/n_c)}] = [(1085.9 - 2187.4) - 2.101\,(1475.89)\sqrt{0.1}, (1085.9 - 2187.4) + 2.101\,(1475.89)\sqrt{0.1}] = [-1101.5 - 980.57, -1101.5 + 980.57] = [-2082.07, -120.93]$, since $\overline{X}_t = 1085.9$ and $\overline{X}_c = 2187.4$. In Chapter 9 (on hypothesis testing), you will learn that because the interval does not contain 0, you are able to reject the hypothesis of no difference in average blood loss.

We note that if we had chosen a 90% confidence interval $C = 1.7341$ (based on the tables for Student's t distribution), the resulting interval would be $[(1085.9 - 2187.4) - 1.7341(1475.89)\sqrt{0.1}, (1085.9 - 2187.4) + 1.7341(1475.89)\sqrt{0.1}] = [-1101.5 - 809.33, -1101.5 + 809.33] = [-1910.83, -292.17]$.

Now let us look at the result obtained from assuming unequal variances, a more realistic assumption (refer to Display 8.6). The confidence interval would then be $[(\bar{X}_t - \bar{X}_c) - C\sqrt{(S_t^2/n_t) + (S_c^2/n_c)}, (\bar{X}_t - \bar{X}_c) + C\sqrt{(S_t^2/n_t) + (S_c^2/n_c)}]$, where C is obtained from a Student's t distribution with ν degrees of freedom and

$$\nu = \frac{\{(S_t^2/n_t) + (S_c^2/n_c)\}^2}{[1/(n_c - 1)](S_c^2/n_c)^2 + [1/(n_t - 1)](S_t^2/n_t)^2}$$

Using $S_t = 717.12$ and $S_c = 1824.27$, we obtain $\nu = 11.717$. Note that we cannot look up C in the t table since the degrees of freedom (ν) are not an integer. Interpolation of results for 11 and 12 degrees of freedom (a linear approximation for degrees of freedom between 11 and 12) could be used as an approximation to C. It can also be calculated numerically. For 11 degrees of freedom $C = 2.201$. For 12 degrees of freedom $C = 2.1788$. The interpolation formula is as follows:

$$\frac{(12 - 11.717)}{(12 - 11)} = \frac{(2.1788 - x)}{(2.1788 - 2.201)}$$

We solve for x as the interpolated value for C. The simple way to remember the change in degrees of freedom from 12 to 11.717 is to define the change in degrees of freedom from 12 to 11 as the change in C from the value for 12 degrees of free-

---

Display 8.6.   A 95% Confidence Interval for a Difference Between two Population Means (Different Unknown Population Variances)

$$[(\bar{X}_t - \bar{X}_c) - C\sqrt{(S_t^2/n_t) + (S_c^2/n_c)}, (\bar{X}_t - \bar{X}_c) + C\sqrt{(S_t^2/n_t) + (S_c^2/n_c)}]$$

where:
n_t is the sample size for the treatment group
S_t^2 is the sample estimate of variance for the treatment group
n_c is the sample size for the control group
S_c^2 is the sample estimate of variance for the control group
C is the 97.5 percentile of the t distribution with ν degrees of freedom with ν given by

$$\nu = \frac{\{(S_t^2/n_t) + (S_c^2/n_c)\}^2}{[1/(n_c - 1)](S_c^2/n_c)^2 + [1/(n_t - 1)](S_t^2/n_t)^2}$$

dom to the interpolated value of the change in C from 12 degrees of freedom to 11 degrees of freedom. So $0.283/1 = (2.1788 - x)/-0.0222$ or $-0.283(0.0222) = 2.1788 - x$ or $x = 2.1788 + 0.283(0.0222) = 2.1788 + 0.0063 = 2.1851$.

So taking $C = 2.185$, the 95% confidence interval is $[(1085.9 - 2187.4) - 2.185\sqrt{332796.1}, (1085.9 - 2187.4) + 2.185\sqrt{332796.1}] = [-1101.5 - 1260.49, -1101.5 + 1260.49] = [-2361.99, 158.99]$.

We note that this interval is different from the previous calculation for the common variance estimate and perhaps more realistic. The conclusion is also qualitatively different from the previous calculation because in this case the interval contains 0, whereas under the equal variance assumption it did not!

8.8   BOOTSTRAP PRINCIPLE

In Chapter 2, we introduced the concept of bootstrap sampling and told you that it was a nonparametric technique for statistical inference. We also explained the mechanism for generating bootstrap samples and showed how that mechanism is similar to the one used for simple random sampling. In this section, we will describe and use the bootstrap principle to show a simple and straightforward method to generate confidence intervals for population parameters based on the bootstrap samples. Reviewing Chapter 2, the difference between bootstrap sampling and simple random sampling is

1. Instead of sampling from a population, a bootstrap sample is generated by sampling from a sample.
2. The sampling is done with replacement instead of without replacement.

Bootstrap sampling behaves similarly to random sampling in that each bootstrap sample is a sample of size n drawn at random from the empirical distribution F_n, a probability distribution that gives equal weight to each observed data point (i.e., with each draw, each observation has the same chance as any other observation of being the one selected). Similarly, random sampling can be viewed as drawing a sample of size n but from a population distribution F (in which F is an unknown distribution). We are interested in parameters of the distribution that help characterize the population. In this chapter, we are considering the population mean as the parameter that we would like to know more about.

The bootstrap principle is very simple. We want to draw an inference about the population mean through the sample mean. If we do not make parametric assumptions (such as assuming the observations have a normal distribution) about the sampling distribution of the estimate, we cannot specify the sampling distribution for inference (except approximately through the central limit theorem when the estimate is a sample mean).

In constructing confidence intervals, we have considered probability statements about quantities such as Z or t that have the form $(\overline{X} - \mu)/\sigma_{\overline{X}}$ or $(\overline{X} - \mu)/S_{\overline{X}}$, where $\sigma_{\overline{X}}$ is the standard deviation or $S_{\overline{X}}$ is the estimated standard deviation for the sampling distribution (standard error) of the estimated $\overline{X}$. The bootstrap principle attempts to mimic this process of constructing quantities such as Z and t and forming confidence intervals. The sample estimate $\overline{X}$ is replaced by its bootstrap analog $\overline{X}^*$, the mean of a bootstrap sample. The parameter μ is replaced by $\overline{X}$.

Since the parameter μ is unknown, we cannot actually calculate $\overline{X} - \mu$, but from a bootstrap sample we can calculate $\overline{X}^* - \overline{X}$. We then approximate the distribution of $\overline{X}^* - \overline{X}$ by generating many bootstrap samples and computing many $\overline{X}^*$ values. By making the number B of bootstrap replications large, we allow the random generation of bootstrap samples (sometimes called the Monte Carlo method) to approximate as closely as we want the bootstrap distribution of $\overline{X}^* - \overline{X}$. The histogram of bootstrap samples provides a replacement for the sampling distribution of the Z or t statistic used in confidence interval calculations. The histogram also replaces the normal or t distribution tables that we used in the parametric approaches.

The idea behind the bootstrap is to approximate the distribution of $\overline{X} - \mu$. If this mimicking process achieves that approximation, then we are able to draw inferences about μ. We have no particular reason to believe that the mimicking process actually works.

The bootstrap statistical theory, developed since 1980, shows that under very general conditions, mimicking works as the sample size n becomes large. Other empirical evidence from simulation studies has shown that mimicking sometimes works well even with small to moderate sample sizes (10–100). The procedure has been modified and generalized to work for a wide variety of statistical estimation problems.

The bootstrap principle is easy to remember and to apply in general. You mimic the sampling from the population by sampling from the empirical distribution. Wherever the unknown parameters appear in your estimation formulae, you replace them by their estimates from the original sample. Wherever the estimates appear in the formulae, you replace them with their bootstrap estimates. The sample estimates and bootstrap estimates can be thought of as actors. The sample estimates take on the role of the parameters and the bootstrap estimates play the role of the sample estimates.

8.9   BOOTSTRAP PERCENTILE METHOD CONFIDENCE INTERVALS

Now that you have learned the bootstrap principle, it is relatively simple to generate percentile method confidence intervals for the mean. The advantages of the bootstrap confidence interval are that (1) it does not rely on any parametric distributional assumptions; (2) there is no reliance on a central limit theorem; and (3) there are no complicated formulas to memorize. All you need to know is the bootstrap principle. Suppose we have a random sample of size 10. Consider the pig blood loss data (treatment group) shown in Table 8.2, which reproduces the treatment data from Table 8.1.

TABLE 8.2. Pig Blood Loss Data (ml)

Pig Index	Treatment Group Pigs
1	543
2	666
3	455
4	823
5	1716
6	797
7	2828
8	1251
9	702
10	1078
	Sample mean = 1085.90
	Sample Standard deviation = 717.12

Let us use the method in Section 8.4 based on the t statistic to generate a parametric 95% confidence interval for the mean. Then we will show you how to generate a bootstrap percentile method confidence interval based on just 20 bootstrap samples. We will then show you a better approximation based on 10,000 bootstrap samples. The result based on 10,000 bootstrap samples requires intensive computing, which we do using the software package Resampling Stats.

Recall that the parametric confidence interval based on t is $[\overline{X} - C(S/\sqrt{n}), \overline{X} + C(S/\sqrt{n})]$, where S is the sample standard deviation, $\overline{X}$ is the sample mean, and C is the constant taken from the t distribution with $n - 1$ degrees of freedom, where n is the sample size and C satisfies the relationship $P(-C \leq t \leq C) = 0.95$. In this case, $n = 10$ and $df = n - 1 = 9$. From the table of Student's t we see that $C = 2.2622$.

Now, in our example, $\overline{X} = 1085.90$ ml and $s = 717.12$ ml. So the confidence interval is $[1085.9 - 2.2622(717.12/\sqrt{10}, 1085.9 + 2.2622(717.12/\sqrt{10}] = [1085.9 - 513.01, 1085.9 + 513.01] = [572.89, 1598.91]$. Similarly, for a 90% interval the value for C is 1.8331; hence, the 90% interval is $[1085.9 - 415.7, 1085.9 + 415.7] = [670.2, 1501.6]$.

Now let us generate 20 bootstrap samples of size 10 and calculate the mean of each bootstrap sample. We first list the samples based on their pig index and then we will compute the bootstrap sample values and estimates. To generate 20 bootstrap samples of size 10 we need 200 uniform random numbers. The following 10 × 20 table (Table 8.3) provides the 200 uniform random numbers. Each row represents a bootstrap sample. The pig indices are obtained as follows:

If the uniform random number U is in [0.0, 0.1), the pig index I is 1.
If the uniform random number U is in [0.1, 0.2), the pig index I is 2.
If the uniform random number U is in [0.2, 0.3), the pig index I is 3.
If the uniform random number U is in [0.3, 0.4), the pig index I is 4.

TABLE 8.3. Bootstrap Sample Uniform Random Numbers

1	0.00858	0.04352	0.17833	0.41105	0.46569	0.90109	0.14713	0.15905	0.84555	0.92326
2	0.69158	0.38683	0.41374	0.17028	0.09304	0.10834	0.61546	0.33503	0.84277	0.44800
3	0.00439	0.81846	0.45446	0.93971	0.84217	0.74968	0.62758	0.49813	0.13666	0.12981
4	0.29676	0.37909	0.95673	0.66757	0.72420	0.40567	0.81119	0.87494	0.85471	0.81520
5	0.69386	0.71708	0.88608	0.67251	0.22512	0.00169	0.58624	0.04059	0.05557	0.73345
6	0.68381	0.61725	0.49122	0.75836	0.15368	0.52551	0.54604	0.61136	0.51996	0.19921
7	0.19618	0.87653	0.18682	0.22917	0.56801	0.81679	0.93285	0.68284	0.11203	0.47990
8	0.16264	0.39564	0.37178	0.61382	0.51274	0.89407	0.11283	0.77207	0.90547	0.50981
9	0.40431	0.28106	0.28655	0.84536	0.71208	0.47599	0.36136	0.46412	0.99748	0.76167
10	0.69481	0.57748	0.93003	0.99900	0.25413	0.64661	0.17132	0.53464	0.52705	0.69602
11	0.80142	0.64567	0.38915	0.40716	0.76797	0.37083	0.53872	0.30022	0.43767	0.60257
12	0.25769	0.28265	0.26135	0.52688	0.11867	0.05398	0.43797	0.45228	0.28086	0.84568
13	0.61763	0.77188	0.54997	0.28352	0.57192	0.22751	0.82470	0.92971	0.29091	0.35441
14	0.54302	0.81734	0.15723	0.10921	0.20123	0.02787	0.97407	0.02481	0.69785	0.58025
15	0.80089	0.48271	0.45519	0.64328	0.48167	0.14794	0.07440	0.53407	0.32341	0.30360
16	0.60138	0.40435	0.75526	0.35949	0.84558	0.13211	0.29579	0.30084	0.47671	0.44720
17	0.56644	0.52133	0.55069	0.57102	0.67821	0.54934	0.66318	0.35153	0.36755	0.88011
18	0.97091	0.42397	0.08406	0.04213	0.52727	0.08328	0.24057	0.78695	0.91207	0.18451
19	0.71447	0.27337	0.62158	0.25679	0.63325	0.98669	0.16926	0.28929	0.06692	0.05049
20	0.18849	0.96248	0.46509	0.56863	0.27018	0.64818	0.40938	0.66102	0.65833	0.39169

Source: taken with permission from Table 2.1 of Kuzma (1998).

If the uniform random number U is in [0.4, 0.5), the pig index I is 5.
If the uniform random number U is in [0.5, 0.6), the pig index I is 6.
If the uniform random number U is in [0.6, 0.7), the pig index I is 7.
If the uniform random number U is in [0.7, 0.8), the pig index I is 8.
If the uniform random number U is in [0.8, 0.9), the pig index I is 9.
If the uniform random number U is in [0.9, 1.0), the pig index I is 10.

In Table 8.4, the indices replace the random numbers from Table 8.3. Then in Table 8.5, the treatment group values from Table 8.2 replace the indices. The rows in Table 8.5 show the bootstrap sample averages with the bottom row showing the average of the 20 bootstrap samples.

Note in Table 8.5 the similarity of the overall bootstrap estimates to the sample estimates. For the original sample the sample, mean was 1085.9 and the estimate of its standard error was 226.77. By comparison, the bootstrap estimate of the mean is 1159.46 and its bootstrap estimated standard error is 251.25. The standard error is obtained by computing a sample standard deviation for the 20 bootstrap sample estimates in Table 8.4.

Bootstrap percentile confidence intervals are obtained by ordering the bootstrap estimates from smallest to largest. For an approximate 90% confidence interval, the 5th percentile and the 95th percentile are taken as the endpoints of the interval. Because there are 20 estimates, the interval is from the second smallest to the

TABLE 8.4. Random Pig Indices Based on Table 8.3

1	1	1	2	5	5	10	2	2	9	10
2	7	4	5	2	1	2	7	4	9	5
3	1	9	5	10	9	8	7	5	2	2
4	3	4	10	7	8	5	9	9	9	9
5	7	8	9	7	3	1	6	1	1	8
6	7	7	5	8	2	6	6	7	6	2
7	2	9	2	3	6	9	10	7	2	5
8	2	4	4	7	6	9	2	8	10	6
9	5	3	3	9	8	5	4	5	10	8
10	7	6	10	10	3	7	2	6	6	7
11	9	7	4	5	8	4	6	4	5	7
12	3	3	3	6	2	1	5	5	3	9
13	7	8	6	3	6	3	9	10	3	4
14	6	9	2	2	3	1	10	1	7	6
15	9	5	5	7	5	2	1	6	4	4
16	7	5	8	4	9	2	3	4	5	5
17	6	6	6	6	7	6	7	4	4	9
18	10	5	1	1	6	1	3	8	10	2
19	8	3	7	3	7	10	2	3	1	1
20	2	10	5	6	3	7	5	7	7	4

next to largest, as 5% of the observations are below the second smallest (1/20) and 5% are above the second largest (1/20). Consequently, the 90% bootstrap percentile method confidence interval for the mean is obtained by inspecting Table 8.6, which orders the bootstrap mean estimates.

Since observation number 2 in increasing rank order is 796.0 and observation 19 in rank order is 1517.4, the confidence interval is [796.0, 1517.4]. Compare this to the parametric 90% interval of [670.2, 1501.6]. This difference between the two calculations could be due to the nonnormality of the data.

We will revisit the results for a random sample of 200 after computing the more precise estimates based on 10,000 bootstrap samples. Using 10,000 bootstrap samples, we will also be able to compute and compare the 95% confidence intervals. These procedures will require the use of the computer program Resampling Stats.

Resampling Stats is a product of the company of the same name founded by Julian Simon and Peter Bruce to provide software tools to teach and perform statistical calculations by bootstrap and other resampling methods. Their software is discussed further in Chapter 16.

Using the Resampling Stats software, we created the following program (displayed in italics) in the Resampling Stats language:

data (543 666 455 823 1716 797 2828 1251 702 1078) bdloss
maximize z 15000
mean bdloss mb
stdev bdloss sigb

TABLE 8.5. Bootstrap Sample Blood Loss Values and Averages Based on Pig Indices from Table 8.4

	1	2	3	4	5	6	7	8	9	10	Bootstrap Sample Average
1	543	543	666	1716	1716	1078	666	666	702	1078	937.4
2	2828	823	1716	666	543	666	2828	823	702	1716	1331.1
3	543	702	1716	1078	702	1251	2828	1716	666	666	1186.8
4	455	823	1078	2828	1251	1716	702	702	702	702	1095.9
5	2828	1251	702	2828	455	543	797	543	543	1251	1449.2
6	2828	2828	1716	1251	666	797	797	2828	797	666	1517.4
7	666	702	666	455	797	702	1078	2828	666	1716	1027.6
8	666	823	823	2828	797	702	666	1251	1078	797	1043.1
9	1716	455	455	702	1251	1716	823	1716	1078	1251	1116.3
10	2828	797	1078	1078	455	2828	666	797	797	2828	1415.2
11	702	2828	823	1716	1251	823	797	823	1716	2828	1430.7
12	455	455	455	797	666	543	1716	1716	455	702	796.0
13	2828	1251	797	455	797	455	702	1078	455	823	964.1
14	797	702	666	666	455	543	1078	543	2828	797	627.2
15	702	1716	1716	2828	1716	666	543	797	823	823	1233.0
16	2828	1716	1251	823	702	666	455	823	1716	1716	1269.6
17	797	797	797	797	2828	797	2828	823	823	702	1198.9
18	1078	1716	543	543	797	543	455	1251	1078	666	867.0
19	1251	455	2828	455	2828	1078	666	455	543	543	1110.2
20	666	1078	1716	797	455	2828	1716	2828	2828	823	1573.5
Average of twenty bootstrap samples											1159.46

```
print mb sigb
repeat 10000
        sample 10 bdloss bootb
        mean bootb mbs$
        stdev bootb sigbs$
        score mbs$ z
end
histogram z
percentile z (2.5 97.5) k
print mb k
```

The first line of the code is the data statement. An array is a collection or vector of values stored under a common name and indexed from 1 to n, where n is the array size. It takes the 10 blood loss values for the pigs and stores it in an array called bdloss; *bdloss* is an array of size $n = 10$.

The next line is the *maxsize* statement. This statement specifies an array size of

TABLE 8.6. Bootstrap Estimates of Mean Blood Loss in Increasing Order

Ordered Value	Bootstrap Mean
1	627.2
2	796.0
3	867.0
4	937.4
5	964.1
6	1027.6
7	1043.1
8	1095.9
9	1110.2
10	1116.3
11	1186.8
12	1198.9
13	1233.0
14	1269.6
15	1331.3
16	1415.2
17	1430.7
18	1449.2
19	1517.4
20	1573.5

15,000 for the array *z*. By default, arrays are normally limited to be 1000 in length. So the *n* = 15,000 for the array *z*. We will be able to generate up to 15,000 bootstrap samples (i.e., *B* = 10,000 for the number of bootstrap samples in this application, but the number could have been as large as 15,000).

The next two statements, *mean* and *stdev*, compute the sample mean and sample standard deviation, respectively, for the data in the *bdloss* array. The results are stored in the variables *mb* and *sigb* for the mean and standard deviation, respectively. The *print* statement tells the computer to print out the results.

The *repeat* statement then tells the computer how many times to repeat the next several statements. It starts a loop (like a *do* loop in Fortran). The *sample* statement tells the computer how to generate the bootstrap samples. The number *10* tells it to sample with replacement 10 times.

The array *bdloss* appears in the position to tell the computer to sample from the data in the *bdloss* array. Then the name *bootb* is the array to store the bootstrap sample. The next two statements produce the sample means and standard deviations for the bootstrap samples. The *score* statement tells the computer to keep the results for the means in a vector called *z*. The *end* statement indicates the end of the loop that does the calculations for each of the 10,000 bootstrap samples.

The *histogram* statement then takes the results in z and creates a histogram, automatically choosing the number of bins (i.e., intervals for the histogram), the bin width and the center of each bin. The *percentile* statement tells the computer to list the specified set of percentiles from the distribution determined by the array of bootstrap means that are stored in z (like the last column in Table 8.5 from the sample of 20 bootstrap estimates of mean blood loss).

When we choose 2.5 and 97.5, these values will represent the endpoint of a bootstrap percentile method confidence interval at the 95% confidence level for the mean based on 10,000 bootstrap samples. The final *print* statement prints the sample mean of the original sample and the endpoints of the bootstrap confidence interval. In real time, the program took 1.5 seconds to execute; the results (in bold face) appeared exactly as follows:

MB = 1085.9
SIGB = 717.12
Vector no. 1: Z

Bin Center	Freq	Pct	Cum Pct __
600	156	1.6	1.6
800	1887	18.9	20.4
1000	3579	35.8	56.2
1200	2806	28.1	84.3
1400	1195	11.9	96.2
1600	321	3.2	99.4
1800	47	0.5	99.9
2000	8	0.1	100.0
2200	1	0.0	100.0

Note: Each bin covers all values within 100 of its center.

MB = 1085.9
K = 727.1   1558.9

Interpreting the output, **MB** represents the sample mean for the original data and **SIGB** the standard deviation for the original data. The histogram is for **Vector no. 1,** the array **Z** of bootstrap sample means. **K** is an array of size $n = 2$ with its first element the 2.5 percentile from the histogram of bootstrap means and the second element the 97.5 percentile from that histogram.

Using 10,000 random samples, the bootstrap percentile method 95% confidence interval is [727.1, 1558.9]. Notice that this is much different from the confidence interval we obtained by assuming a normal distribution. Recall that that interval was [572.89, 1598.91], which is much wider than the interval produced by the bootstrap percentile method. This result is due to the fact that the distribution for the in-

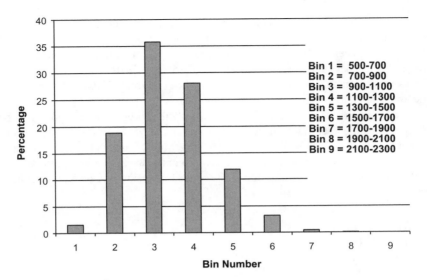

Figure 8.3. Histogram of bootstrap means for the pig treatment group blood loss used for 95% bootstrap percentile method confidence interval.

dividual observations is not normal and the sample size of 10 is too small for the central limit theorem to apply to the sample mean.

Not only does the bootstrap give a tighter interval than the normal approximation, but also the resulting interval is more realistic based on the sample we observed! Figure 8.3 shows the bootstrap histogram that indicates a skewed distribution for the sampling distribution of the mean.

To obtain a 90% bootstrap confidence interval using Resampling Stats, we need only change the percentile statement above to the following:

percentile z (5.0 95.0) k

The resulting interval is [727.1, 1558.9]. Recall that, based on only 20 bootstrap samples, we found [796.0, 1517.4] and from normal distribution theory [670.2, 1501.6]. Again, the two bootstrap results are not only different from the results obtained by using the normal distribution, but also are more realistic. We see that 20 samples do not yield an adequate bootstrap interval estimate.

There is a large difference between 20 bootstrap samples and 10,000 bootstrap samples. The histogram from the Monte Carlo approximation provides a good approximation to the bootstrap distribution only as the number of Monte Carlo iterations (B) becomes large. For B as high as 10,000, this distribution and the resulting confidence interval will not change much if we continue to increase B.

However, when B is only 20 this result will not be the case. We chose a small value of 20 for B so that we could demonstrate all the steps of the bootstrap interval estimate without having to resort to the computer. But to produce an accurate inter-

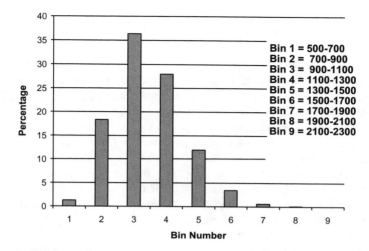

Figure 8.4. Second histogram of bootstrap means for the pig treatment group blood loss. Used for 90% bootstrap percentile method confidence interval.

val, we did need a large B and resorted to the Resampling Stats program.

Subsequently, we found an estimate for the 90% bootstrap confidence interval by using a different set of 10,000 bootstrap samples; hence, the histogram (refer to Figure 8.4) is slightly different from that produced for the 95% confidence interval. The results for this Monte Carlo approximation are as follows (shown in bold face type):

MB = 1085.9
SIGB = 717.12
Vector no. 1: Z

Bin Center	Freq	Pct	Cum Pct
600	128	1.3	1.3
800	1833	18.3	19.6
1000	3634	36.3	56.0
1200	2796	28.0	83.9
1400	1195	11.9	95.9
1600	345	3.5	99.3
1800	60	0.6	99.9
2000	9	0.1	100.0
2200	1	0.0	100.0

Note: Each bin covers all values within 100 of its center.

8.10 SAMPLE SIZE DETERMINATION FOR CONFIDENCE INTERVALS

When conducting an experiment or a clinical trial, cost is an important practical consideration. Often, the number of tests in an engineering experiment or the number of patients enrolled in a clinical trial has a major impact on the cost of the experiment or trial. We have seen that the variance of the sample mean decreases by a factor of $1/n$ with an increase in the sample size from 1 to n. This statement implies that in order to obtain precise confidence intervals for the population mean, the larger the sample the better.

But, because of the cost constraints, we may need to trade off precision of our estimate with the cost of the test. Also, with clinical trials, the number of patients who are enrolled can have a major impact on the time it will take to complete the trial. Two of the main factors that are impacted by sample size are precision and cost; thus, sample size also affects the feasibility of a clinical trial.

The real question we must ask is: "How precise an estimate do I need in order to have useful results?" We will show you how to address this question in order to determine a minimum acceptable value for n. Once this minimum n is determined, we can see what this n implies about the feasibility of the experiment or trial. In many epidemiological and other health-related studies, sample size estimation is also of crucial importance. For example, epidemiologists need to know the minimum sample size required in order to detect differences in occurrences of diseases, health conditions, and other characteristics by subpopulations (e.g., smokers versus nonsmokers), or in the effects of different exposures or interventions.

In Chapter 9, we will revisit this issue from the perspective of hypothesis testing. The issues in hypothesis testing are the same and the methods of evaluation are very similar to those for sample size estimation based on confidence interval width that we will now describe.

Let us first consider the simplest case of estimating a population mean when the variance σ^2 is known. In Section 8.4, we saw that a 95% confidence interval is given by $[\overline{X} - 1.96\sigma/\sqrt{n}, \overline{X} + 1.96\sigma/\sqrt{n}]$. If we subtract the lower endpoint of the interval from the upper endpoint, we see that the width of the interval is $\overline{X} + 1.96\sigma/\sqrt{n} - \overline{X} + 1.96\sigma/\sqrt{n} = 2(1.96\sigma/\sqrt{n})$ or $3.92\sigma/\sqrt{n}$.

The way we determine sample size is to put a constraint on the width $3.92\sigma/\sqrt{n}$ or the half-width $1.96\sigma/\sqrt{n}$. The half-width represents the greatest distance a point in the interval can be away from the point estimate. So it is a meaningful quantity to constrain. When the main objective is an accurate confidence interval for the parameter the half-width of the interval is a very natural choice. Other objectives such as power of a statistical test can also be used. We specify a maximum value d for this half-width. The quantity d is very much dependent on what would be a meaningful interval in the particular trial or experiment. Requiring the half-width to be no larger than d leads to the inequality $1.96\ \sigma/\sqrt{n} \leq d$. Using algebra, we see that $\sqrt{n} \geq 1.96\sigma/d$ or $n \geq 3.8416\ \sigma^2/d^2$. To meet this requirement with the smallest possible integer n, we calculate the quantity $3.8416\ \sigma^2/d^2$ and let n be the next integer larger than this quantity. Display 8.7 summarizes the sample size formula using the half-width d of a confidence interval.

**Display 8.7.   Sample Size Formula Using the
Half-Width d of a Confidence Interval**

Take n as the next integer larger than $(C)^2\sigma^2/d^2$; e.g., for the 95% confidence interval for the mean, take n as the next integer larger than $(1.96)^2\sigma^2/d^2$.

Let us consider the case where we are sampling from a normal distribution with a known standard deviation of 5, and let us assume that we want the half-width of the 95% confidence interval to be no greater than 0.5. Then $d = 0.5$ and $\sigma = 5$ in this case. Now the quantity 3.8416 σ^2/d^2 is $3.8416(5/0.5)^2 = 3.8416\ (10)^2 = 3.8416(100) = 384.16$. So the smallest integer n that satisfies the required inequality is 385.

In order to solve the foregoing problem we needed to know σ, which in most practical situations will be unknown. Our alternatives are to find or guess at an upper bound for σ, to estimate σ from a small pilot study, or to refer to the literature for studies that may publish estimates of σ.

Estimating the sample size for the difference between two means is a problem similar to estimating the sample size for a single mean but requires knowing two variances and specifying a relationship between the two sample sizes n_t and n_c.

Recall from Section 8.6 that the 95% confidence interval for the difference between two means of samples selected from two independent normal distributions with known and equal variances is given by $[(\bar{X}_t - \bar{X}_c) - 1.96\ \sigma\sqrt{(1/n_t) + (1/n_c)}, (\bar{X}_t - \bar{X}_c) + 1.96\ \sigma\sqrt{(1/n_t)+(1/n_c)}]$. The half-width of this interval is $1.96\ \sigma\sqrt{(1/n_t) + (1/n_c)}$. Assume $n_t = kn_c$ for some proportionality constant $k \geq 1$. The proportionality constant k adjusts for the differences in sample sizes used in the treatment and control groups, as explained in the next paragraph. Let d be the constraint on the half-width. The inequality becomes $1.96\ \sigma\sqrt{\{1/(kn_c)\} + \{1/(n_c)\}} = 1.96\sigma\sqrt{\{1/(kn_c)\} + \{1/(n_c)\}} = 1.96\ \sigma\sqrt{(k + 1)/(kn_c)} \leq d$ or $kn_c/(k + 1) \geq 3.8416\ \sigma^2/d^2$ or $n_c \geq 3.8416(k + 1)\sigma^2/(kd^2)$. If $n_c = 3.8416\ (k + 1)\sigma^2/(kd^2)$, then $n_t = kn_c = 3.8416\ (k + 1)\sigma^2/d^2$. In Display 8.8 we present the sample size formula using the half-width d of a confidence interval for the difference between two population means.

Note that if $k = 1$, then $n_c = n_t = 3.8416\ (2\sigma^2/d^2)$. Taking k greater than 1 increases n_t while it lowers n_c, but the total sample size $n_t + n_c = (k + 1)^2\ 3.8416\ \sigma^2/(kd^2)$.

**Display 8.8.   Sample Size Formula Using the Half-Width d
of a Confidence Interval (Difference Between Two Population
Means When the Sample Sizes Are n and kn, where $k > 1$)**

Take n as the next integer larger than $(C)^2(k + 1)\sigma^2/(kd^2)$; e.g., for the 95% confidence interval for the mean, take n as the next integer larger than $(1.96)^2(k + 1)\sigma^2/(kd^2)$.

For $k > 1$, the result is larger than 4 ($3.8416\sigma^2/d^2$), the result for $k = 1$ [since $(1 + 1)^2 = 4$]. This calculation shows without loss of generality that $k = 1$ minimizes the total sample size. However, in clinical trials there may be ethical reasons for wanting n_t to be larger than n_c.

For example, in 1995 Chernick designed a clinical trial (the Tendril DX study) to show that steroid eluting pacing leads were effective in reducing capture thresholds for patients with pacemakers. (For more details, see Chernick, 1999, pp. 63–67). Steroid eluting leads have steroid in the tip of the lead that slowly oozes out into the tissue. This medication is intended to reduce inflammation. The capture threshold is the minimum required voltage for the electrical shock from the lead into the heart that causes the heart to contract (a forced pacing beat). Lower capture thresholds conserve the pacemaker battery and thus allow a longer period before replacement of the pacemaker. The pacing leads are connected from a pacemaker that is implanted in the patient's chest and run through part of the circulatory system into the heart where they provide an electrical stimulus to induce pacing heart beats (beats that restore normal heart rhythm).

The investigator chose a value of $k = 3$ for the study because competitors had demonstrated reductions in capture thresholds for their steroid leads that were approved by the FDA based on similar clinical trials. Factors for k such as 2 and 3 were considered because the company and the investigating physicians wanted a much greater percentage of the patients to receive the steroid leads but did not want k to be so large that the total number of patients enrolled would become very expensive. Consequently, the physicians who were willing to participate in the trial wanted to give the steroid leads to most of their patients, as they perceived it to be the better treatment than the use of leads without the steroid.

Chernick actually planned the Tendril DX trial (assuming thresholds were normally distributed) so that he could reject the null hypothesis of no difference in capture threshold versus an alternative hypothesis (i.e., that the difference was at least 0.5 volts with statistical power of 80% as the alternative). In Chapter 9, when we consider sample size for hypothesis testing, we will look again at these assumptions (e.g., statistical power) and requirements.

For now, to illustrate sample size calculations based on confidence intervals, let us assume that we want the half-width of a 95% confidence interval for the mean difference to be no greater than $d = 0.2$ volts. Assume that both leads have the same standard deviation of 0.8 volts. Then, since $n_t = 3.8416 [(k + 1)\sigma^2/d^2] = 3.8416[4(0.64/0.04)] = 245.86$ or 246 (rounding to the next integer) and $n_c = n_t/3 = 82$, this gives a total sample size of 328.

Without changing assumptions, suppose we were able to let $k = 1$. Then $n_t = n_c = 3.8416[2\sigma^2/d^2] = 3.8416[2(0.64/0.04)] = 122.93$ or 123. This modification gives a much smaller total sample size of 246. Note that by going to a 3:1 randomization scheme (i.e., $k = 3$), n_t increased by a factor of 2 or a total of 123, while n_c decreased by only 41. We call it a 3:1 randomization scheme because the probability is 0.75 that a patient will receive the steroid lead and 0.25 that a patient will receive the nonsteroid lead.

Formulae also can be given for more complex situations. However, in some cases iterative procedures by computer are needed. Currently, there are a number of soft-ware packages available to handle differing confidence sets and hypothesis testing problems under a variety of assumptions. We will describe some of these software packages in Section 16.3. See the related references in Section 8.12 and Section 16.5.

8.11 EXERCISES

8.1 In your own words define the following terms:
  a. Descriptive statistics
  b. Inferential statistics
  c. Point estimate of a population parameter
  d. Interval (confidence interval) estimate of a population parameter
  e. Type I error
  f. Biased estimator of a population parameter
  g. Mean square error

8.2 What are the desirable properties of an estimator of a population parameter?

8.3 What are the advantages and disadvantages of using point estimates for sta-tistical inference?

8.4 What are the desirable properties of a confidence interval? How do sample size and the level of confidence (e.g., 90%, 95%, 99%) affect the width of a confidence interval?

8.5 State the advantages and disadvantages of using confidence intervals for sta-tistical inference.

8.6 Two situations affect the choice of a calculation of a confidence interval: (1) the population is known; (2) the population variance is unknown. How would you calculate a confidence interval given these two different circumstances?

8.7 Explain the bootstrap principle. How can it be used to make statistical infer-ences?

8.8 How can bootstrap confidence intervals be generated? Name the simplest form of a bootstrap confidence interval. Are bootstrap confidence intervals exact?

8.9 Suppose we randomly select 20 students enrolled in an introductory course in biostatistics and measure their resting heart rates. We obtain a mean of 66.9 ($S = 9.02$). Calculate a 95% confidence interval for the population mean and give an interpretation of the interval you obtain.

8.10 Suppose that a sample of pulse rates gives a mean of 71.3, as in Exercise 8.9, with a standard deviation that can be assumed to be 9.4 (close to the estimate observed in exercise 8.9). How many patients should be sampled to obtain a 95 % confidence interval for the mean that has half-width 1.2 beats per minute?

8.11 In a sample of 125 experimental subjects, the mean score on a postexperimental measure of aggression was 55 with a standard deviation of 5. Construct a 95% confidence interval for the population mean.

8.12 Suppose the sample size in exercise 8.11 is 169 and the mean score is 55 with a standard deviation of 5. Construct a 99% confidence interval for the population mean.

8.13 Suppose you want to construct a 95% confidence interval for mean aggression scores as in Exercise 8.11, and you can assume that the standard deviation of the estimate is 5. How many experimental subjects do you need for the half-width of the interval to be no larger than 0.4?

8.14 What would the number of experimental subjects have to be under the assumptions in Exercise 8.13 if you want to construct a 99% confidence interval with half-width no greater then 0.4? Under the same criteria we decide that *n* should be large enough so that a 95% confidence interval would have this half-width of 0.4. Which confidence interval requires the larger sample size and why? What is *n* for the 95% interval?

8.15 The mean weight of 100 men in a particular heart study is 61 kg with a standard deviation of 7.9 kg. Construct a 95% confidence interval for the mean.

8.16 The standard hemoglobin reading for normal males of adult age is 15 g/100 ml. The standard deviation is about 2.5 g/100 ml. For a group of 36 male construction workers, the sample mean was 16 g/100 ml.
   a. Construct a 95% confidence interval for the male construction workers. What is your interpretation of this interval relative to the normal adult male population?
   b. What would the confidence interval have been if the above results were obtained based on 49 construction workers?
   c. Repeat *b* for 64 construction workers.
   d. Do fixed-level confidence intervals shrink or widen as the sample size increases (all other factors remaining the same)? Explain your answer.
   e. What is the half-width of the confidence interval that you would obtain for 64 workers?

8.17 Repeat Exercise 8.16 for 99% confidence intervals.

8.18 The mean diastolic blood pressure for 225 randomly selected individuals is 75 mmHg with a standard deviation of 12.0 mmHg. Construct a 95% confidence interval for the mean.

8.19 Change exercise 8.18 to assume there are 400 randomly selected individuals with a mean of 75 and standard deviation of 12. Construct a 99% confidence interval for the mean.

8.20 In Exercise 8.18, how many individuals must you select to obtain the half-width of a 99% confidence interval no larger than 0.5 mmHg?

8.12 ADDITIONAL READING

1. Arena, V. C. and Rockette, H. E. (2001). "Software" *in Biostatistics in Clinical Trials, Redmond, C. and Colton, T.* (editors), pp. 424–437. John Wiley and Sons, Inc., New York.

2. Borenstein, M., Rothstein, H., Cohen, J., Schoefeld, D., Berlin, J., and Lakatos, E. (2001). Power and Precision™. Biostat Inc., Englewood, New Jersey.

3. Chernick, M. R. (1999). *Bootstrap Methods: A Practitioner's Guide.* Wiley, New York.

4. Davison, A. C. and Hinkley D.V. (1997). *Bootstrap Methods and Their Applications.* Cambridge University Press, Cambridge.

5. Efron, B. and Tibshirani, R. (1993). *An Introduction to the Bootstrap.* Chapman and Hall, London.

6. Elashoff, J. D. (2000). *nQuery Advisor® Release 4.0 Users Guide.* Statistical Solutions, Boston.

7. Hintze, J. L. (2000). *PASS User's Guide: PASS 2000 Power Analysis and Sample Size for Windows.* NCSS Inc., Kaysville.

8. Hogg, R. V. and Tanis, E. A. (1997). *Probability and Statistical Inference,* Sixth Edition. Prentice Hall, Upper Saddle River, New Jersey.

9. Kuzma, J. W. (1998). *Basic Statistics for the Health Sciences,* Third Edition. Mayfield Publishing Company, Mountain View, California.

10. O'Brien, R. G. and Muller, K. E. (1993). "Unified Power Analysis for *t*-Tests Through Multivariate Hypotheses," in *Applied Analysis of Variance in Behavioral Science,* Edwards, L. K. (editor), pp. 297–344. Marcel Dekker, Inc., New York.

11. StatXact5 for Windows (2001): *Statistical Software for Exact Nonparametric Inference User Manual.* CYTEL: Cambridge, Massachusetts.

CHAPTER 9

Tests of Hypotheses

If the fresh facts which come to our knowledge all fit themselves
into the scheme the hypothesis may gradually become a solution.
—Sherlock Holmes in Sir Arthur Conan Doyle's *The Complete Sherlock Holmes,*
The Adventure of Wisteria Lodge

9.1 TERMINOLOGY

Hypothesis testing is a formal scientific process that accounts for statistical uncertainty. As such, the process involves much new statistical terminology that we now introduce. A hypothesis is a statement of belief about the values of population parameters. In hypothesis testing, we usually consider two hypotheses: the null and alternative hypotheses. The null hypothesis, denoted by H_0, is usually a hypothesis of no difference. Initially, we will consider a type of H_0 that is a claim that there is no difference between the population parameter and its hypothesized value or set of values. The hypothesized values chosen for the null hypothesis are usually chosen to be uninteresting values. An example might be that in a trial comparing two diabetes drugs, the mean values for fasting plasma glucose are the same for the two treatment groups.

In general, the experimenter is interested in rejecting the null hypothesis. The alternative hypothesis, denoted by H_1, is a claim that the null hypothesis is false; i.e., the population parameter takes on a value different from the value or values specified by the null hypothesis. The alternative hypothesis is usually the scientifically interesting hypothesis that we would like to confirm. By using probability theory, our goal is to lend credence to the alternative hypothesis by rejecting the null hypothesis. In the diabetes example, an interesting alternative might be that the fasting plasma glucose mean is significantly (both statistically and clinically) lower for patients with the experimental drug as compared to the mean for patients with the control drug.

Because of statistical uncertainty regarding inferences about population parameters based on sample data, we cannot prove or disprove either the null or the alternative hypotheses. Rather, we make a decision based on probability and accept a probability of making an incorrect decision.

Introductory Biostatistics for the Health Sciences, by Michael R. Chernick
and Robert H. Friis. ISBN 0-471-41137-X. Copyright © 2003 Wiley-Interscience.

The type I error is defined as the probability of falsely rejecting the null hypothesis; i.e., to claim on the basis of data from a sample that the true parameter is not a value specified by the null hypothesis when in fact it is. In other words, a type I error occurs when the null hypothesis is true but we incorrectly reject H_0. The other possible mistake we can make is to not reject the null hypothesis when the true parameter value is specified by the alternative hypothesis. This kind of error is called a type II error.

Based on the observed data, we form a statistic (called a test statistic) and consider its sampling distribution in order to define critical values for rejecting the null hypothesis. For example, the Z and t statistics covered previously (refer to Chapter 8) can serve as test statistics for those population parameters. A statistician uses one or more cutoff values for the test statistic to determine when to reject or not to reject the null hypothesis.

These cutoff values are called critical values; the set of values for which the null hypothesis would be rejected is called the critical region, or rejection region. The other values of the test statistic form a region that we will call the nonrejection region. We are tempted to call the nonrejection region the acceptance region; however, we hesitate to do so because the Neyman–Pearson approach to hypothesis testing chooses the critical value to control the type I error, but the type II error then depends on the specific value of the parameter when the alternative is true. In the next section, we will discuss this point in detail as well as the Neyman–Pearson approach.

The probability of observing a value in the critical region when the null hypothesis is correct is called the significance level; the hypothesis test is also called a test of significance. The significance level is denoted by α, which often is set at a low value such as 0.01 or 0.05. These values also can be termed error levels; i.e., we are acknowledging that it is acceptable to be wrong one time out of 100 tests or five times out of 100 tests, respectively. The symbol α is also the probability of a type I error; the symbol β is used to denote the probability of a type II error, as explained in Section 9.7.

Given a test statistic and an observed value, one can compute the probability of observing a value as extreme or more extreme than the observed value when the null hypothesis is true. This probability is called the p-value. The p-value is related to the significance level in that if we had chosen the critical value to be equal to the observed value of the test statistic, the p-value would be equal to the significance level.

9.2 NEYMAN–PEARSON TEST FORMULATION

In the previous section, we introduced the notion of hypothesis testing and defined the terms null hypothesis and alterative hypothesis, and type I error and type II error. These terms are attributed to Jerzy Neyman and Egon Pearson, who were the developers of formal statistical hypothesis testing in the 1930s. Earlier, R. A. Fisher developed what he called significance testing, but his description was vague and followed a theory of inference called fiducial inference that now appears to have been discredited. The Neyman and Pearson approach has endured but is also challenged by the Bayesian approach to inference (covered in Section 9.16).

In the Neyman and Pearson approach, we construct the null and alternative hypotheses and choose a test statistic. We need to keep in mind the test statistic, the sample size, and the resulting sampling distribution for the test statistic under the null hypothesis (i.e., the distribution when the null hypothesis is assumed to be true). Based on these three factors, we determine a critical value or critical values such that the type I error never exceeds a specified value for α when the null hypothesis is true.

Sometimes, the null hypothesis specifies a unique sampling distribution for a test statistic. A unique sampling distribution for the null hypothesis occurs when the following criteria are met: (1) we hypothesize a single value for the population mean; (2) the variance is assumed to be known; and (3) the normal distribution is assumed for the population distribution. Under these circumstances, the sampling distribution of the test statistic is unique. The critical values can be determined based on this unique sampling distribution; i.e., for a two-tailed (two-sided) test, the 5th percentile and the 95th percentile of the sampling distribution would be used for the critical values of the test statistic; the 10th percentile or the 90th percentile would be used for a one-tailed (one-sided) test depending on which side of the test is the alternative. In Section 9.4, one-sided tests will be discussed and contrasted with two-sided tests.

However, in two important situations the sampling distribution of the test statistic is not unique. The first situation occurs when the population variance (σ^2) is unknown; in this instance, σ^2 is called a nuisance parameter because it affects the sampling distribution but otherwise is not used in the hypothesis test. Nevertheless, even when the population variance is unknown, σ^2 may influence the sampling distribution of the test statistic. For example, σ^2 is relevant to the Behrens–Fisher problem, in which the distribution of the mean difference depends on the ratio of two population variances. (See the article by Robinson on the Behrens–Fisher problem in Johnson and Kotz, 1982). An exception that would not require σ^2 is the use of the t statistic in a one-sample hypothesis test, because the t distribution does not depend on σ^2.

A second situation in which the sampling distribution of the test statistic is not unique occurs during the use of a composite null hypothesis. A composite null hypothesis is one that includes more than one value of the parameter of interest for the null hypothesis. For example, in the case of a population mean, instead of considering only the value 0 for the null hypothesis, we might consider a range of small values; all values of μ such that $|\mu| < 0.5$ would be uninteresting and, hence, included in the null hypothesis.

To review, we have indicated two scenarios: (1) when the sampling distribution depends on a nuisance parameter, and (2) when the hypothesized parameter can take on more than one value under the null hypothesis. For either situation, we consider the distribution that is "closest" to the alternative in a set of distributions for parameter values in the interval for the null hypothesis. The critical values determined for that "closest" distribution would have a significance level higher than those for any other parameter values under the null hypothesis. That significance level is defined to be the level of the overall test of significance. However, this issue is beyond the scope of this text and, hence, will not be elaborated further.

In summary, the Neyman–Pearson approach controls the type I error. Regardless of the sample size, the type I error is controlled so that it is less than or equal to α for any value of the parameters under the null hypothesis. Consequently, if we use the Neyman–Pearson approach, as we will in Sections 9.3, 9.4, 9.9, and 9.10, we can be assured that the type I error is constrained so as to be as small or smaller than the specified α. If the test statistic falls in the rejection region, we can reject the null hypothesis safely, knowing that the probability that we have made the wrong decision is no greater than α.

However, the type II error is not controlled by the Neyman–Pearson approach. Three factors determine the probability of a type II error (β): (1) the sample size, (2) the choice of the test statistic, and (3) the value of the parameter under the alternative hypothesis. When the values for the alternative hypothesis are close to those for the null hypothesis, the type II error can be close to $1 - \alpha$, which defines the region of nonrejection for the null hypothesis. Thus, the probability of a type II error increases as the difference between the mean for the null hypothesis and the mean at the alternative decreases. When this difference between these means becomes large, β becomes small, i.e., closer to α, which defines the significance level of the test as well as its rejection region.

For example, suppose we have a standard normal distribution with mean $\mu = 0$ and variance of the sampling distribution of the sample mean $\sigma_{\bar{X}}^2 = 1$ under the null hypothesis for a sample size $n = 5$. By algebra, we can determine that the population has a variance of $\sigma^2 = 5$ (i.e., $\sigma_{\bar{X}}^2 = (\sigma^2/\sqrt{5}) = 1$). We choose a two-sided test with significance level 0.05 for which the critical values are -1.96 and 1.96. Under the alternative hypothesis, if the mean $\mu = 0.1$ and variance $\sigma^2 = 1$, then the power of the test (defined to be $1 -$ the type II error) is the probability that the sample mean is greater than 1.96 or less than -1.96. But this probability is the same as the probability that the Z value for the standard normal distribution is greater than 1.86 or less than -2.06. Note that we find the values 1.86 and -2.06 by subtracting 0.1 (μ under the alternative hypothesis) from $+1.96$ and -1.96.

From the table of the standard normal distribution (Appendix E), we see that $P[Z < -2.06] = 0.5 - 0.4803 = 0.0197$ and $P[Z > 1.86] = 0.5 - 0.4686 = 0.0314$. The power of the test at this alternative is $0.0197 + 0.0314 = 0.0511$. This mean is close to zero and the power is not much higher than the significance level 0.05. On the other hand, if $\mu = 2.96$ under the alternative with a variance $\sigma^2 = 1$, then the power of the test at this alternative is $P[Z < -4.92\} + P[Z > -1]$. Since $P\{Z < -4.92]$ is almost zero, the power is nearly equal to $P[Z > -1] = 0.5 + P[0 > Z > -1] = 0.5 + P[0 < Z < 1] = 0.5 + 0.3413 = 0.8413$. So as the alternative moves relatively far from zero, the power becomes large. The relationship between the alternative hypothesis and the power of a test will be illustrated in Figures 9.1 and 9.2 later in the chapter.

Consequently, when we test hypotheses using the Neyman–Pearson approach, we do not say that we accept the null hypothesis when the test statistic falls in the nonrejection region; there may be reasonable values for the alternative hypothesis when the type II error is high.

In fact, since we select α to be small so that we have a small type I error, $1 - \alpha$ is large. Some values under the alternative hypothesis have a high type II error, indicating that the test has low power at those alternatives.

In Section 9.12, we will see that the way to control the type II error is to be interested only in alternatives at least a specified distance (such as d) from the null value(s). In addition, we will require that the sample size is large enough so that the power at those alternatives is reasonably high. By alternatives we mean the alternative distribution closest to the null distribution, which is called the least favorable distribution. By reasonably high we mean at least a specified value, such as β. The symbol β (β error) refers to the probability of committing a type II error.

9.3 TEST OF A MEAN (SINGLE SAMPLE, POPULATION VARIANCE KNOWN)

The first and simplest case of hypothesis testing we will consider is the test of a mean (H_0: $\mu = \mu_0$). In this case, we will assume that the population variance is known; thus, we are able to use the Z statistic. We perform the following steps for a two-tailed test (in the next section we will look at both one-tailed and two-tailed tests):

1. State the null hypothesis H_0: $\mu = \mu_0$ versus the alternative hypothesis H_1: $\mu \neq \mu_0$.
2. Choose a significance level $\alpha = \alpha_0$ (often we take $\alpha_0 = 0.05$ or 0.01).
3. Determine the critical region, that is, the region of values of Z in the upper and lower $\alpha/2$ tails of the sampling distribution for Z when $\mu = \mu_0$ (i.e., the sampling distribution when the null hypothesis is true).
4. Compute the Z statistic: $Z = (\overline{X} - \mu_0)/(\sigma/\sqrt{n})$ for the given sample and sample size n.
5. Reject the null hypothesis if the test statistic Z computed in step 4 falls in the rejection region for this test; otherwise, do not reject the null hypothesis.

As an example, consider the study that used blood loss data from pigs (refer to Table 8.1). Take $\mu_0 = 2200$ ml (a plausible amount of blood to lose for a pig in the control group). In this case, the sensible alternative would be one-sided; we would assume $\mu < 2200$ for the alternative with the treatment group, because we expect the treatment to reduce and not to increase blood loss.

However, if we are totally naïve about the effectiveness of the drug, we might consider the two-sided alternative, namely, H_1: $\mu_0 \neq 2200$. In this section we are illustrating the two-sided test, so we will look at the two-sided alternative. We will use the sample data given in Section 8.9 and assume that the standard deviation σ is known to be 720. The sample mean is 1085.9 and the sample size $n = 10$. We now have enough information to carry out the test. The five steps are as follows:

1. State the null hypothesis: The null hypothesis is H_0: $\mu = \mu_0 = 2200$ versus the alternative hypothesis H_1: $\mu \neq \mu_0 = 2200$.
2. Choose a significance level $\alpha = \alpha_0 = 0.05$.
3. Determine the critical region, that is, the region of values of Z in the upper and lower 0.025 tails of the sampling distribution for Z when $\mu = \mu_0$ (i.e., when the null hypothesis is true). For $\alpha_0 = 0.05$, the critical values are $Z = \pm 1.96$ and the critical region includes all values of $Z > 1.96$ or $Z < -1.96$.
4. Compute the Z statistic: $Z = (\overline{X} - \mu_0)/(\sigma/\sqrt{n})$ for the given sample and sample size $n = 10$. We have the following data: $n = 10$; the sample mean ($\overline{X}$) is 1085.9; $\sigma = 720$; and $\mu_0 = 2200$. $Z = (1085.9 - 2200)/(720/\sqrt{10}) = -1114.1/227.684 = -4.893$.
5. Since 4.893 (the absolute value of the test statistic) is clearly larger than 1.96, we reject H_0 at the 5% level; i.e., $-4.893 < -1.960$. Therefore, we conclude that the treatment was effective in reducing blood loss, as the calculated Z is negative, implying that $\mu < \mu_0$.

9.4   TEST OF A MEAN (SINGLE SAMPLE, POPULATION VARIANCE UNKNOWN)

In the case of a test of a mean (H_0: $\mu = \mu_0$) when the population variance is unknown, we estimate the population variance by using s^2 and apply the t distribution to define rejection regions. We perform the following steps for a two-tailed test:

1. State the null hypothesis H_0: $\mu = \mu_0$ versus the alternative hypothesis H_1: $\mu \neq \mu_0$. Note: This hypothesis set is exactly as stated in Section 9.3.
2. Choose a significance level $\alpha = \alpha_0$ (often we take $\alpha_0 = 0.05$ or 0.01).
3. Determine the critical region for the appropriate t distribution, that is, the region of values of t in the upper and lower $\alpha/2$ tails of the sampling distribution for Student's t distribution with $n - 1$ degrees of freedom when $\mu = \mu_0$ (i.e., the sampling distribution when the null hypothesis is true).
4. Compute the t statistic: $t = (\overline{X} - \mu_0)/(s/\sqrt{n})$ for the given sample and sample size n where $\overline{X}$ is the sample mean and s is the sample standard deviation.
5. Reject the null hypothesis if the test statistic t computed in step 4 falls in the rejection region for this test; otherwise, do not reject the null hypothesis.

For example, reconsider the pig treatment data; take $\mu_0 = 2200$ ml (a plausible amount of blood to lose for a pig in the control group). In this case, because the sensible alternative would be one-sided, we could assume $\mu < 2200$ for the alternative with the treatment group, as we expect the treatment to reduce blood loss and not to increase it. However, again assume we are totally naïve about the effectiveness of the drug; so we consider the two-sided alternative hypothesis, namely, H_1: $\mu_0 \neq 2200$.

In this section, we are illustrating the two-sided test, so we will look at the two-sided alternative hypothesis. We will use the sample data given in Section 8.9 but this time use the standard deviation $s = 717.12$. The sample mean is 1085.9 and the sample size $n = 10$. We now have enough information to run the test.

The five steps for hypothesis testing yield the following:

1. State the null hypothesis. The null hypothesis is H_0: $\mu = \mu_0 = 2200$ versus the alternative hypothesis H_1: $\mu \neq \mu_0 = 2200$.
2. Choose a significance level $\alpha = \alpha_0 = 0.05$.
3. Determine the critical region, that is, the region of values of t in the upper and lower 0.025 tails of the sampling distribution for t (Student's t distribution with 9 degrees of freedom) when $\mu = \mu_0$ (i.e., the sampling distribution when the null hypothesis is true). For $\alpha_0 = 0.05$, the critical values are $t = \pm 2.2622$; the critical region includes all values of $t > 2.2622$ or $t < -2.2622$.
4. Compute the t statistic: $t = (\overline{X} - \mu_0)/(s/\sqrt{n})$ for the given sample and sample size $n = 10$; since $n = 10$, the sample mean ($\overline{X}$) is 1085.9, $s = 717.12$, and $\mu_0 = 2200$. Then $t = (1085.9 - 2200)/(717.12/\sqrt{10}) = -1114.1/226.773 = -4.913$.
5. Given that 4.913 (the absolute value of the t statistic) is clearly larger than 2.262, we reject H_0 at the 5% level.

Later, in Section 9.6, we will see that a more meaningful quantity than the 5% level would be a specific p-value, which gives us more information as to the degree of significance of the test. In Section 9.6, we will calculate the p-value for a hypothesis test.

9.5 ONE-TAILED VERSUS TWO-TAILED TESTS

In the previous section, we pointed out that when determining the significance level of a test we must specify either a one-tailed or a two-tailed test. The decision should be based on the context of the problem, i.e., the outcome that we wish to demonstrate. We must consider the relevant research hypothesis, which becomes the alternative hypothesis.

For example, in the Tendril DX trial, we have strong prior evidence from other studies that the steroid (treatment group) leads tend to provide lower capture thresholds than the nonsteroid (control group) leads. Also, we are interested in marketing our product only if we can claim, as do our competitors, that our lead reduces capture thresholds by at least 0.5 volts as compared to nonsteroid leads.

Because we would like to assert that we are able to reduce capture thresholds, it is natural to look at a one-sided alternative. In this case, the null hypothesis H_0 is $\mu_1 - \mu_0 \geq 0$ versus the alternative H_1 that $\mu_1 - \mu_0 < 0$, where μ_1 = the population mean for the treatment group and μ_0 = the population mean for the control group. In Section 9.8, we will see that the appropriate t statistic (under the normality assumption) would have a critical value determined by $t < -t_\alpha$ where t_α is the $100(1 - \alpha)$ percentile of Student's t distribution with $n_c + n_t - 2$ degrees of freedom, n_c is the number of observations in the control group, and n_t is the number of observations in the treatment group.

In the real application, Chernick and associates took $n_t = 3n_c$ and chose the values for n_c and n_t such that the power of the test was at least 80% when $\mu_1 - \mu_0 < -0.5$; α was set at 0.05. We will calculate the sample size for this example in Section 9.8 after we introduce the power function.

In other applications, we may be trying to show only equivalence in medical effectiveness of a new treatment compared to an old one. For medical devices or pharmaceuticals, this test of equivalence may occur when the current product (the control) is an effective treatment and we want to show that the new product is equally effective. However, the new product may be preferred for other reasons, such as ease of application. One example might be the introduction of a simpler needle (called a pen in the industry) to inject the insulin that controls sugar levels for diabetic patients, as compared to a standard insulin injection.

In such cases, the null hypothesis is $\mu_1 - \mu_0 = 0$, versus the alternative $\mu_1 - \mu_0 \neq 0$. Here, we wish to control the type II error. To do this for β error, we must specify a δ so that we have a good chance of rejecting equivalence if $|\mu_1 - \mu_0| > \delta$. Often, δ is chosen to be some clinically relevant difference in the means. The sample size would be chosen so that when $|\mu_1 - \mu_0| > \delta$, the probability that the test statistic is large enough to reject H_0 is high (80% or 90% or 95%), corresponding to a low type II error (20% or 10% or 5%, respectively). For this problem, H_0 is rejected when $|t| > t_{\alpha/2}$ for $t_{\alpha/2}$ equal to the $100(1 - \alpha/2)$ percentile of the t distribution with $n_c + n_t - 2$ degrees of freedom; the value n_c is the number of observations in the control group; n_t is the number of observations in the treatment group.

However, such a test is really backwards because the scientific hypothesis that we want to confirm is the null hypothesis rather than the alternative. It is for this reason that Blackwelder and others (Blackwelder, 1982) have recommended, for equivalence testing (defined in the foregoing example) and also for noninferiority testing (a one-sided form of equivalence), that we really want to "prove the null hypothesis" in the Neyman–Pearson framework.

Hence, Blackwelder advocates simply switching the null and alternative hypotheses so that rejecting the null hypothesis becomes rejection of equivalence and accepting the alternative is acceptance of equivalence. Switching the null and alternative hypotheses allows us to control, through type I error, the probability of falsely claiming equivalence. When we set the type I (α) and type II (β) errors (i.e., the type II error at $|\mu_1 - \mu_0| = \delta$) to be equal, the distinction between α and β errors becomes unimportant. The reason the distinction is unimportant is that if the $\alpha = \beta$, both formulations yield the same required sample size for a specified power. When $|\mu_1 - \mu_0| = \delta$ but $\alpha \neq \beta$, the test results are different from those when $\alpha = \beta$. Because it is common to choose $\alpha < \beta$, the Blackwelder approach often is preferred, particularly by the Food and Drug Administration. For more details see Blackwelder's often-cited article (Blackwelder, 1982).

Now let us look step by step at a one-tailed (left-tail) test procedure for the pig blood loss data considered in the previous section. A left-tailed test means that we reject H_0 if we can show that $\mu < \mu_0$. Alternatively, a right-tailed test denotes rejecting H_0 if we can show that $\mu > \mu_0$.

1. State the null hypothesis H_0: $\mu = \mu_0$ versus the alternative hypothesis H_1: $\mu < \mu_0$.
2. Choose a significance level $\alpha = \alpha_0$ (often we take $\alpha_0 = 0.05$ or 0.01).
3. Determine the critical region, i.e., the region of values of t in the lower (left-tail) tail of the sampling distribution for Student's t distribution with $\alpha_0 = 0.05$ and $n - 1$ degrees of freedom when $\mu = \mu_0$ (i.e., the sampling distribution when the null hypothesis is true).
4. Compute the t statistic: $t = (\overline{X} - \mu_0)/(s/\sqrt{n})$ for the given sample and sample size n, where $\overline{X}$ is the sample mean and s is the sample standard deviation.
5. Reject the null hypothesis if the test statistic t (computed in step 4) falls in the rejection region for this test; otherwise, do not reject the null hypothesis.

Again we will use the sample data given in Section 8.9 but this time use the standard deviation $s = 717.12$. The sample mean is 1085.9 and the sample size $n = 10$. We now have enough information to do the test.

We have the following five steps:

1. The null hypothesis is H_0: $\mu = \mu_0 = 2200$ (H_0: $\mu = 2200$) versus the alternative hypothesis H_1: $\mu < \mu_0 = 2200$ (H_1: $\mu < 2200$).
2. Choose a significance level $\alpha = \alpha_0 = 0.05$.
3. Determine the critical region, that is, the region of values of t in the lower 0.05 tail of the sampling distribution for t (Student's t distribution with 9 degrees of freedom) when $\mu = \mu_0$ (i.e., the sampling distribution when the null hypothesis is true). For $\alpha_0 = 0.05$ the critical value is $t = -1.8331$; therefore, the critical region includes all values of $t < -1.8331$.
4. Compute the t statistic: $t = (\overline{X} - \mu_0)/(s/\sqrt{n})$ for the given sample and sample size $n = 10$. We know that $n = 10$, the sample mean is 1085.9, $s = 717.12$, and $\mu_0 = 2200$. $t = (1085.9 - 2200)/(717.12/\sqrt{10}) = -1114.1/226.773 = -4.913$.
5. Since -4.913 is clearly less than -1.8331, we reject H_0 at the 5% level.

In the previous example, if it were appropriate to use a one-tailed (right tail) test the procedure would change as follows:

In step 1, we would take H_1: $\mu > \mu_0 = 2200$.
In step 3, we would consider the upper α tail of the sampling distribution for t (Student's t distribution with 9 degrees of freedom) when $\mu = \mu_0$ (i.e., the sampling distribution when the null hypothesis is true).
In step 5, the rejection region would be values of $t > 1.8331$.

9.6   *p*-VALUES

The *p*-value is the probability of the occurrence of a value for the test statistic as extreme as or more extreme than the actual observed value, under the assumption that the null hypothesis is true. By more extreme we mean a value in a direction farther from the center of the sampling distribution (under the null hypothesis) than what was observed.

For a one-tailed (right-tailed) *t* test, this statement means the probability that a statistic T with a Student's t distribution satisfies $T > |t|$, where t is the observed value of the test statistic. For a one-tailed (left-hand tail) *t* test, this statement means the probability that a statistic T with a Student's t distribution satisfies $T < -|t|$, where t is the observed value of the test statistic. For a two-tailed *t* test, it means the probability that a statistic T with a Student's t distribution satisfies $|T| > |t|$ (i.e., $T > |t|$ or $T < -|t|$) where t is the observed value of the test statistic.

Now let us now compute the two-sided *p*-value for the test statistic in the pig blood loss example from Section 9.4. Recall that the standard deviation $s = 717.12$, the sample mean $\overline{X} = 1085.9$, the hypothesized value $\mu_0 = 2200$, and the sample size $n = 10$. From this information, we see that the t statistic is $t = (1085.9 - 2200)/(717.12/\sqrt{10}) = -1114.1/226.773 = -4.913$.

To find the two-sided *p*-value we must compute the probability that $T > 4.913$ and add the probability that $T < -4.913$. This combination is equal to $2P(T > 4.913)$. The probability $P(T > 4.913)$ is the one-sided right-tail *p*-value; it is also equal to the one-sided left-tail *p*-value, $P(T < -4.913)$. The table of Student's t distribution shows us that with 9 degrees of freedom, $P(T < 4.781) = 0.9995$. So $P(T > 4.781) = 0.0005$.

Since $P(T > 4.913) < P(T > 4.781)$, we see that the one-sided *p*-value $P(T > 4.913) < 0.0005$; hence, the two-sided *p*-value is less than 0.001. This observation is more informative than just saying that the test is significant at the 5% level. The result is so significant that even for a two-sided test, we would reject the null hypothesis at the 0.1% level.

Most standard statistical packages (e.g., SAS) present *p*-values when providing information on hypothesis test results, and major journal articles usually report *p*-values for their statistical tests. SAS provides *p*-values as small as 0.0001, and anything smaller is reported simply as 0.0001. So when you see a *p*-value of 0.0001 in SAS output, you should interpret it to mean that the *p*-value for the test is actually less than or equal to 0.0001 (sometimes it can be considerably smaller).

9.7   TYPE I AND TYPE II ERRORS

In Section 9.1, we defined the type I error α as the probability of rejecting the null hypothesis when the null hypothesis is true. We saw that in the Neyman–Pearson formulation of hypothesis testing, the type I error rate is fixed at a certain low level. In practice, the choice is usually 0.05 or 0.01. In Sections 9.3 through 9.5, we saw examples of how critical regions were defined based on the distribution of the test statistic under the null hypothesis.

Also in Section 9.1, we defined the type II error as β. The type II error is the probability of not rejecting the null hypothesis when the null hypothesis is false. It depends on the "true" value of the parameter under the alternative hypothesis.

For example, suppose we are testing a null hypothesis that the population mean $\mu = \mu_0$. The type II error depends on the value of $\mu = \mu_1 \neq \mu_0$ under the alternative hypothesis. In the next section, we see that the power of a test is defined as $1 - \beta$. The term "power" refers to the probability of correctly rejecting the null hypothesis when it is in fact false. Given that β depends on the value of μ_1 in the context of testing for a population mean, the power is a function of μ_1; hence, we refer to a power function rather than a single number.

In sample size determination (Section 9.13), we will see that analogous to choosing a width d for a confidence interval, we will select a distance δ for $|\mu_1 - \mu_0|$ such that we achieve a specific high value for the power at that δ. Usually, the value for $1 - \beta$ is chosen to be 0.80, 0.90, or 0.95.

9.8   THE POWER FUNCTION

The power function depends on the significance level of a test and the sampling distribution of the test statistic under the alternative values of the population parameters. For example, when a Z or t statistic is used to test the hypothesis (H_0) that the population mean μ equals μ_0, the power function equals α at $\mu_1 = \mu_0$ and increases as μ moves away from μ_0. The power function approaches 1 as μ_1 gets very far from μ_0. Figure 9.1 shows a plot of the power function for a population mean in the

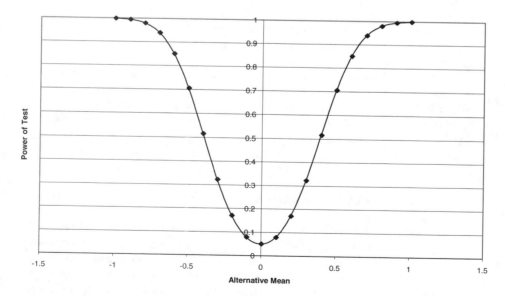

Figure 9.1. Power function for a test that a normal population has mean zero versus a two-sided alternative when the sample size $n = 25$ and the significance level $\alpha = 0.05$.

simple case when $\mu_0 = 0$ and σ is known, the sample size $n = 25$, and the population distribution is assumed to be a normal distribution. In this case, $Z = (\overline{X} - \mu_1)/(\sigma/\sqrt{n}) = (\overline{X} - \mu_1)/(\sigma/5) = 5(\overline{X} - \mu_1)/\sigma$ and Z has a standard normal distribution. This distribution depends on μ_1 and σ. We know the value of σ and can take $\sigma = 1$, recognizing that although the power depends on μ_1 for the curve in Figure 9.1, to be more general we would replace μ_1 with μ_1/σ for other values of σ. The power is the probability of observing Z in the acceptance region that is $P(-C < Z < C)$, where C is the critical value; consequently, the power depends on the sample size and significance level through C as well as the sample size n through the formula for Z.

Figure 9.2 displays, on the same graph used for $n = 25$, the comparable results for a sample size $n = 100$. We see how the power function changes with increased sample size.

9.9   TWO-SAMPLE t TEST (INDEPENDENT SAMPLES WITH A COMMON VARIANCE)

Recall from Section 8.5 the use of the appropriate t statistic for a confidence interval under the following circumstances: the parent populations have normal distribu-

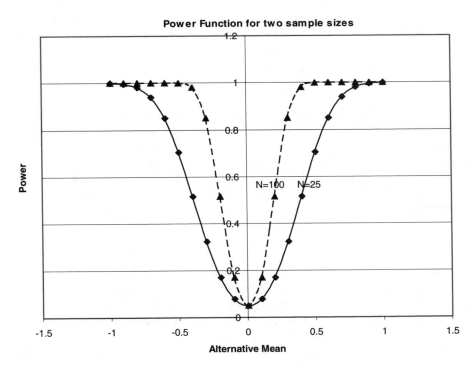

Figure 9.2. Power function for a test that a normal population has mean zero versus a two-sided alternative when the sample size $n = 25$, $n = 100$, and the significance level $\alpha = 0.05$.

tions and common variance that is unknown. In this situation, we used the pooled variance estimate, s_p^2, calculated by the formula $S_p^2 = \{S_t^2(n_t - 1) + S_c^2(n_c - 1)\}/[n_t + n_c - 2]$.

Suppose we want to evaluate whether the means of two independent samples selected from two parent populations are significantly different. We will use a t test with s_p^2 as the pooled variance estimate. The corresponding t statistic is $t = \{(\overline{X}_t - \overline{X}_c) - (\mu_t - \mu_c)\}/[S_p\sqrt{(1/n_t) + (1/n_c)}]$. The formula for t is obtained by replacing the common σ in the formula for the two sample Z test with the pooled estimate S_p. The resulting statistic has Student's t distribution with $n_t + n_c - 2$ degrees of freedom. This sample t statistic is used for hypothesis testing. For a two-sided test the steps are as follows:

1. State the null hypothesis H_0: $\mu_t = \mu_c$ versus the alternative hypothesis H_1: $\mu_t \neq \mu_c$.
2. Choose a significance level $\alpha = \alpha_0$ (often we take $\alpha_0 = 0.05$ or 0.01).
3. Determine the critical region, that is, the region of values of t in the upper and lower $\alpha/2$ tails of the sampling distribution for Student's t distribution with $n_t + n_c - 2$ degrees of freedom when $\mu_t = \mu_c$ (i.e., the sampling distribution when the null hypothesis is true).
4. Compute the t statistic: $t = \{(\overline{X}_t - \overline{X}_c) - (\mu_t - \mu_c)\}/[S_p\sqrt{(1/n_t) + (1/n_c)}]$ for the given sample and sample sizes n_t and n_c, where $\overline{X}_t$ is the sample mean for the treatment group, $\overline{X}_c$ is the sample mean for the control group, and S_p is the pooled sample standard deviation.
5. Reject the null hypothesis if the test statistic t (computed in step 4) falls in the rejection region for this test; otherwise, do not reject the null hypothesis.

We will apply these steps to the pig blood loss data from Section 8.7, Table 8.1. Recall that $S_p^2 = \{S_t^2(n_t - 1) + S_c^2(n_c - 1)\}/[n_t + n_c - 2] = \{(717.12)^2\,9 + (1824.27)^2\,9\}/18$, since $n_t = n_c = 10$, $S_t = 717.12$, and $S_c = 1824.27$. So $S_p^2 = 2178241.61$ and taking the square root we find $S_p = 1475.89$. As the degrees of freedom are $n_t + n_c - 2 = 18$, we find that the constant C from the table of the Student's t distribution is 2.101. Applying steps 1–5 to the pig blood loss data for a two-tailed (two-sided) test, we have:

1. State the null hypothesis H_0: $\mu_t = \mu_c$ versus the alternative hypothesis H_1: $\mu_t \neq \mu_c$.
2. Choose a significance level $\alpha = \alpha_0 = 0.05$.
3. Determine the critical region, that is, the region of values of t in the upper and lower 0.025 tails of the sampling distribution for Student's t distribution with 18 degrees of freedom when μ_t/μ_c (i.e., the sampling distribution when the null hypothesis is true).
4. Compute the t statistic: $t = \{(\overline{X}_t - \overline{X}_c) - (\mu_t - \mu_c)\}/[S_p\sqrt{(1/n_t) + (1/n_c)}]$. We are given that the sample sizes are $n_t = 10$ and $n_c = 10$, respectively. Under the null hypothesis, $\mu_t - \mu_c = 0$ and $\overline{X}_t - \overline{X}_c = 1085.9 - 2187.4 = -1101.5$ and s_p,

the pooled sample standard deviation, is 1475.89. Since $\sqrt{(1/n_t) + (1/n_c)]} = \sqrt{2/20} = \sqrt{0.1} = 0.316$, $t = -1101.5/(1475.89)0.316 = -2.362$.

5. Now, since $-2.362 < -C = -2.101$, we reject H_0.

9.10   PAIRED *t* TEST

Previously, we covered statistical tests (e.g., the independent groups Z test and t test) for assessing differences between group means derived from independent samples. In some medical applications, we use measures that are paired; examples are comparison of pre–post test results from the same subject, comparisons of twins, and comparisons of littermates. In these situations, there is an expected correlation (relationship) between any pair of responses. The paired t test looks at treatment differences in medical studies that have paired observations.

The paired t test is used to detect treatment differences when measurements from one group of subjects are correlated with measurements from another. You will learn about correlation in more detail in Chapter 12. For now, just think of correlation as a positive relationship. The paired t test evaluates within-subject comparisons, meaning that a subject's scores collected at an earlier time are compared with his own scores collected at a later time. The scores of twin pairs are analogous to within-subject comparisons.

The results of subjects' responses to pre- and posttest measures tend to be related. To illustrate, if we measure children's gains in intelligence over time, their later scores are related to their initial scores. (Smart children will continue to be smart when they are remeasured.) When such a correlation exists, the pairing can lead to a mean difference that has less variability than would occur had the groups been completely independent of each other. This reduction in variance implies that a more powerful test (the paired t test) can be constructed than for the independent case. Similarly, paired t tests can allow the construction of more precise confidence intervals than would be obtained by using independent groups t tests.

For the paired t test, the sample sizes n_t and n_c must be equal, which is one disadvantage of the test. Paired tests often occur in crossover clinical trials. In such trials, the patient is given one treatment for a time, the outcome of the treatment is measured, and then the patient is put on another treatment (the control treatment). Usually, there is a waiting period, called a washout period, between the treatments to make sure that the effect of the first treatment is no longer present when the second treatment is started.

First, we will provide background information about the logic of the paired t test and then give some calculation examples using the data from Tables 9.1 and 9.2. Matching or pairing of subjects is done by patient; i.e., the difference is taken between the first treatment for patient A and the second treatment for patient A, and so on for patient B and all other patients. The differences are then averaged over the set of n patients.

As implied at the beginning of this section, we do not compute differences between treatment 1 for patient A and treatment 2 for patient B. The positive correlation between the treatments exists because the patient himself is the common factor. We wish to avoid mixing patient-to-patient variability with the treatment effect in the computed paired difference. As physicians enjoy saying, "the patient acts as his own control."

Order effects refer to the order of the presentation of the treatments in experimental studies such as clinical trials. Some clinical trials have multiple treatments; others have a treatment condition and a control or placebo condition. Order effects may influence the outcome of a clinical trial. In the case in which a patient serves as his own control, we may not think that it matters whether the treatment or control condition occurs first. Although we cannot rule out order effects, they are easy to minimize; we can minimize them by randomizing the order of presentation of the experimental conditions. For example, in a clinical trial that has a treatment and a control condition, patients could be randomized to either leg of the trial so that one-half of the patients would receive the treatment first and one-half the control first.

By looking at paired differences (i.e., differences between treatments A and B for each patient), we gain precision by having less variability in these paired differences than with an independent-groups model; however, the act of pairing discards the individual observations (there were $2n$ of them and now we are left with only n paired differences). We will see that the resulting t statistic will have only $n - 1$ degrees of freedom rather than the $2n - 2$ degrees of freedom as in the t test for differences between means of two independent samples.

Although we have achieved less variability in the sample differences, the paired t test cuts the sample size by a factor of two. When the correlation between treatments A and B is high (and consequently the variability is reduced considerably), pairing will pay off for us. But if the observations being paired were truly independent, the pairing could actually weaken our analysis.

A paired t-test (two-sided test) consists of the following steps:

1. Form the paired differences.
2. State the null hypothesis H_0: $\mu_t = \mu_c$ versus the alternative hypothesis H_1: $\mu_t \neq \mu_c$. (As H_0:$\mu_t = \mu_c$, we also can say H_0: $\mu_t - \mu_c = 0$; H_1: $\mu_t - \mu_c \neq 0$.)
3. Choose a significance level $\alpha = \alpha_0$ (often we take $\alpha_0 = 0.05$ or 0.01).
4. Determine the critical region; that is, the region of values of t in the upper and lower $\alpha/2$ tails of the sampling distribution for Student's t distribution with $n - 1$ degrees of freedom when μ_t/μ_c (i.e., the sampling distribution when the null hypothesis is true) and when $n = n_t = n_c$.
5. Compute the t statistic: $t = \{\bar{d} - (\mu_t - \mu_c)\}/[S_d/\sqrt{n}]$ for the given sample and sample size n for the paired differences, where $\bar{d}$ is the sample mean difference between groups and s_d is the sample standard deviation for the paired differences.
6. Reject the null hypothesis if the test statistic t (computed in step 4) falls in the rejection region for this test; otherwise, do not reject the null hypothesis.

Now we will now look at an example of how to perform a paired t test. A striking example where the correlation between two groups is due to a seasonal effect follows. Although it is a weather example, these kinds of results can occur easily in clinical trial data as well. The data are fictitious but are realistic temperatures for the two cities at various times during the year. We are considering two temperature readings from stations that are located in neighboring cities such as Washington, D.C., and New York. We may think that it tends to be a little warmer in Washington, but seasonal effects could mask a slight difference of a few degrees.

We want to test the null hypothesis that the average daily temperatures of the two cities are the same. We will test this hypothesis versus the two-sided alternative that there is a difference between the cities. We are given the data in Table 9.1, which shows the mean temperature on the 15th of each month during a 12-month period.

Now let us consider the two-sample t test as though the data for the cities were independent. Later we will see that this is a faulty assumption. The means for Washington $(\overline{X}_1)$ and New York $(\overline{X}_2)$ equal 56.16°F and 52.5°F, respectively. Is the difference (3.66) between these means statistically significant? We test H_0: $\mu_1 - \mu_2 = 0$ against the alternative H_1: $\mu_1 - \mu_2 \neq 0$, where μ_1 is the population mean temperature for Washington and μ_2 is the population mean temperature for New York. The respective sample standard deviations, S_1 and S_2, equal 23.85 and 23.56. These sample standard deviations are close enough to make plausible the assumption that the population standard deviations are equal.

Consequently, we use the pooled variance $S_p^2 = \{S_1^2(n_1 - 1) + S_2^2(n_2-1)\}/[n_1 + n_2 - 2]$. In this case, $S_p^2 = [11(23.85)^2 + 11 (23.56)^2]/22$. These data yield $S_p^2 = 561.95$ or $S_p = 23.71$. Now the two-sample t statistic is $t = (56.16 - 52.5)/\sqrt{561.95(2/12)} = 3.66/\sqrt{561.95/6} = 3.66/9.68 = 0.378$. Clearly, $t = 0.378$ is not significant. From the table for the t distribution with 22 degrees of freedom, the critical value even for α

TABLE 9.1. Daily Temperatures in Washington and New York

Day	Washington Mean Temperature (°F)	New York Mean Temperature (°F)
1 (January 15)	31	28
2 (February 15)	35	33
3 (March 15)	40	37
4 (April 15)	52	45
5 (May 15)	70	68
6 (June 15)	76	74
7 (July 15)	93	89
8 (August 15)	90	85
9 (September 15)	74	69
10 (October 15)	55	51
11 (November 15)	32	27
12 (December 15)	26	24

= 0.10 would be 1.7171. So it seems to be convincing that the difference is not significant.

But let us look more closely at the data. The independence assumption does not hold. We can see that temperatures are much higher in summer months than in winter months for both cities. We see that the month-to-month variability is large and dominant over the variability between cities for any given day. So if we pair temperatures on the same days for these cities we will remove the effect of month-to-month variability and have a better chance to detect a difference between cities. Now let us follow the paired t test procedure based on data from Table 9.2.

Here we see that the mean difference $\bar{d}$ is again 3.66 but the standard deviation $S_d = 1.614$, which is a dramatic reduction in variation over the pooled estimate of 23.71! (You can verify these numbers on your own by using the data from Table 9.2.)

We are beginning to see the usefulness of pairing: $t = (\bar{d} - (\mu_1 - \mu_2))/(S_d/\sqrt{n}) = (3.66 - 0)/(1.614/\sqrt{12}) = 3.66/0.466 = 7.86$. This t value is highly significant because even for an alpha of 0.001 with a t of 11 degrees of freedom ($n - 1 = 11$), the critical value is only 4.437!

This outcome is truly astonishing! Using an unpaired test with this temperature data we were not even close to a statistically significant result, but with an appropriate choice for pairing, the significance of the paired differences between the cities is extremely high. These two opposite findings indicate how wrong one can be when using erroneous assumptions.

There is no magic to statistical methods. Bad assumptions lead to bad answers. Another indication that it was warmer in Washington than in New York is the fact that the average temperature in Washington was higher for all twelve days.

In Section 14.4, we will consider a nonparametric technique called the sign test. Under the null hypothesis that the two cities have the same mean temperatures each

TABLE 9.2. Daily Temperatures for Two Cities and Their Paired Differences

Day	Washington Mean Temperature (°F)	New York Mean Temperature (°F)	Paired Difference #1 – #2
1 (January 15)	31	28	3
2 (February 15)	35	33	2
3 (March 15)	40	37	3
4 (April 15)	52	45	7
5 (May 15)	70	68	2
6 (June 15)	76	74	2
7 (July 15)	93	89	4
8 (August 15)	90	85	5
9 (September 15)	74	69	5
10 (October 15)	55	51	4
11 (November 15)	32	27	5
12 (December 15)	26	24	2

day of the year, the probability of Washington being warmer than New York would be 0.5 on each day. In the sample, this outcome occurs 12 days in a row. According to the sign test, the probability of this outcome under the null hypothesis is $(0.50)^{12}$ = 0.00024.

Finally, let us go through the six steps for the paired t test using the temperature data:

1. Form the paired differences (the far right column in Table 9.2).
2. State the null hypothesis H_0: $\mu_1 = \mu_2$ or $\mu_1 - \mu_2 = 0$ versus the alternative hypothesis H_1: $\mu_1 \neq \mu_2$ or $\mu_1 - \mu_2 \neq 0$.
3. Choose a significance level $\alpha = \alpha_0 = 0.01$.
4. Determine the critical region, that is, the region of values of t in the upper and lower 0.005 tails of the sampling distribution for Student's t distribution with $n - 1 = 11$ degrees of freedom when $\mu_1 = \mu_2$ (i.e., the sampling distribution when the null hypothesis is true) and when $n = n_1 = n_2$.
5. Compute the t statistic: $t = \{\bar{d} - (\mu_1 - \mu_2)\}/[S_d/\sqrt{n}]$ for the given sample and sample size n for the paired differences, where $\bar{d} = 3.66$ is the sample mean difference between groups and $S_d = 1.614$ is the sample standard deviation for the paired differences.
6. Reject the null hypothesis if the test statistic t (computed in step 5) falls in the rejection region for this test; otherwise, do not reject the null hypothesis. For a t with 11 degrees of freedom and $\alpha = 0.01$, the critical value is 3.1058. Because the test statistic t is 7.86, we reject H_0.

9.11 RELATIONSHIP BETWEEN CONFIDENCE INTERVALS AND HYPOTHESIS TESTS

Hypothesis tests and confidence intervals have a one-to-one correspondence. This correspondence allows us to use a confidence interval to form a hypothesis test or to use the critical regions defined for a hypothesis test to construct a confidence interval. Up to this point, we have not needed this relationship, as we have constructed hypothesis tests and confidence intervals independently. However, in the next section we will exploit this relationship for bootstrap tests. With the bootstrap, it is natural to construct confidence intervals for parameters. We will use the one-to-one correspondence between hypothesis tests and confidence intervals to determine a bootstrap hypothesis test based on a bootstrap confidence interval (refer to Section 9.12).

The correspondence works as follows: Suppose we want to test the null hypothesis that a parameter $\theta = \theta_0$, versus the alternative hypothesis that $\theta \neq \theta_0$ at the $100\alpha\%$ significance level; we have a method to obtain a $100(1 - \alpha)\%$ confidence interval for θ. Then we test the null hypothesis $\theta = \theta_0$ as follows: If θ_0 is contained in the $100(1 - \alpha)\%$ confidence interval for θ, then do not reject H_0; if θ_0 lies outside the region, then reject H_0. Such a test will have a significance level of $100\alpha\%$. By $100\alpha\%$ significance we mean the same thing as an α level but express α as a percentage.

On the other hand, suppose we have a critical region defined for the test of a null hypothesis that $\theta = \theta_0$, against a two-sided alternative at the $100\alpha\%$ significance level. Then, the set of all values of θ_0 that would lead to not rejecting the null hypothesis form a $100(1 - \alpha)\%$ confidence region for θ.

As an example let us consider the one sample test of a mean with the variance known. Suppose we have a sample of size 25 with a standard deviation of 5. The sample mean $\overline{X}$ is 0.5, and we wish to test $\mu = 0$ versus the alternative that $\mu \neq 0$. A 95% confidence interval for μ is then $[\overline{X} - 1.96\ \sigma/\sqrt{n}, \overline{X} + 1.96\sigma/\sqrt{n}] = [0.5 - 1.96, 0.5 + 1.96] = [-1.46, 2.46]$, since $\sigma = 5$ and $\sqrt{n} = 5$. Thus, values of the sample mean that fall into this interval are in the nonrejection region for the 5% significance level test based on the one-to-one correspondence between hypothesis tests and confidence intervals. In our case with $\overline{X} = 0.5$, we do not reject H_0, because 0 is contained in the interval The same would be true for any value in the interval. The nonrejection region for the 5% level two-sided test contains the values of $\overline{X}$ such that 0 lies inside the interval, and the rejection region is the set of $\overline{X}$ values such that 0 lies outside the interval, which is formed by $\overline{X} + 1.96 < 0$ or $\overline{X} - 1.96 > 0$ or $\overline{X} < -1.96$ or $\overline{X} > 1.96$ or $|\overline{X}| > 1.96$.

Note that had we constructed the 5% two-sided test directly, using the procedure we developed in Section 9.3, we would have obtained the same result.

Also, by taking the critical region defined by $|\overline{X}| > 1.96$ that we obtain directly in Section 9.3, the one-to-one correspondence gives us a 95% confidence interval $[0.5 - 1.96, 0.5 + 1.96] = [-1.46, 2.46]$, exactly the confidence interval we would get directly using the method of Section 8.4. In the formula for the two-sided test, we replace $\overline{X}$ with 0.5 and $\sigma/\sqrt{n}$ with 1.0.

9.12   BOOTSTRAP PERCENTILE METHOD TEST

Previously, we considered one of the simplest forms for approximate bootstrap confidence intervals, namely, Efron's percentile method. Although there are many other ways to generate bootstrap type confidence intervals, such methods are beyond the scope of this text. Some methods have better properties than the percentile method. To learn more about them, see Chernick (1999), Efron and Tibshirani (1993), or Carpenter and Bithell (2000). However, the relationship given in the previous section tells us that for any such confidence interval we can construct a hypothesis test through the one-to-one correspondence principle. Here we will demonstrate bootstrap confidence intervals for the bootstrap percentile method.

Recall that in Section 8.9 we had the following ten values for blood loss for the pigs in the treatment group: 543, 666, 455, 823, 1716, 797, 2828, 1251, 702, and 1078. The sample mean was 1085.9. Using the Resampling Stats software, we found (based on 10,000 bootstrap samples) that an approximate two-sided percentile method 95% confidence interval for the population mean μ was [727.1, 1558.9].

From this information, we can construct a bootstrap hypothesis test of the null hypothesis that the mean $\mu = \mu_0$, versus the two-sided alternative that $\mu \neq \mu_0$. The test rejects the null hypothesis if the hypothesized $\mu_0 < 727.1$ or if the hypothesized $\mu_0 > 1558.9$. We will know μ_0 and the result depends on whether or not μ_0 is in the confidence interval. Recall we reject H_0 if μ_0 is outside the interval.

9.13 SAMPLE SIZE DETERMINATION FOR HYPOTHESIS TESTS

In Section 8.10, we showed you how to determine the required sample size based on a criterion for confidence intervals, namely, to require the half-width or width of the confidence interval to be less than a specified δ. For hypothesis testing, one can also set up a criterion for sample size. Recall from Section 9.8 that we defined and illustrated in a particular example the power function for a two-sided test. We showed that if the level of a two-sided test (such as for a population mean or mean difference) is α, then the power of the test at the null hypothesis value (e.g., μ_0 for a population mean) is equal to α and increases as we move away from the null hypothesis value.

We learned that the power function is symmetric about the null hypothesis value and increases to 1 as we move far away from that value. We also saw that when the sample size is increased, the power function increases rapidly. This information suggests that we could specify a level of power (e.g., 90%) and a separation δ such that for a true mean μ satisfying $|\mu - \mu_0| > \delta$, the power of the test at that value of μ is at least 90%.

For a given δ, this will not be achieved for small sample sizes; however, as the sample size increases there will be eventually a minimum value n at which the power will exceed 90% for the given δ. Various software packages including nQuery Advisor, PASS 2000, and Power and Precision enable you to calculate the required n or to determine the power that can be achieved at that δ for a specified n.

In the Tendril DX clinical trial, Chernick and associates calculated the difference between the treatment and control group means using an unpaired t test; the sample size was $n_t = 3n_c$, where n_t was the sample size for the treatment group and n_c was the sample size for the control group. In this problem, Chernick took $\delta = 0.5$ volts, set the power at 80%, and assumed a common σ tested at the 0.10 significance level for a two-sided test. The resulting calculations required a sample size of 99 for the treatment group and 33 for the control group, leading to a total sample size of 132. Note that if instead we required $n_t = n_c$, then the required value for n_t is 49 for a total sample size of 98. Table 9.3 shows the actual table output from nQuery. In most cases, you can rely on the software to give you the solution. In some cases, there is not a simple formula, but in other cases simple sample size formulas can be obtained similar to the ones we derived in Chapter 8 for fixed-width confidence intervals.

TABLE 9.3. nQuery Advisor 4.0 Table for 3:1 and 1:1 Sample Size Ratios for Tendril DX Trial Design

Test significance level α	0.100	0.100
1 or 2 sided test?	2	2
Group 1 mean μ_1	1.000	1.000
Group 2 mean μ_2	0.500	0.500
Difference in means, $\mu_1 - \mu_2$	0.500	0.500
Common standard deviation, σ	0.980	0.980
Effect size, $\delta = |\mu_1 - \mu_2|/\sigma$	0.510	0.510
Power (%)	80	80
n_1	33	49
n_2	99	49
Ratio: n_2/n_1	3.000	1.000
$N = n_1 + n_2$	132	98

9.14   SENSITIVITY AND SPECIFICITY IN MEDICAL DIAGNOSIS

Screening tests are used to identify patients who should be referred for diagnostic evaluation. The validity of screening tests is evaluated by comparing their screening results with those obtained from a "gold standard." The gold standard is the definitive diagnosis for the disease. However, it should be noted that screening is not the same thing as diagnosis; it is a method applied to a population of apparently healthy individuals in order to identify those who may have unrecognized or subclinical conditions. In designing a screening test, physicians need to identify a particular cutoff measurement from a set of measurements in order to discriminate between healthy and "diseased" persons.

These measurements for healthy individuals can have a range of normal values that overlap with values for patients having the disease. Also, the very nature of measurement leads to some amount of error. For some illnesses, there is no ideal screening measure that perfectly discriminates between the patients who are free from disease and those with the disease. As a result, there is a possibility that the screening test will classify a patient with a disease as normal and a patient without the disease as having the disease.

An example is blood glucose screening test for diabetes. Blood sugar measurements for diabetic and normal persons form two overlapping curves. Some high normal blood sugar values overlap the lower end of the distribution for diabetic patients. If we declare that a blood glucose value of 120 should form the cutoff between normal and diabetic persons, we will unwittingly include a few nondiabetic persons with diabetic individuals.

If we formulated the screening test as a statistical hypothesis testing problem, we would see that these two types of error could be the type I and type II errors for the hypothesis test. In medical diagnosis, however, we use special terminology. Refer to Table 9.4 and the discussion that follows the table for the definitions of these terms.

Suppose we applied a screening test to n patients and out of the n patients ob-

TABLE 9.4. Sensitivity and Specificity in Diagnostic Testing

Test Results	True Condition of the Patient According to the Gold Standard		Total
	Diseased	Not Diseased	
Disease Present	a	b	$a + b = s$
Disease Absent	c	d	$c + d = n - s$
Total	$a + c = m$	$B + d = n - m$	$a + b + c + d = n$

tained the following outcomes. The test screens s of the patients as positive (indicating the presence of the disease) and $n - s$ as negative (indicating the absence of the disease). In reality, if we knew the truth (according to the gold standard or otherwise), there are m patients with the disease and $n - m$ patients without the disease.

The s patients diagnosed with the disease include a patients who actually have it and b patients who do not. So $s = a + b$. Now, of the m patients who actually have the disease, a were diagnosed with it from the test and c were not. So $m = a + c$. This leaves d patients who do not have the disease and are diagnosed as not having it. So $d = n - s - c = n - s - m + a$. The results are summarized in Table 9.4.

The off-diagonal terms b and c represent the number of "false positives" and "false negatives," respectively. The ratio b/n is an estimate of the probability of a false positive, and c/n is an estimate of the probability of a false negative.

Also of interest are the conditional error rates, estimated by $b/(n - m) = b/(b + d)$ and $c/m = c/(c + a)$, which represent, respectively, the conditional probability of a positive test result given that the patient does not have the disease and the conditional probability of a negative test result given that the patient does have the disease.

Related to these conditional error rates are the conditional rates of correct classification known as specificity and sensitivity, the definitions of which follow.

Sensitivity is the probability that the screening test identifies the patient as having the disease (a positive test result) given that he or she does in fact have the disease. The name comes about because a test that has a high probability of correct detection is thought to be highly sensitive. An estimate of sensitivity from Table 9.4 is $a/(a + c) = 1 - c/(a + c) = 1 - c/m$. This is 1 minus the conditional probability of a false positive.

Specificity is the probability that a screening test declares the patient well (a negative test result), given that he or she does not have the disease. From Table 9.4, specificity is estimated by $d/(b + d) = 1 - b/(b + d) = 1 - b/(n - m)$. This is 1 minus the conditional probability of a false negative.

Ideally, a screening test should have high sensitivity and high specificity; i.e., the specificity and the sensitivity should be as close to 1 as possible. However, measurement error and imperfect discriminators make it impossible for either value to be 1. Recall that in hypothesis testing if we are given the test statistic for a fixed sample size, we can change the type I error by changing the cutoff value that determines the critical region. But any change that decreases the type I error will increase the type II error, so we have a trade-off between the two error rates. The same trade-off is true regarding the conditional error rates; consequently, increasing sensitivity will decrease specificity and vice versa. For a further discussion of screening tests, consult Friis and Sellers (1999).

9.15   META-ANALYSIS

Two problems often occur regarding clinical trials:

1. Often, clinical studies do not encompass large enough samples of patients to reach definitive conclusions.
2. Two or more studies may have conflicting results (possibly because of type I and type II errors).

A technique that is being used more and more frequently to address these problems is meta-analysis. Meta-analyses are statistical techniques for combining data, summary statistics, or p-values from various similar tests to reach stronger and more consistent conclusions about the results from clinical trials and other empirical studies than is possible with a single study.

Care is required in the selection of the trials to avoid potential biases in the process of combining results. Several excellent books address these issues, for example, Hedges and Olkin (1985). The volume edited by Stangl and Berry (2000) presents several illustrations that use the Bayesian hierarchical modeling approach. The hierarchical approach puts a Bayesian prior distribution on the unknown parameters. This prior distribution will depend on other unknown parameters called hyperparameters. Additional prior distributions are specified for the hyperparameters, thus establishing a hierarchy of prior distributions. It is not important for you to understand the Bayesian hierarchical approach, but if you are interested in the details, see Stangl and Berry (2000). We will define prior and posterior distributions and Bayes rule in the next section. Bayesian hierarchical models are also used in an inferential approach called the empirical Bayes method. You might encounter this terminology if you study some of the literature.

In this section, we will show you two real-life examples in which Chernick used a particular method, Fisher's test, which R. A. Fisher (1932) and K. Pearson (1933) developed for combining p-values in a meta-analysis. These illustrations will give you some appreciation of the value of meta-analysis and will provide you with a simple tool that you could use, given an appropriate selection of studies.

The rationale for Fisher's test is as follows: The distribution theory for a test statistic proposed that under the null hypothesis each study would have a p-value that comes from a uniform distribution on the interval $[0, 1]$. Denote a particular p-value by the random variable U. Let L also refer to a random variable. Now consider the transformation $L = -2 \ln(U)$ where ln is the logarithm to the base e. It can be shown mathematically that the random variable L has a chi-square distribution with 2 degrees of freedom. (You will encounter a more general discussion of the chi-square distribution in Chapter 11.)

Suppose we have k independent trials to be combined and $U_1, U_2, U_3, \ldots, U_k$ are the random variables denoting the p-values for the k independent trials. Now consider the variable $L_k = -2 \ln(U_1, U_2, U_3, \ldots, U_k) = -2 \ln(U_1) - 2 \ln(U_2) - 2 \ln(U_3) - \ldots - 2 \ln(U_k)$; then L_k is the sum of k independent chi-square random variables each with 2 degrees of freedom. It is known that the sum of independent chi-square random variables is a chi-square random variable with degrees of freedom equal to the sum of the degrees of freedom for the individual chi-square random variables in the summation. Therefore, L_k is a chi-square variable with $2k$ degrees of freedom.

The chi-square with $2k$ degrees of freedom is, therefore, the reference distribution that holds under the null hypothesis of no effect. We will see in the upcoming examples that the alternative of a significant difference should produce p-values that are concentrated closer to zero rather than being uniformly distributed. Lower values of the U's lead to higher values of L_k. So we select a cutoff based on the upper tail of the chi-square with $2k$ degrees of freedom. The critical value is determined, of course, by the significance level α that we specify for Fisher's test.

In the first example, one of us (Chernick) was consulting for a medical device company that manufactured an instrument called a cutting balloon for use in angioplasty procedures. The company conducted a controlled clinical trial in Europe and in the United States to show a reduction in restenosis rate for the cutting balloon angioplasty procedure over conventional balloon angioplasty. Other studies indicated that conventional angioplasty had a restenosis rate near 40%.

The manufacturer had seen that procedures with the cutting balloon were achieving rates in the 20%–25% range. They powered the trial to detect at least a 10% improvement (i.e., reduction in restenosis). However, results were somewhat mixed, possibly due to physicians' differing angioplasty practices and differing patient selection criteria in the various countries.

Example 8.5.2 in Chernick (1999) presents the clinical trial results using the bootstrap for a comparative country analysis. The results of the meta-analysis, not reported there, are given in Table 9.5. Countries A, B, C, and D are European countries, and country E is the United States.

The difficulty for the manufacturer was that although the rate of 22% in the United States was statistically significantly lower than the 40% that is known for con-

TABLE 9.5. Balloon Angioplasty Restenosis Rates by Country

Country	Restenosis Rate % (failures/# of patients)
A	40% (18/45)
B	41% (58/143)
C	29% (20/70)
D	29% (51/177)
E	22% (26/116)

ventional balloon angioplasty, the values in countries A and B were not lower, and the combined results for all countries were not statistically significantly lower than 40%. Some additional statistical analyses gave indications about variables that explained the differences. These explanations led to hypotheses about the criteria for selection of patients.

However, these data were not convincing enough for the regulatory authorities to approve the procedure without some labeling restrictions on the types of patients eligible for it. The procedure did not create any safety issues relative to conventional angioplasty. The company was aware of several other studies that could be combined with this trial to provide a meta-analysis that might be more definitive. Chernick and associates conducted the meta-analysis using Fisher's method for combining p-values.

In the analysis, Chernick considered six peer-reviewed studies of the cutting balloon along with the combined results for the clinical trial already mentioned (referred to as GRT). In the latter study, sensitivity analyses also were conducted regarding the choice of studies to include with the GRT. The other six studies are referred to by the name of the first listed author of each study. (Refer to Table 9.6.)

The variable CB ratio refers to the restenosis rate for the cutting balloon, whereas PTCA ratio is the corresponding restenosis rate for conventional balloon-angioplasty-treated patients. Table 9.6 shows the results for these studies and the combined Fisher test. Here $k = 7$ (the number of independent trials), so the reference chi-square distribution has 14 ($2k$) degrees of freedom.

The table provides the individual p-values (the U's for the Fisher chi-square test) that are based on a procedure called Fisher's exact test for comparing two proportions (see Chapter 11). Note that we have two test procedures here; both are called Fisher's test because they were devised by the same famous statistician, R. A. Fisher. However, there is no need for confusion. Fisher's exact test is applied in each study to compare the restenosis rates and calculate the individual p-values. Then we use these seven p-values to compute Fisher's chi-square statistic in order to determine their combined p-value. Note that the most significant test was Suzuki with a p-value of 0.001, and the least significant was the GRT itself with a p-value equal to 0.7455. However, the combined p-value is a convincing 0.000107.

TABLE 9.6. Meta-Analysis for Combined p-values in Balloon Angioplasty Studies

Study	CB Ratio	PTCA Ratio	p-Value	$-2\ln(U)$
GRT	173/551	170/559	0.7455	0.5874
Molstad	5/30	8/31	0.5339	1.2551
Inoue	7/32	13/32	0.1769	3.4643
Kondo	22/95	40/95	0.0083	9.5830
Ergene	14/51	22/47	0.0483	6.0606
Nozaki	26/98	40/93	0.022	7.6334
Suzuki	104/357	86/188	0.001	13.8155
Combined	—	—	0.000107	42.3994

TABLE 9.7. Comparison of Blood Loss Studies with Combined Meta-Analysis

Name	Test #	p-Value	$-2 \ln(p)$
Lynn_01	1	0.44	1.641961
Lynn_02	2	0.029	7.080919
Martinowitz_01	3	0.0947	4.714083
Schreiber_01	4	0.371	1.983106
Scheiber_02	5	0.0856	4.91614
	Total		20.33621
	Combined p-value	0.026228379	

In the next example, we look at animal studies of blood loss in pigs when comparing the use of Novo Nordisk's clotting agent NovoSeven® with conventional treatment. Three investigators performed five studies; the results of the individual tests for mean differences and Fisher's chi-square test are given in Table 9.7.

It is interesting to note here that although in all studies we used the Wilcoxon test for differences, it does not matter what tests are used to obtain the individual p-values. All we need is that the individual p-values have a uniform distribution under the null hypothesis and be independent of the other tests. Generally, these conditions are met for a large variety of parametric and nonparametric tests. We could have mixed t tests with Wilcoxon or with any other test of the null hypotheses.

9.16 BAYESIAN METHODS

The Bayesian paradigm provides an approach to statistical inference that is different from the methods we have considered thus far. Although the topic is not commonly taught in introductory statistical courses, we believe that Bayesian methods deserve coverage in this text. Despite the fact that the basic idea goes back to Thomas Bayes' treatise written more that 200 years ago, the use of the Bayesian idea as a tool of inference really took place mostly in the 20th century. There are now many books on the subject, even though it was not previously in favor among mainstream statisticians.

In the 1990s, Bayesian methods had a rebirth in popularity with the advent of fast computational techniques (especially the Markov chain Monte Carlo approaches), which allowed computation of general posterior probability distributions that had been difficult or impossible to compute (or approximate) previously. Posterior distributions will be defined shortly. Bayesian hierarchical methods now are being used in medical device submissions to the FDA.

A good introductory text that provides the Bayesian prospective was authored by Berry (1996). Bayesian hierarchical models also are used as a method for doing meta-analyses (as described from the frequentist approach in the previous section). An excellent treatment of use of meta-analyses (Bayesian approaches) in many medical applications is given in Stangl and Berry (2000), which we mentioned in the previous section.

Basically, in the Bayesian approach to inference, the unknown parameters are treated as random quantities with probability distributions to describe their uncertainty. Prior to collecting data, a distribution called the prior distribution is chosen to describe our belief about the possible values of the parameters.

Although Bayesian analysis is simple when there is only one parameter, often we are interested in more than one parameter. In addition, one or more nuisance parameters may be involved, as is the case in frequentist inference about a mean when the variance is unknown. In this instance, the mean is the parameter of interest and the variance is a nuisance parameter. In frequentist analysis, we estimate the variance from the data and use it to form a t statistic whose frequency distribution does not depend on the nuisance parameter. In the Bayesian approach, we determine a bivariate prior distribution for the mean and variance; we use Bayes' rule and the data to construct a bivariate posterior distribution for the mean and variance; then we integrate over the values for the variance to obtain a marginal posterior distribution for the mean.

Bayes' rule is simply a mathematical formula that says that you find the posterior distribution for a parameter θ by taking the prior distribution for θ and multiplying it by the likelihood for the data given a specified value of θ. For the mean, this likelihood can be regarded as the sample distribution for $\overline{X}$ when the population variance is assumed to be known and the population mean is a specified μ. We know by the central limit theorem that this distribution is approximately normal with mean μ and variance σ^2/n, where σ^2 is the known variance and n is the sample size. The density function for this normal distribution is the likelihood. We multiply the likelihood by the prior density for μ to get the posterior density, called the posterior density of μ given the sample mean $\overline{X}$.

There is controversy among the schools of statistical inference (Bayesian and frequentist). With respect to the Bayesian approach, the controversy involves the treatment of μ as a random quantity with a prior distribution. In the discrete case, it is a simple law of conditional probabilities that if X and Y are two random quantities, then $P[X = x | Y = y] = P[X = x, Y = y]/P[Y = y] = P[Y = y | X = x]P[X = x]/P[Y = y]$. Now, $P[Y = y] = \Sigma_x P[Y = y, X = x]$. This leads to Bayes' rule, the uncontroversial mathematical result that $P[X = x | Y = y] = P[Y = y | X = x]P[X = x]/\Sigma_x P[Y = y, X = x]$.

In the problem of a population mean, the Bayesian followers take X to be the population mean and Y the sample estimate. The left-hand side of the above equation $\{P[X = x | Y = y]\}$ is the posterior distribution (or density) for X, and the right-hand side is the appropriately scaled likelihood for Y, given X ($P[Y = y | X = x]/\Sigma_x P[Y = y, X = x]$) multiplied by the prior distribution (or density) for X at x (namely, $P[X = x]$). The formula applies for continuous or discrete random quantities but is derived more easily in the discrete case. The mathematics cannot be disputed, but one can question philosophically the existence of a prior distribution for X when X is an unknown parameter of a probability distribution.

Point estimates of parameters usually are obtained by taking the mode of the posterior distribution (but means or medians also can be used). The analog to the confidence interval is called a credible region and is obtained by finding points a and b such that the posterior probability that the parameter μ falls in the interval $[a,$

b] is set at a value such as 0.95. Points *a* and *b* are not unique and generally are chosen on grounds of symmetry. Sometimes the points are selected optimally in order to make the width of the interval as short as possible.

For hypothesis testing, one constructs an odds ratio for the alternative hypothesis relative to the null hypothesis as a prior distribution and then applies Bayes' rule to construct a posterior odds ratio given the test data. That is, we have a distribution for the ratio of the probability that the alternative is true to the probability that the null hypothesis is true. Before collecting the data, one specifies how large this ratio should be in order to reject the null hypothesis. See Berry (1996) for more details and examples.

Markov chain Monte Carlo methods now have made it computationally feasible to choose realistic prior distributions and solve hierarchical Bayesian problems. This development has led to a great deal of statistical research using the Bayesian approach to solve problems. Most researchers are using the software Winbugs and associated diagnostics to solve Bayesian problems. Developed in the United Kingdom, this software is free of charge. See Chapter 16 for details on Winbugs.

9.17 GROUP SEQUENTIAL METHODS

In the hypothesis testing problems that we have studied, the critical value of the test statistic and the power of the test are based on predetermined sample sizes. In some clinical trials, the sample size may not be fixed but allowed to be determined as the data are collected. When decisions are made after each new sample, such procedures are called sequential methods. More practical than making decisions after each new sample is to allow decisions to be made in steps as specified groups of samples are collected.

The statistical theory that underlies these techniques was developed in Great Britain and the United States during World War II. It was used extensively in quality assurance testing during the war. The goal was to waste as little ammunition as possible during testing.

In clinical trials, group sequential methods are used to stop trials early for either lack of efficacy or for safety reasons, or if medication is found to be highly effective. Sequential methods have advantages over fixed-sample-size trials in that they can lead to trials that tend to have smaller sample sizes than their fixed-sample-size counterparts. Since the actual sample size is unknown at the beginning of the trial, we can determine only a mean or a distribution of possible sample sizes that could result from the outcome of the trial.

Another reason for taking such a stepwise approach is that we may not have a good estimate of the population variances for the data prior to the trial. The accrual of some data enables us to estimate unknown parameters such as these variances; these data help us to determine more accurately the sample size we really need. If a bad initial guess in a fixed sample size trial gives too small a variance, we will have less power than we had planned for. On the other hand, if we conservatively overestimate the variance, our fixed sample size test will use more samples than we actually need and thus cost more than is really necessary. Two-stage sampling and group sequential sampling provide methodology to overcome such problems.

In recent years, statistical software has been developed to design group sequential trials. EaSt by Cytel, S + SeqTrial by Insightful Corporation (producers of Splus), and PEST by John Whitehead are representative packages that are discussed in Chapter 16. Among the texts that describe sequential and group sequential methods, one of the best recent ones is by Jennison and Turnbull (2000).

9.18 MISSING DATA AND IMPUTATION

In the real world of clinical trials, protocols sometimes are not completed, or patients may drop out of the trial for reasons of safety or for obvious lack of efficacy. Loss of subjects from follow-up studies sometimes is called censoring. The missing data are referred to as censored observations. Dropout creates problems for statistical inference, hypothesis testing, or other modeling techniques (including analysis of variance and regression, which are covered later in this text). One approach, which ignores the missing data and does the analysis on just the patients with complete data, is not a good solution when there is a significant amount of missing data.

One problem with ignoring the missing data is that the subset of patients considered (called completers) may not represent a random sample from the population. In order to have a representative random sample, we would like to know about all of the patients who have been sampled. Selection bias occurs when patients are not missing at random. Typically, when patients drop out, it is because the treatment is not effective or there are safety issues for them.

Many statistical analysis tools and packages require complete data. The complete data are obtained by statistical methods that use information from the available data to fill in or "impute" values to the missing observations. Techniques for doing this include: (1) last observation carried forward (LOCF), (2) multiple imputation, and (3) techniques that model the mechanism for the missing data.

After imputation, standard analyses are applied as if the imputed data represented real observations. Most techniques attempt to adjust for bias, and some deal with the artificial reduction in variance of the estimates. The usefulness of the methods depends greatly on the reasonableness of the modeling assumptions about how the data are missing. Little and Rubin (1987) provide an authoritative treatment of the imputation approaches and the statistical issues involved.

A second problem arises when we ignore cases with partially censored data: a significant proportion of the incomplete records may have informative data even though they are incomplete. Working only with completers throws out a lot of potentially useful data.

In a phase II clinical study, a pharmaceutical company found that patient dropout was a problem particularly at the very high and very low doses. At the high doses, safety issues relating to weight gain and lowering of white blood cell counts caused patients to drop out. At the low doses, patients dropped out because the treatment was ineffective.

In this case, the reason for missing data was related to the treatment. Therefore, some imputation techniques that assume data are missing in a random manner are not appropriate. LOCF is popular at pharmaceutical companies but is reasonable only if there is a slow trend or no trend in repeated observations over time. If there is a sharp downward trend, the last observation carried forward would tend to over-estimate the missing value. Similarly, a large upward trend would lead to a large underestimate of the missing value. Note that LOCF repeats the observation from the previous time point and thus implicitly assumes no trend.

Even when there is no trend over time, LOCF can grossly underestimate the variability in the data. Underestimation of the variability is a common problem for many techniques that apply a single value for a missing observation. Multiple impu-tation is a procedure that avoids the problem with the variance but not the problem of correlation between the measurement and the reason for dropout.

As an example of the use of a sophisticated imputation technique, we consider data from a phase II study of patients who were given an investigational drug. The study examined patients' responses to different doses, including any general health effects. One adverse event was measured in terms of a laboratory measurement and low values led to high dropouts for patients. Most of these dropouts occurred at the higher doses of the drug.

To present the information on the change in the median of this laboratory mea-surement over time, the statisticians used an imputation technique called the incre-mental means method. This method was not very reliable at the high doses; there were so few patients in the highest dose group remaining in the study at 12 weeks that any estimate of missing data was unreliable. All patients showed an apparent sharp drop that might not have been real. Other methods exaggerated the drop even more than the incremental means method. The results are shown in Figure 9.3. The

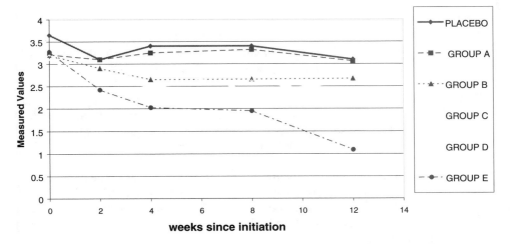

Figure 9.3. Laboratory measurements (median over time) imputed.

groups are labeled placebo and from A to E in order of increasing dose. The figure shows that laboratory measurements apparently remained stable over time in four of the treatment groups in comparison to the placebo group, with the exception of the highest dose group (Group E), which showed an apparent decline. However, the decline is questionable because of the small number of patients in that group who were observed at 12 weeks.

9.19   EXERCISES

9.1   The following terms were discussed in Chapter 9. Give definitions of them in your own words:
   a. Hypothesis test
   b. Null hypothesis
   c. Alternative hypothesis
   d. Type I error
   e. Type II error
   f. *p*-value
   g. Critical region
   h. Power of a test
   i. Power function
   j. Test statistic
   k. Significance level

9.2   Chapters 8 and 9 discussed methods for calculating confidence intervals and testing hypotheses, respectively. In what manner are parameter estimation and hypothesis testing similar to one another? In what manner are they different from one another?

9.3   In a factory where he conducted a research study, an occupational medicine physician found that the mean blood lead level of clerical workers was 11.2. State the null and alternative hypotheses for testing that the population mean blood lead level is equal to 11.2. What is the name for this type of hypothesis test?

9.4   Using the data from Exercise 9.3, state the hypothesis set (null and alternative hypotheses) for testing whether the population mean blood lead level exceeds 11.2. What is the name for this type of hypothesis test?

9.5   In the example cited in Exercise 9.3, the physician measures the blood lead levels of smelter workers in the same factory and finds their mean blood lead level to be 15.3. State the hypothesis set (null and alternative hypotheses) for testing whether the mean blood lead level of clerical workers differs from that of smelter workers.

9.6   Using the data from Exercise 9.5, state the hypothesis set (null and alternative hypotheses) for testing whether the mean blood lead level of smelter workers exceeds that of clerical workers.

9.7   The Orange County Public Health Department was concerned that the mean daily fecal coliform level in a particular month at Huntington Beach, California, exceeded a safe level. Let us call this level "*a.*" State the appropriate hypothesis set (null and alternative) for testing whether the mean coliform level exceeded a safe standard.

9.8   Suppose we would like to test the hypothesis that mean cholesterol levels of residents of Kalamazoo and Ann Arbor, Michigan, are the same. We know that both populations have the same variance. State the appropriate hypothesis set (null and alternative). What test statistic should be used?

9.9   Consider a sample of size 5 from a normal population with a variance of 5 and a mean of zero under the null hypothesis. Find the critical values for a 0.05 two-sided significance test of the mean equals zero versus the mean differs from zero.

9.10 Use the test in Exercise 9.9 (i.e., critical values) to determine the power of the test when the mean is 1.0 under the alternative hypothesis, the variance is 5, and the sample size is 5.

9.11 Again use the test in Exercise 9.9 to determine the power when the mean is 1.5 under the alternative hypothesis and the variance is again 5.

9.12 We suspect that the average fasting blood sugar level of Mexican Americans is 108. A random sample of 225 clinic patients (all Mexican American) yields a mean blood sugar level of 119 ($S^2 = 100$). Test the hypothesis that $\mu = 108$.
   a. What is the hypothesis set for a two-tailed test?
   b. Find the estimated s.e.m.
   c. Find the Z statistic.
   d. What decision should we make, i.e., reject or fail to reject H_0 at the $\alpha = 0.05$ level; reject or fail to reject H_0 at the $\alpha = 0.01$ level?
   e. What type of test is this: exact or approximate?

9.13 In the previous exercise there were two possible outcomes; reject the null hypothesis or fail to reject the null hypothesis. Explain in your own words what is meant by these outcomes.

9.14 Test the hypothesis that a normally distributed population has a mean blood glucose level of 100 ($\sigma^2 = 100$). Suppose we select a random sample of 30 individuals from this population ($\overline{X} = 98.1$, $S^2 = 126$).

    a. What is the hypothesis set (null and alternative) for a two-tailed test?
    b. Find the estimated s.e.m.
    c. Find the Z statistic.
    d. What decision should we make, i.e., reject or fail to reject H_0 at the $\alpha = 0.05$ level; reject or fail to reject H_0 at the $\alpha = 0.01$ level?
    e. What type of test is preferable to run in this situation, exact or approximate? Explain your answer.

9.15 Describe the differences between a one-tailed and a two-tailed test. Give examples of when it would be appropriate to use a two-tailed test and when it would be appropriate to use a one-tailed test.

9.16 Redo Exercise 9.14 but use a one-tailed (left-tail) test.

9.17 Recent advances in DNA testing have helped to confirm guilt or innocence in many well-publicized criminal cases. Let us consider the DNA test results to be the gold standard of guilt or innocence and a jury trial to be the test of a hypothesis. What types of errors are committed in the following two situations?
    a. The jury convicts a person of murder who later is found to be innocent by DNA testing.
    b. The jury exonerates a person who later is found to be guilty by DNA testing.

9.18 Find the area under the t-distribution between zero and the following values:
    a. 2.62 with 14 degrees of freedom
    b. −2.85 with 20 degrees of freedom
    c. 3.36 with 8 degrees of freedom
    d. 2.04 with 30 degrees of freedom
    e. −2.90 with 17 degrees of freedom
    f. 2.58 with 1000 degrees of freedom

9.19 Find the critical values for t that correspond to the following:
    a. $n = 12$, $\alpha = 0.05$ one-tailed (right)
    b. $n = 12$, $\alpha = 0.01$ one-tailed (right)
    c. $n = 19$, $\alpha = 0.05$ one-tailed (left)
    d. $n = 19$, $\alpha = 0.05$ two-tailed
    e. $n = 28$, $\alpha = 0.05$ one-tailed (left)
    f. $n = 41$, $\alpha = 0.05$ two-tailed
    g. $n = 8$, $\alpha = 0.10$ two-tailed
    h. $n = 201$, $\alpha = 0.001$ two-tailed

9.20 Consider the paired t test that was used with the data in Table 9.1, what would the power of the test be if the alternative is that the mean temperature differs by 3 degrees between the cities? What is the power at a difference of 5 degrees? Why does the power depend on the assumed true difference in means?

9.21 Suppose you are planning another experiment like the one in Exercise 9.20. Based on that data: (1) you are willing to assume that the standard deviation of the difference in means is 1.5°F, and (2) you anticipate that the average temperature in New York tends to be 3°F lower than the corresponding temperature in Washington on the same day.
   a. For such a one-sided paired t-test test, how many test days do you need to obtain 95% power at the specified alternative?
   b. How many do you need for 99% power?
   c. How many do you need for 80% power?

9.22 What is a meta-analysis? Why are meta-analyses performed?

9.23 What is Bayes' theorem? Define prior distribution. What is a posterior distribution?

9.24 How do Bayesians treat parameters? How do frequentists treat parameters? Are the two approaches different from one another?

9.25 Why can missing data be a problem in data analysis? What is imputation?

9.26 Define sensitivity and specificity. How do they relate to the type I and type II errors in hypothesis testing?

9.27 Here are some questions about hypothesis testing:
   a. Describe the one sample test of a mean when the variance is unknown and when the variance is known.
   b. Describe the use of a two-sample t test (common variance estimate).
   c. Describe when it is appropriate to use a paired t test.

9.20 ADDITIONAL READING

1. Berry, D. (1996). *Statistics: A Bayesian Perspective.* Duxbury Press, Belmont, California.
2. Blackwelder, W. (1982). "Proving the null hypothesis" in clinical trials. *Controlled Clinical Trials* **3**, 345–353.
3. Carpenter, J. and Bithell, J. (2000). Bootstrap confidence intervals: when, which, what? A practical guide for medical statisticians. *Statistics in Medicine* **19**, 1141–1164.
4. Chernick, M. R. (1999). *Bootstrap Methods: A Practitioner's Guide.* Wiley, New York.
5. Efron, B. and Tibshirani, R. (1993). *An Introduction to the Bootstrap.* Chapman and Hall, London.
6. Fisher, R. (1932). *Statistical Methods for Research Workers,* 4th Edition. Oliver and Boyd, London.

7. Friis, R. H. and Sellers, T. A. (1999). *Epidemiology for Public Health Practice,* 2nd Edition. Aspen, Gaithersburg, Maryland.

8. Hedges, L. and Olkin, I. (1985). *Statistical Methods for Meta-Analysis.* Academic Press, Orlando, Florida.

9. Jennison, C. and Turnbull B. (2000). *Group Sequential Methods with Applications to Clinical Trials.* CRC Press, Boca Raton, Florida.

10. Kotz, S and Johnson, N. editors (1982). *Encyclopedia of Statistical Sciences, Volume 1. Behrens–Fisher Problem,* pp. 205–209. Wiley, New York.

11. Little, R. and Rubin, D. (1987). *Statistical Analysis with Missing Data.* Wiley, New York.

12. McClave, J. and Benson, P. (1991). *Statistics for Business and Economics,* 5th Edition. Dellen, San Francisco.

13. Pearson, K. (1933). On a method of determining whether a sample of a given size n supposed to have been drawn from a parent population having a known probability integral has probably been drawn at random. *Biometrika* **25,** 379–410.

14. Stangl, D. and Berry, D., (editors). (2000). *Meta-Analysis in Medicine and Health Policy.* Marcel Dekker, New York.

CHAPTER 10

Inferences Regarding Proportions

*A misunderstanding of Bernoulli's theorem is responsible for one
of the commonest fallacies in the estimation of probabilities, the
fallacy of the maturity of chances. When a coin has come down
heads twice in succession, gamblers sometimes say that it is more
likely to come down tails next time because "by the law of averages" (whatever that may mean) the proportion of tails must be
brought right some time.*

—W. Kneale *Probability and Induction*, p. 140

10.1 WHY ARE PROPORTIONS IMPORTANT?

Chapter 9 covered statistical inferences with variables that represented interval or
ratio-level measurement. Now we will discuss inferences with another type of variable—a proportion, which was introduced in Chapter 5. Let us review some of the
terminology regarding variables, including a random variable, continuous and discrete variables, and binomial variables.

A random variable is a type of variable for which the specific value of each observation is determined by chance. For example, the systolic blood pressure measurement for each patient is a random value. Variables can be categorized further as
continuous or discrete. Continuous variables can have an infinite number of values
within a specified range. For example, weight is a continuous variable because it always can be measured more precisely, depending on the precision of the measurement scale used. Discrete variables form data that can be arranged into specific
groups or sets of values, e.g., blood type or race.

Bernoulli variables are discrete random variables that have only two possible
values, e.g., success or failure. The binomial random variable is the number of successes in n trials. It can take on integer values from 0 to n. Let n = the number of objects in a sample and p = the population proportion of a binomial characteristic, also
known as a "success," i.e., the proportion of successes; then, $1 - p$ = the proportion
of failures. There are numerous examples of medical outcomes that represent binomial variables. Also, sometimes it is convenient to create a dichotomy from a continuous variable. For example, we could look at the proportion of diabetic patients

Introductory Biostatistics for the Health Sciences, by Michael R. Chernick
and Robert H. Friis. ISBN 0-471-41137-X. Copyright © 2003 Wiley-Interscience.

with hemoglobin A1C measurements above 7.5% versus the proportion with hemoglobin A1C below 7.5%.

Proportions are very important in medical studies, especially in research that uses dichotomous outcomes such as dead or alive, responding or not responding to a drug, or survival/nonsurvival for 5 years after treatment for a disease. Another example is the use of proportions to measure customer or patient satisfaction, for measures that have dichotomous responses: satisfied versus dissatisfied, yes/no, agree/disagree.

For example, a manufacturer of drugs to treat diabetes studied patients, physicians and nurses to see how well patients complied with their prescribed treatment and to see how well they understood the chronic nature of the disease. For this survey, proportions of patients who gave certain responses in particular subgroups of the population were of primary interest. To illustrate, the investigators queried subjects as to complications from type II diabetes. Respondents' knowledge about each type of complication—renal disease, retinopathy, peripheral neuropathy—was scored according to a yes/no format.

At medical device companies, the primary endpoint may be the success of a particular medical or surgical procedure. The proportion of patients with successful outcomes may be a primary endpoint and that proportion for the treatment group may be compared to a proportion for a control group (i.e., a group that receives either a placebo no treatment, or a competitor's treatment). The groups receiving the treatment from a sponsoring company are generally referred to as the treatment groups and the group receiving the competitor's treatment are called the active control groups. The term active control distinguishes them from control groups that receive placebo.

The sample proportion of successes is the number of successes divided by the number of patients who are treated. If we denote the total number of successes by S, then the estimated proportion $\hat{p} = S/n$, where n is the total number of patients treated. This proportion in a clinical trial can be viewed as an estimate of a probability, namely, the probability of a success in the patient population being sampled. Detailed examples from clinical trials will be discussed later in this chapter.

The binomial model is usually appropriate for inferences that involve the use of clinical trial outcomes expressed as proportions. We can assume that patients have been selected randomly from a population of interest. We can view the success or failure of each patient's treatment as the result of a Bernoulli trial with success probability equal to the population success probability p. In Chapter 5, a Bernoulli distribution was defined as a type of probability distribution associated with two mutually exclusive and exhaustive outcomes. Each patient can be viewed as being independent of the other patients. As we discussed in Section 5.6, the sample number of successes out of n patients then has a binomial distribution with parameters n and p.

10.2 MEAN AND STANDARD DEVIATION FOR THE BINOMIAL DISTRIBUTION

In Chapter 4, we discussed the mean and variance of a continuous variable (μ, σ^2 and $\overline{X}$, S^2) for the parameters and their respective sample estimates. It is possible to compute analogs for a dichotomous variable. As shown in Chapter 5, the binomial distribution is used to describe the distribution of dichotomous outcomes such as heads or tails or "successes and failures." The mean and variance of the binomial distribution are functions of the parameters n and p, where n refers to the number in the population and p to the proportion of successes. This relationship between the parameters n and p and the binomial distribution affects the way we form test statistics and confidence intervals for the proportions when using the normal approximation that we will discuss in Section 10.3. The mean of the binomial is np and the variance is $np(1 - p)$, as we will demonstrate.

Recall (see Section 5.7) that for a binomial random variable X with parameters n and p, X can take on the values 0, 1, 2, . . . , n with $P\{X = k\} = C(n, k) \, p^k(1 - p)^{n-k}$ for $k = 0, 1, 2, \dots , n$. Recall that $P\{X = k\}$ is the probability of k successes in the n Bernoulli trials and $C(n, k)$ is the number of ways of arranging k successes and $n - k$ failures in the sequence of n trials. From this information we can show with a little algebra that the mean or expected value for X denoted by $E(X)$ is np. This fact is given in Equation 10.1. The proof is demonstrated in Display 10.1 (see page 220).

The algebra becomes a little more complicated than for the proof of $E(X) = np$ shown in Display 10.1; using techniques similar to those employed in the foregoing proof, we can demonstrate that the variance of X, denoted Var(X), satisfies the equation Var$(X) = np(1 - p)$. Equations 10.1 and 10.2 summarize the formulas for the expected value of X and the variance of X.

For a binomial random variable X

$$E(X) = np \tag{10.1}$$

where n is the number of Bernoulli trials and p is the population success probability.

For a binomial random variable X

$$\text{Var}(X) = np(1 - p) \tag{10.2}$$

where n is the number of Bernoulli trials and p is the population success probability.

To illustrate the use of Equations 10.1 and 10.2, let us use a simple example of a Bernouilli trial in which $n = 3$ and $p = 0.5$. An illustration would be an experiment involving three tosses of a fair coin; a head will be called a success. Then the possible number of successes on the three tosses is 0, 1, 2, or 3. Applying Equation 10.1, we find that the mean number of successes is $np = 3 \, (0.5) = 1.5$; applying Equation 10.2, we find that the variance of the number of successes is $np(1 - p) = 3(0.5)(1 - 0.5) = 1.5(.5) = 0.75$. Had we not obtained these two simple formulas by algebra, we could have performed the calculations from the definitions in Chapter 5 (summarized in Display 10.1 and Formula D10.1).

To apply Formula D10.1, we compute the probability of each of the successes (outcomes 0, 1, 2, and 3), multiply each of these probabilities by the number of successes (0, 1, 2, and 3) and then sum the results, as shown in the next paragraph.

The probability of 0 successes is $C(3, 0)p^0(1 - p)^3$; when we replace p by (0.5), the term $C(3, 0)(0.5)^0(1 - 0.5)^3 = (1)(1)(0.5)^3 = 0.125$. As there are 0 successes,

---

Display 10.1. Proof that $E(X) = np$

To conduct this proof, we will use the formula presented in Chapter 5, Section 5.7, in which the probability of r successes in n trials was defined as $P(Z = r) = C(n, r)p^r(1 - p)^{n-r}$. For the proof, we replace r by k (the number of trials) and sum over the k trials; this sum equals 1, as shown below:

$$\Sigma_k C(n, k)p^k(1 - p)^{n-k} = 1 \qquad (D10.1)$$

This equation holds for any positive integer n and proportion $0 < p < 1$ when the summation is taken over $0 \le k \le n$. Assume $k \ge 2$ for the following argument. The mean denoted by $E(X)$ is by definition

$$\sum_{k=0}^{n} kC(n, k)p^k(1 - p)^{n-k} = \sum_{k=0}^{n} k\{n!/[k!(n - k)!]\}p^k(1 - p)^{n-k}$$

$$= \sum_{k=1}^{n} \{n!/[(k - 1)!(n - k)!]\}p^k(1 - p)^{n-k}$$

$$= np \sum_{k=1}^{n} \{(n - 1)!/[(k - 1)!(n - k)!]\}p^{k-1}(1 - p)^{n-k}$$

$$= np \sum_{j=0}^{n-1} \{(n - 1)!/[(j)!(n - 1 - j)!]\}p^j(1 - p)^{n-1-j}$$

$$= np \sum_{j=0}^{n-1} C(n - 1, j)p^j(1 - p)^{n-1-j}$$

Remember that by applying formula D10.1, with $n - 1$ in place of n in the formula

$$\sum_{j=0}^{n-1} C(n - 1, j)p^j(1 - p)^{n-1-j}$$

since $n - 1$ is a positive integer (recall that $n \ge 2$, implying that $n - 1 \ge 1$). So for $n \ge 2$, $E(X = np$. For $n = 1$, $E(X) = 0(1 - p) + 1(p) = p = np$ also. So we have shown for any positive integer n, $E(X) = np$.

---

we multiply 0.125 by 0 and obtain 0. Consequently, the contribution of 0 successes to the mean is 0. Next, we calculate the probability of 1 success by using $C(3, 1)p(1 - p)^2$, which is the number of ways of arranging 1 success and 2 failures in a row multiplied by the probability of a particular arrangement that has 1 success and 2 failures. $C(3, 1) = 3$, so the resulting probability is $3p(1 - p)^2 = 3(0.5)(0.5)^2 = 3(0.125) = 0.375$. We multiply that result by 1, since it corresponds to 1 success and we find that 1 success contributes 0.375 to the mean of the distribution. The probability of 2 successes is $C(3, 2)p^2(1 - p)$, which is the number of ways of arranging 2 successes and 1 failure in a row multiplied by the probability of any one such arrangement. $C(3, 2) = 3$, so the probability is $3p^2(1 - p) = 3(0.5)^2(0.5) = 0.375$. We then multiply 0.375 by 2, as we have 2 successes, which contribute 0.750 to the mean. To obtain the final term, we compute the probability of 3 successes and then multiply the resulting probability by 3. The probability of 3 successes is $C(3, 3) = 1$ (since all three places have to be successes, there is only one possible arrangement) multiplied by $p^3 = (0.5)^3 = 0.125$. We then multiply 0.125 by 3 to obtain the contribution of this term to the mean. In this case the contribution to the mean is 0.375.

In order to obtain the mean of this distribution, we add the four terms together. We obtain the mean = $0 + 0.375 + 0.750 + 0.375 = 1.5$. Our long computation agrees with the result from Equation 10.1. For larger values of n and different values of p, the direct calculation is even more tedious and complicated, but Equation 10.1 is simple and easy to perform, a statement that also holds true for the variance calculation. Note that in our present example, if we apply the formula for the variance (Equation 10.2), we obtain a variance of $np(1 - p) = 3(0.5)(0.5) = 0.750$.

10.3 NORMAL APPROXIMATION TO THE BINOMIAL

Let $W = X/n$, where X is a binomial variable with parameters n and p. Then, since W is just a constant times X, $E(W) = p$ and $\text{Var}(W) = p(1 - p)/n$. W represents the proportion of successes when X is the number of successes. Because often we wish to estimate the proportion p, we are interested in the mean and variance of W (the sample estimate for the proportion p). In the example where $n = 3$ and $p = 0.5$, $E(W) = 0.5$ and $\text{Var}(W) = 0.5(0.5)/3 = 0.25/3 = 0.0833$.

The central limit theorem applied to the sample mean of n Bernoulli trials tells us that for large n the random variable W, which is the sample mean of the n Bernoulli trials, has a distribution that is approximately normal, with mean p and variance $p(1 - p)/n$. As p is unknown, the common way to normalize to obtain a statistic that has an approximate standard normal distribution for a hypothesis test would be $Z = (W - p_0)/\sqrt{p_0(1 - p_0)/n}$, where p_0 is the hypothesized value of p under the null hypothesis. Sometimes W itself is used in place of p_0 in the denominator, since $W(1 - W)$ is a consistent estimate of the Bernoulli variance $p(1 - p)$ for a single trial. Multiplying both the numerator and denominator by n we see that algebraically Z is also equal to $(X - np_0)/\sqrt{n[p_0(1 - p_0)]}$.

Because the binomial distribution is discrete and the normal distribution is continuous, the approximation can be improved by using what is called the continuity correction. We simply make $Z = (X - np_0 - 1/2)/\sqrt{n[p_0(1 - p_0)]}$. The normal approximation to the binomial works fairly well with the continuity correction when $n \geq 30$, provided that $0.3 < p < 0.7$. However, in clinical trials we are often interested in $p > 0.90$; these cases require n to be several hundred before the Z approximation works well. For this reason and because of the computational speed of modern computers, exact binomial methods commonly are used now, even for fairly large sample sizes such as $n = 1000$

To express Z in terms of W in the continuity corrected version, we divide both the numerator and denominator by n. The result is $Z = (W - p_0 - 1/\{2n\})/\sqrt{p_0(1 - p_0)/n}$.

We use this form for Z as it provides a better approximation to expressions such as $P(W \leq a)$ or $P(W > a)$. On the other hand, if we consider $P(W < a)$ or $P(W \geq a)$, then we should use $Z = (X - np_0 + 1/2)/\sqrt{n[p_0(1 - p_0)]}$ or, equivalently, $Z = (W - p_0 + 1/\{2n\})/\sqrt{p_0(1 - p_0)/n}$.

10.4 HYPOTHESIS TEST FOR A SINGLE BINOMIAL PROPORTION

To test the hypothesis that the parameter p of a binomial distribution equals a hypothesized value p_0, versus the alternative that it differs from p_0, we can use the approximate normal quantities given in Section 10.3 either with or without continuity correction. This statement means that we want to test the hypothesis that the proportion (p) obtained from a sample is equivalent to some hypothesized value for the population proportion (p_0). The continuity correction is particularly important when the sample size n is small. However, exact methods are now used instead; such methods involve computing cumulative binomial probabilities for various values of p. With the speed of modern computers, these calculations that used to be very lengthy can now be computed rather rapidly.

A mathematical relationship between the integral of a beta function and the cumulative binomial allows these binomial probabilities to be calculated by a numerical integration method rather than by direct summation of the terms of the binomial distribution. The numerical integration method is a mathematical identity that expresses the sum of binomial probabilities as an integral of a particular function. The advantage of numerical integration is that an integral can be calculated relatively quickly by numerical methods, whereas the summation method is computationally slower. This approach, presented by Clopper and Pearson (1934), consequently helps speed up the computation of the binomial probabilities needed to identify the endpoints of a confidence interval. Hahn and Meeker (1991) show how to use this method to obtain exact binomial confidence intervals.

The test procedures that use exact methods are always preferable to the normal approximation but carry the disadvantage that they do not have a simple form for an easy table lookup. Consequently, we have to rely on the computer to provide us with p-values for the hypothesis test or to compute an exact confidence interval for p.

Fortunately, though, there are relatively inexpensive software packages such as StatXact that do this work for you. StatXact–5, Power and Precision, UnifyPow, PASS2000, and nQuery 4.0 are packages that will determine power or sample size requirements for hypothesis tests and/or confidence intervals for binomial proportions or differences between two binomial proportions. See Chernick and Liu (2002) for a comparison of these products and a discussion of the peculiar saw-toothed nature of the power function. We also discuss these packages briefly in Chapter 16.

Equation 10.3 shows the continuity-corrected test statistic used for the normal approximation:

$$Z = \frac{(X - np_0 - 1/2)}{\sqrt{n[p_0(1 - p_0)]}}$$ (10.3)

where X is a binomial random variable with parameters n and p_0. Alternatively,

$$Z = \frac{(W - p_0 - 1/\{2n\})}{\sqrt{p_0(1 - p_0)/n}}$$

where $W = X/n$. Z has approximately a standard normal distribution and is used in this form when approximating $P(W \leq a)$ or $P(W > a)$.

For large sample sizes, the continuity correction is not necessary; Equation 10.4 shows the test statistic in that case:

$$Z = \frac{(X - np_0)}{\sqrt{n[p_0(1 - p_0)]}}$$ (10.4)

where X is a binomial random variable with parameters n and p_0. Alternatively,

$$Z = \frac{(W - p_0)}{\sqrt{p_0(1 - p_0)/n}}$$

where $W = X/n$. Z has approximately a standard normal distribution.

Here is an example of how clinical trials use proportions. A medical device company produces a catheter used to perform ablations for fast arrhythmias called supraventricular tachycardia (SVT). In order to show the location of cardiac electrical activity associated with SVT, a map of the heart is constructed. The company has developed a new heart mapping system that uses a catheter with a sensor on its tip. Relatively simple ablation procedures (i.e., cutting nerve pathways) for SVT have been carried out sufficiently often for us to know that current practice produces a 95% acute success rate. Acute success is no recurrence for a short period (usually one or two days) before the patient is sent home. Companies also define a parameter called chronic success, which requires that a recurrence not happen for at least six months after the procedure. The new mapping system is expected to produce about the same success rate as that of the present procedure but will have the advantage of quicker identification of the location to ablate and, hence, an expected reduction in procedure time.

Most of the reduction in procedure time will be attributed to the reduction in the so-called fluoroscopy time, the amount of time required for checking the location of the catheter by using fluoroscopy. Shortening this time reduces the amount of radiation the patient receives; physicians and the FDA view such a reduction as a benefit to the patient. This reduction in fluoroscopy time is a valid reason for marketing the new device if the manufacturer also can show that the device is as efficacious as current methods.

Consequently, the manufacturer decides to conduct a clinical trial to demonstrate a reduction in fluoroscopy time. The manufacturer also wants to demonstrate the device's equivalence (or, more precisely, lack of inferiority) with respect to acute success rate.

All patients will be treated with the new device and mapping system; their success rate will be compared to the industry standard, $p_0 = 0.95$. (The proportion under the null hypothesis will be set at 0.95.) The one-sample binomial test described in this section will be used at the end of the trial.

Now let us consider what happened in an actual test of the device. Equivalence testing as explained in Section 9.5 was used in the test. The company eventually received approval for the device to treat SVT. A slightly modified version of the device was available; the company sought approval of it as a mapping system to treat VT (ventricular tachycardia). Mapping procedures for VT are more complicated than those for SVT and have less than a 50% chance of success. With the mapping system, the company expected to improve the acute success rate to above 50% and also reduce procedure time. In order to show superiority in acute success rate, they tested the null hypothesis that $p = p_0 \leq 0.50$ versus the alternative that $p > 0.50$. We refer to this example as a one-sided test in which we are trying to show superiority of the new method. Later, we will see the use of a one-sided test to show a statistically significant decrement in performance, i.e., $p = p_0 \geq .0.50$ versus $p < 0.50$.

10.5   TESTING THE DIFFERENCE BETWEEN TWO PROPORTIONS

In testing the difference between two proportions, we have at our disposal exact binomial methods. The software companies listed in the previous section also provide solutions to this problem. In addition, we can use Fisher's exact test (described in Chapter 14). Now, as another solution, we will provide the normal approximations for testing the difference between two proportions and give an example.

Let $W_1 = X_1/n_1$ and $W_2 = X_2/n_2$, where X_1 is binomial with parameters p_1 and n_1 and where X_2 is binomial with parameters p_2 and n_2. Note that p_1 and p_2 refer to population proportions. We are interested in the difference between these two proportions: $p_1 - p_2$. This difference can be estimated by $W_1 - W_2$. Now, the standard deviation for $W_1 - W_2$ is $\sqrt{[p_1(1-p_1)/n_1 + p_2(1-p_2)/n_2]}$ because the variance of $W_1 - W_2$ is the sum of the individual variances. Each of the variance terms under the radical is simply an analog of the variance for a single proportion, as shown previously in Equation 10.4. So a choice for Z would be $Z = \{W_1 - W_2 - (p_1 - p_2)\}/\sqrt{[p_1(1-p_1)/n_1 + p_2(1-p_2)/n_2]}$.

However, this equation is impractical because p_1 and p_2 are unknown. One way to obtain an approximation that will yield a Z that has approximately a standard normal distribution would be to use the unbiased and consistent estimates W_1 and W_2 in place of p_1 and p_2, respectively, everywhere in the denominator. Z is then a pivotal quantity that can be used for hypothesis testing or for confidence intervals.

The usual null hypothesis is that $p_1 = p_2$ or $p_1 - p_2 = 0$. So under H_0: $Z = (W_1 - W_2)/\sqrt{[W_1(1 - W_1)/n_1 + W_2(1 - W_2)/n_2]}$ is the test statistic with an approximately standard normal distribution.

Now, $W_1 = X_1/n_1$ and $W_2 = X_2/n_2$. Under the null hypothesis, $p_1 = p_2 = p$; consequently, W_1 and W_2 have the same binomial parameter p. In this case, it makes sense to combine the data and $X_c = X_1 + X_2$ is binomial with parameters $n_1 + n_2$ and p. Then $W_c = X_c/(n_1 + n_2)$ is a natural estimate for p and has greater precision than either W_1 or W_2. This estimate W_c is reasonable only under the null hypothesis, however. Using this argument, we can make a case that $Z' = (W_1 - W_2)/\sqrt{[W_c(1 - W_c)/n_1 + W_c(1 - W_c)/n_2]}$ is better to use, since the denominator gives a better estimate of the standard error of $W_1 - W_2$ when the null hypothesis is true. It simplifies to $Z' = (W_1 - W_2)/\sqrt{[W_c(1 - W_c)[(1/n_1) + (1/ n_2)]}$. This formula will not apply when we are generating approximate confidence intervals.

The Z test for the difference between two proportions $p_1 - p_2$ is

$$Z' = \frac{(W_1 - W_2)}{\sqrt{W_c(1 - W_c)[(1/n_1) + (1//n_2)]}} \tag{10.5}$$

where H_0: $p_1 = p_2 = p$, $X_c = X_1 + X_2$, and $W_c = X_c/(n_1 + n_2)$.

To illustrate, suppose $n_1 = 10$, $n_2 = 9$, $X_1 = 7$, and $X_2 = 5$. Then $W_1 = 7/10 = 0.700$, $W_2 = 5/9 = 0.556$, and $W_c = 12/19 = 0.632$. Then $Z = (0.700 - 0.556)/(\sqrt{0.632(0.368)[(1/10) + (1/9)]} = 0.134/\sqrt{0.233[19/90]} = 0.134/\sqrt{0.233(0.211)} = 0.134/\sqrt{0.049} = 0.134/0.222 = 0.604$. This difference is not statistically significant. Using the normal approximation we see from the standard normal table that $P[|Z| > 0.604] = 2P[Z > 0.604] = 2(0.5 - P[0 < Z < 0.604]) \approx 2(0.5 - P[0 < Z < 0.6]) = 1 - 2P[0 < Z < 0.6] = 1 - 2(0.2257) = 1 - 0.4514 = 0.5486$. So the p-value is greater than 0.5.

10.6   CONFIDENCE INTERVALS FOR PROPORTIONS

First we will consider a single proportion and the approximate intervals based on the normal distribution. If W is X/n, where X is a binomially distributed random variable with parameters n and p, then by the central limit theorem W is approximately normally distributed with mean p and variance $p(1 - p)/n$. Therefore, $(W - p)/\sqrt{p(1 - p)/n}$ has an approximately standard normal distribution.

Because p is unknown, we cannot normalize W by dividing W by p. Instead, we consider the quantity $U = (W - p)/\sqrt{W(1 - W)/n}$. Since W is a consistent estimate of p, this quantity U converges to a standard normal random variable as the sample size n increases.

Therefore, we use the fact that if U were standard normal, then $P[-1.96 \le U \le 1.96] = 0.95$ or $P[-1.96 \le (W - p)/\sqrt{W(1 - W)/n} \le 1.96] = 0.95$ or, after the usual algebraic manipulations, $P[W - 1.96\sqrt{W(1 - W)/n} \le p \le W + 1.96\sqrt{W(1 - W)/n}]$. So the random interval $[W - 1.96\sqrt{W(1 - W)/n}, W + 1.96\sqrt{W(1 - W)/n}]$ is an approximate 95% confidence interval for a single proportion p.

$$[W - 1.96\sqrt{W(1 - W)/n}, \qquad W + 1.96\sqrt{W(1 - W)/n}] \qquad (10.6)$$

where $W = X/n$ and X is binomially distributed with parameters n and p. For other confidence levels, change 1.96 to the appropriate constant C from the standard normal distribution.

As an example, suppose that we have 16 successes in 20 trials; $X = 16$ and $n = 20$. What would be an approximate 95% confidence interval for the population proportion of successes, p? From Equation 10.6, since $W = 16/20 = 0.80$, we have $[0.80 - 1.96\sqrt{0.8(0.2)/20}, 0.80 + 1.96\sqrt{0.8(0.2)/20}] = [0.80 - 0.1753, 0.80 + 0.1753] = [0.625, 0.975]$. Later we will compare this interval to the exact interval obtained by the Clopper–Pearson method.

Now let us consider two independent estimates of proportions, $W_1 = X_1/n_1$ and $W_2 = X_2/n_2$, where X_1 is a binomial random variable with parameters p_1 and n_1 and X_2 is a binomial random variable with parameters p_2 and n_2. Then, $Z = (W_1 - W_2) - (p_1 - p_2)/\sqrt{[W_1(1 - W_1)/n_1 + W_2(1 - W_2)/n_2]}$ has an approximately standard normal distribution. Therefore, $P[-1.96 \leq Z \leq 1.96]$ is approximately 0.95. After substitution and algebraic manipulations, we have $P[(W_1 - W_2) - 1.96\sqrt{[W_1(1 - W_1)/n_1 + W_2(1 - W_2)/n_2]} \leq (p_1 - p_2) \leq [(W_1 - W_2) + 1.96\sqrt{[W_1(1 - W_1)/n_1 + W_2(1 - W_2)/n_2]}$. The probability that $p_1 - p_2$ lies within this interval is approximately 0.95; hence, the random interval $[(W_1 - W_2) - 1.96\sqrt{[W_1(1 - W_1)/n_1 + W_2(1 - W_2)/n_2]}[(W_1 - W_2) + 1.96\sqrt{[W_1(1 - W_1)/n_1 + W_2(1 - W_2)/n_2]}$ is an approximate 95% confidence interval for $p_1 - p_2$.

An approximate 95% confidence interval for the difference between two proportions $p_1 - p_2$ is

$$[(W_1 - W_2) - 1.96\sqrt{W_1(1 - W_1)/n_1 + W_2(1 - W_2)/n_2},$$

$$(W_1 - W_2) + 1.96\sqrt{W_1(1 - W_1)/n_1 + (W_2(1 - W_2)/n_2)}] \qquad (10.7)$$

where $W_1 = X_1/n_1$ and X_1 is binomially distributed with parameters n_1 and p_1, and $W_2 = X_2/n_2$ and X_2 is binomially distributed with parameters n_2 and p_2. For other confidence levels, change 1.96 to the appropriate constant C from the standard normal distribution.

For a numerical example, suppose n_1 is 100 and n_2 is 50. Suppose $X_1 = 85$ and $X_2 = 26$. We will calculate the approximate 95% and 99% confidence intervals for $p_1 - p_2$ when $W_1 = 85/100 = 0.85$ and $W_2 = 26/50 = 0.52$. In the case of the 95% confidence interval, the constant $C = 1.96$; hence, the interval is $[(0.85 - 0.52) - 1.96\sqrt{0.85(0.15)/100 + 0.52(0.48)/50}, (0.85 - 0.52) + 1.96\sqrt{0.85(0.15)/100 + 0.52(0.48)/50}] = [0.175, 0.485]$.

For exact intervals, the Clopper–Pearson method is used. Clopper and Pearson (1934) provided the results of their method in graphical form. Hahn and Meeker (1991) reprinted Clopper and Pearson's work, along with much detail about confidence intervals. The two-sided interval uses the F distribution with the $100(1 - \alpha)$% interval given by Equation 10.8. We will learn about the F distribution in Chapter 13.

The exact $100(1 - \alpha)\%$ confidence interval for a single binomial proportion is

$$[\{1 + (n - x + 1)F(1 - \alpha/2{:}2n - 2x + 2, 2x)/x\}^{-1},$$
$$\{1 + (n - x)/\{(x + 1)F(1 - \alpha/2{:}2x + 2, 2n - 2x)\}\}^{-1}]$$

where x is the number of successes in n Bernoulli trials and $F(\gamma{:}\ dfn,\ dfd)$ is the 100γth percentile of an F distribution with dfn degrees of freedom for the numerator and dfd degrees of freedom for the denominator. For the lower endpoint, $\gamma = 1 - \alpha/2$, $dfn = 2n - 2x$, and $dfd = 2x$. For the upper endpoint, $\gamma = 1 - \alpha/2$, $dfn = 2x + 2$, and $dfd = 2n{-}2x$.

Now let us revisit the example for approximate confidence intervals where $X = 16$, $n = 20$, and $1 - \alpha/2 = 0.95$. The above equation becomes $[\{1 + 5\ F(0.95{:}\ 10, 32)/16\}^{-1}, \{1 + 4/\{5\ F(0.95{:}\ 34, 8)\}\}^{-1}]$. For now we will take these percentiles by consulting a table for the F distribution. From the table (Appendix A), we see that $F(0.95{:}\ 10, 32) = 2.94$ and $F(0.95{:}\ 34, 8) = 5.16$ (by interpolation between $F(0.95, 30, 8) = 5.20$ and $F(0.95, 40, 8) = 5.11$. Plugging these values into Equation 10.8, we obtain the interval $[0.521, 0.866]$. The value 0.95 tells us the percentile to look up in the table; the two other parameters are the numerator and denominator degrees of freedom, to be defined in Chapter 12.

Compare this new interval to the interval from the normal approximation $[0.625, 0.975]$. Note that the widths of the intervals are about the same, but the normal approximation gives a symmetric interval centered at 0.80. The reason for the difference is that the sample size of 20 is too small for the normal approximation to be very good, as the true proportion is probably close to 0.80; the Binomial distribution, though centered at 0.80, is much more skewed than a normal distribution and has a longer left tail than right tail. In this case, the exact binomial solution is appropriate but the normal approximation is not.

If n were 100, the normal approximation and the exact Binomial distribution would be in much closer agreement. So let us make the comparison when $n = 100$ and $x = 80$. The normal approximation gives $[0.80 - 1.96\ \sqrt{0.8(0.2)/100},\ 0.80 + 1.96\ \sqrt{0.8(0.2)/100}] = [0.722, 0.878]$, whereas the Clopper–Pearson method gives $[\{1 + 21\ F(0.95{:}\ 42, 160)/80\}^{-1}, \{1 + 20/\{81\ F(0.95{:}\ 162, 40)\}\}^{-1}]$. We have $F(0.95{:}\ 42, 160) = 1.72$ (by interpolation in the table, Appendix A) and $F(0.95{:}\ 162, 40) = 1.90$ (also by interpolation in the table). Substituting these values in the equation above gives the interval $[0.689, 0.885]$. We note that the normal approximation, though not as accurate as we would like, is much closer to the exact result when the sample size is 100 as compared to when the sample size is only 20.

10.7   SAMPLE SIZE DETERMINATION—CONFIDENCE INTERVALS AND HYPOTHESIS TESTS

Using the formulas for the normal approximation, sample sizes can be derived in a manner similar to that employed in Chapters 8 and 9. Again, these calculations would be based on the width of the confidence interval or the power of a test at a specific alternative. The resulting formulas are slightly different from those for continuous variables. In the case of variance in the test of a single proportion, or calculating a confidence interval about a proportion, we guess at p to find the necessary standard deviation. We make this estimate because W is $p(1-p)/n$, and we do not know p (the population parameter). We also can be conservative in determining the confidence interval, because for all $0 \le p \le 1$, $p(1-p)$ is largest at $p = 1/2$.

Therefore, the variance of $W = p(1-p)/n \le (1/2)(1/2)/n = 1/(4n)$. This upper bound, $1/(4n)$, on the variance of W can be used in the formulas to obtain a minimum sample size that will satisfy the condition for any value of p. We could not find such a bound for the unknown variance of a normal distribution.

Again, software packages such as the ones reviewed by Chernick and Liu (2002) provide solutions for all the cases (using both exact and approximate methods).

10.8 EXERCISES

10.1 Give definitions of the following terms in your own words:
   a. Sample proportion
   b. Population proportion
   c. Binomial variable
   d. Bernoulli trial
   e. Continuity correction
   f. Confidence interval for a proportion

10.2 Peripheral neuropathy is a complication of uncontrolled diabetes. The number of cases of peripheral neuropathy among a control group of 35 diabetic patients was 12. Among a group of 11 patients who were taking an oral agent to prevent hyperglycemia, there were three cases of peripheral neuropathy. Is the proportion of patients with peripheral neuropathy comparable in both groups? Perform the test at $\alpha = 0.05$.

10.3 Construct exact 95% confidence intervals for the proportion of patients with peripheral neuropathy in the medication group and the proportion of patients in the control group in the previous exercise. Construct two confidence intervals for each proportion, one with correction for continuity and the other without correction for continuity.

10.4 Referring to Exercise 10.2, construct an approximate 95% confidence interval for the difference between the proportions of patients affected by peripheral neuropathy in the control group and in the medication group.

10.5 A dental researcher investigated the occurrence of edentulism (defined in the research study as loss of two or more permanent teeth, not including loss of prophylactically extracted wisdom teeth) in a rural Latin American village. A total of 34 out of 100 sampled adults had lost at least two teeth. A study of a U.S. city found that the rate of loss of at least two teeth was 14%. Was the proportion of persons who had edentulism higher in the Latin American village than in the U.S. city? Conduct the test at the $\alpha = 0.05$ level.

10.6   Calculate an exact 95% confidence interval for the proportion of edentulous persons in the Latin American village (refer to Exercise 10.5.)

10.7   For the data in Exercise 10.5, compute a 99% confidence interval using the normal approximation with continuity correction. Is the result close to the exact interval found in Exercise 10.6? Explain why or why not.

10.8   In a British study of social class and health, a total of 171 out of 402 lower social class persons were classified as overweight. The percent of over-weight persons in the general population was 39%. Based on these findings, would you assert that low social class is related to being overweight? Test this hypothesis at the $\alpha = 0.01$ level.

10.9   A longitudinal study of occupational status and smoking behavior among women reported at baseline that 170 per 1000 professional/managerial women were nicotine dependent. The corresponding rate among blue collar women was 310 per 1000. At the $\alpha = 0.05$ level, determine whether there is a significant difference in nicotine dependence between the proportion of women who are classified as professional/managerial workers in compari-son to those who are classified as blue collar workers. Then compute the ap-proximate 99% confidence interval for the difference between these two proportions.

10.10   An epidemiologic study examined risk factors associated with pediatric AIDS. In a small study of 30 cases and 30 controls, a positive history of substance abuse occurred among 11 of the cases and 6 of the controls. Based on these data, can the investigator assert that substance abuse is sig-nificantly associated with pediatric AIDS at the $\alpha = 0.05$ level? Compute the approximate 95% confidence interval for the difference between the proportions of substance abuse found in the case and control groups.

10.9   ADDITIONAL READING

1. Chernick, M. R. and Liu, C. (2002). The Saw-toothed Behavior of Power versus Sample Size and Software Solutions: Single Binomial Proportion using Exact Methods. *The American Statistician* **56**, 149–155.

2. Clopper, C. J. and Pearson, E. S. (1934). The use of confidence or fiducial limits illustrated in the case of the binomial. *Biometrika* **26**, 404–413.

3. Hahn, G. J. and Meeker, W. Q. (1991). *Statistical Intervals: A Guide for Practitioners.* Wiley, New York.

4. Fleiss, J. L. (1981). *Statistical Methods for Rates and Proportions,* 2nd Edition. Wiley, New York.

CHAPTER 11

Categorical Data and
Chi-Square Tests

*It has become increasingly apparent over a period of several
years that psychologists, taken in the aggregate, employ the
chi-square test incorrectly.*
—Don Lewis and C. J. Burke, The Use and Misuse of the Chi-Square Test,
Psychological Bulletin, 46, 6, 1949, p. 433

The chi-square test is one of the most commonly cited tests in the biomedical literature. Before discussing this statistic, we would like to digress briefly to consider
how it fits into the "big picture" of statistical testing. Previously, we presented the
concepts of measurement systems, levels of measurement, and the appropriate use
of statistics for each type of measurement system.

To review, the four levels of measurement are nominal, ordinal, interval, and ratio. Nominal measures are classifications such as sex (male, female) or race (white,
black, Asian). Ordinal measures refer to rankings, e.g., shoe size (narrow, medium,
wide) or year in college (freshman, sophomore, junior, senior). Both interval and
ratio measures have the property of equal measurement intervals. The measurement
systems are different in that an interval scale does not have a true zero point, whereas a ratio scale has a meaningful zero point.

For example, the Fahrenheit temperature scale is an interval scale; IQ scores also
denote interval measurement. You may see that any two adjacent points on an interval scale have the same distance between them as any other two adjacent points,
i.e., the distance between IQ 60 and 61 is the same as the distance between 120 and
121—one unit. Note that the measurement scale for IQ does not have a true zero
point; there is no such thing as a zero IQ. A ratio scale is also an interval scale but it
has the property of a "true" zero point that means nothing. There are many examples of ratio scales: blood cholesterol level, height, and weight are only a few. You
can see that a cholesterol value of 0 would mean 0 cholesterol. However, a Fahrenheit temperature of 0 does not mean the absence of heat. In the Kelvin scale (a ratio
scale), a temperature of 0 refers to the absence of heat (purely a theoretical concept
that has never been attained).

11.1 UNDERSTANDING CHI-SQUARE

In chapters 8 and 9, we covered the *t* test and *Z* test, which use interval or ratio measures. Now we turn to the chi-square test, which is appropriate for nominal and ordinal measurement. The chi-square test may be used for two specific applications: (1) to assess whether an observed proportion agrees with expectations; (2) to determine whether there is a statistically significant association between two variables (such as variables that represent nominal level measurement or, in some cases, ordinal level measurement).

In the case of testing the association between two or more variables, the data are portrayed as contingency tables. these tables are also known as cross-tabulation tables. For example, the investigator might cross-tabulate the results for a study of gender and smoking status. A chi-square test could be used to determine the association between these two variables. Later, we will give an example of how to set up a contingency table and perform a chi-square test.

The formula for many test statistics with approximate chi-square distributions is:

$$\chi^2 = \sum \frac{(O-E)^2}{E} \tag{11.1}$$

where
O = observed frequency
E = expected frequency

As an example of one of the simplest uses of the foregoing formula, let us perform the chi-square test for a single proportion. (We will see that in some instances, the chi-square test may be used as an alternative to tests of proportion discussed in Chapter 10.) The chi-square test that we will use in this example shall be called a test with an a priori theoretical hypothesis, because the expected frequency of the outcome is known theoretically.

Suppose we run a coin toss experiment with 100 trials and find 70 heads; is this a biased outcome? That is, we want to know whether this is a very unusual event for a fair coin toss. If so, we may decide that the alternative—that the coin is loaded in favor of heads—may be more plausible. The data may be portrayed as shown in Table 11.1.

We would expect a fair coin toss to produce 50% heads and 50% tails in the long run (the theoretical a priori expectation). Table 11.1 lists all of the elements re-

TABLE 11.1. Data from a Coin Toss Experiment

	O	E	$O-E$	$(O-E)^2$	$(O-E)^2/E$
Heads	70	50	20	400	8
Tails	30	50	−20	400	8
Sum (Σ)	100	100	0	800	16

quired by the chi-square formula to calculate the chi-square statistic. This value is shown at the intersection of the last column and last row. Substituting it in the chi-square formula, we obtain:

$$\chi^2 = \Sigma \frac{(O - E)^2}{E} = 16$$

In order to evaluate whether this is a significant chi-square value—i.e., whether the coin toss is unfair—we need to compare the result we have obtained with the value in a chi-square table. We need to know the number of degrees of freedom associated with the coin toss experiment. Degrees of freedom (the term means "free to vary") are denoted by the symbol df. In this case, $df = 1$. (You may surmise that in a given number of coin tosses, once the number of heads is known, then the number of tails is fixed; only one value is free to vary. Let us say that in a small trial of 10 coin tosses, we find six heads; the number of tails *must* be four.)

In our example, we need to do a table lookup to determine the chi-square critical value. As with other statistical tests, the level of significance may be set to $p < 0.05$ or 0.01 or 0.001. We know from a chi-square table that the chi-square critical value is 3.84 for $df = 1$ at $p < 0.05$.

Therefore, the null hypothesis that the coin toss is unbiased would be rejected, as we obtained a chi-square of 16. The coin toss seems to be favoring heads. By the way, it is helpful to memorize this particular chi-square value as it comes up in many situations that have one degree of freedom, such as the 2 × 2 tables (shown in Sections 11.3 and 11.6).

One of the best statistical texts that deals explicitly with categorical data is Agresti (1990). Refer to it if you are interested in more details or aspects of the theory.

11.2   CHI-SQUARE DISTRIBUTIONS AND TABLES

Appendix D provides chi-square values for various degrees of freedom and p values. To use the table, identify the appropriate degrees of freedom (df) and level of significance of the test. The entries reported in the table each indicate the value of x^2 above which a proportion "p" of the distribution falls. Here is an example: For $df = 1$, a x^2 of 3.841 is exceeded by 5% of the distribution at $p = 0.05$.

11.3   TESTING INDEPENDENCE BETWEEN TWO VARIABLES

In testing independence between two variables, we do not assume an a priori expected outcome or theoretical (alternative) hypothesis. For example, we might want to know whether men differ from women in their preference for Western medicine or alternative medicine for treatment of stress-related medical problems. In this example, we assume that subjects can select only a single preference such as Western

TABLE 11.2. Gender and Preference for Medical Care

	Type of medical care preference		
Gender	Western	Alternative	Total
Men	49 (39.5) a	51 (60.5) b	100 $(a + b)$
Women	30 (39.5) c	70 (60.5) d	100 $(c + d)$
Total	79 $(a + c)$	121 $(b + d)$	200
			Grand total (n)

Note: Expected frequencies are shown in parentheses.

or alternative, but not both types. Our null hypothesis will be that the proportions in each category do not differ. There are a total of 200 subjects, equally divided between men and women as shown in Table 11.2; this is called a contingency table or cross-tabulation of two variables.

The table presents the observed frequencies from a survey of a research sample. Now we need to compute the expected frequencies for each of the four cells. This calculation uses the formula $[(a + b)(a + c)]/n$ for cell a. The formula is based on the null hypothesis that assumes no difference between men and women. This is the same as saying that the rows and columns are statistically independent. So the expected proportion of men who prefer Western medicine should be the population total n multiplied by the probability of being a man preferring Western medicine. The probability of being a man is estimated by the frequency $(a + b)/n$, the proportion of men in the table (sample). The probability of preferring Western medicine is estimated by $(a + c)/n$, the proportion of people favoring Western medicine in the table. The independence assumption lead to multiplication of these two probabilities, namely $[(a + b)/n]$ $[(a + c)/n]$ or $(a + b)(a + c)/n^2$. The foregoing formula is then obtained in a manner similar to that for an expectation for a binomial total; i.e., np, where in this case $p = (a + b)(a + c)/n^2$. So the expected total for the cell is $n\{(a + b)(a + c)/n^2\} = (a + b)(a + c)/n$. This same idea can be applied to obtain the expectations for the other three cells.

To calculate the expected frequency for cell a, we first determine the proportion of males and females $(100/200 = 0.5)$ and then multiply this result by the respective column totals (e.g., the expected frequency for men who prefer Western medicine is $0.5 \times 79 = (39.5)$ The general formula for the expected frequency in each cell is as follows:

$$E(a) = [(a + b)/n](a + c) = \frac{(a + b)(a + c)}{n}$$

$$E(b) = [(a + b)/n](b + d) = \frac{(a + b)(b + d)}{n}$$

$$E(c) = [(c + d)/n](a + c) = \frac{(c + d)(a + c)}{n}$$

$$E(d) = [(c + d)/n](b + d) = \frac{(c + d)(b + d)}{n}$$

$$\text{chi-square} = \frac{(49 - 39.5)^2}{39.5} + \frac{(30 - 39.5)^2}{39.5} + \frac{(51 - 60.5)^2}{60.5} + \frac{(70 - 60.5)^2}{60.5} = 7.55$$

where $df = 1$, χ^2 critical value = 3.84, and $\alpha = 0.05$. In contingency tables, degrees of freedom $(df) = (\# \text{ rows} - 1)(\# \text{ columns} - 1)$. For example, in this table, the chi-square critical value = 3.84, $\alpha = 0.05$, $df = 1$ $[df = (r - 1)(k - 1) = 1]$. We have obtained chi-square = 7.55, which exceeds the critical value. The result is statistically significant, suggesting that there are gender differences in preference for alternative medicine treatments for stress-related illnesses.

Now, in the next example (refer to Table 11.3), we will consider a chi-square test for a table that has more than two columns or rows. This type of table is called an $r \times c$ contingency table because there can be r rows and c columns. We will limit our example to a 3×3 table, i.e., one that has three rows and three columns. By extension, it will be possible to apply this example to tables that have r and c rows and columns.

Each cell in the contingency table is given an "address" depending on where it is located. Note that the first cell is $n_{1,1}$. The first subscripted number refers to the row and the second to the column; the last cell is $n_{3,3}$. The notations for the respective row and column totals are shown in the table.

The expected frequencies are computed as follows:

$$E(n_{1,1}) = \frac{(\Sigma n_1.)(\Sigma n_{.1})}{n}$$

$$E(n_{2,1}) = \frac{(\Sigma n_2.)(\Sigma n_{.1})}{n}$$

$$E(n_{3,3}) = \frac{(\Sigma n_3.)(\Sigma n_{.3})}{n}$$

There may be delays in participating in breast cancer screening programs according to racial group membership. As a result, some racial groups may tend to present with more advanced forms of breast cancer. Data from a hypothetical breast cancer staging study are shown in Table 11.4. We wish to test the hypothesis that

TABLE 11.3. Notation Used in a 3 × 3 Contingency Table

Variable X	Variable Y			
	$n_{1,1}$	$n_{1,2}$	$n_{1,3}$	$\Sigma n_1.$
	$n_{2,1}$	$n_{2,2}$	$n_{2,3}$	$\Sigma n_2.$
	$n_{3,1}$	$n_{3,2}$	$n_{3,3}$	$\Sigma n_3.$
	$\Sigma n_{.1}$	$\Sigma n_{.2}$	$\Sigma n_{.3}$	Total $= n$

TABLE 11.4. Computation Example—the Association between Race/Ethnicity and Breast Cancer Stage in a Sample of Tumor Registry Patients

	Breast cancer stage			
Race	In situ	Local	Regional/distant	Total
White	124 (232.28)	761 (663.91)	669 (657.81)	1554
African American	36 (83.85)	224 (239.67)	301 (237.47)	561
Asian	221 (64.87)	104 (185.42)	109 (183.71)	434
Total	381	1089	1079	2549

Note: Expected values are shown in parentheses.

the proportions of each racial classification by stage of breast cancer are equal. The expected frequencies shown in parentheses in Table 11.4 have been computed by using the foregoing formulas. For example, cell (1, 1): $(1554 \times 381)/2549 = 232.2770$. Then we compute $(O - E)^2/E$. These values are reported in Table 11.5.

Referring to Table 11.5, you can see that chi-square is 552.0993. The degrees of freedom are $(r - 1)(c - 1) = (3 - 1)(3 - 1) = 4$. At the 0.001 level, a chi-square value of 16.266 would be statistically significant. Thus, we may conclude that cancer diagnoses are not equally distributed by proportion across the contingency table.

11.4   TESTING FOR HOMOGENEITY

A chi-square test for homogeneity is used in empirical investigations when the marginal totals for one condition have been fixed at certain values and the totals for the other condition may vary at random. This situation might occur when an investigator has assigned a fixed number of subjects to a study design and then determines how the subjects are distributed according to a second variable, such as an exposure factor for a disease.

Table 11.6 provides an example of the possible association between smoking and chronic cough. Suppose that a researcher who is studying adult factory workers recruits 250 smokers and a comparison group of 300 nonsmokers. The researcher

TABLE 11.5. Values of $|O - E|^2/E$ for the Association between Race and Cancer Stage

	Breast cancer stage			
Race	In situ	Local	Regional/distant	Total
White	50.4738	14.1985	0.1902	
African American	27.3085	1.0250	16.9942	
Asian	375.7743	35.7499	30.3849	
Total	453.5566	50.9743	47.5694	552.0993

TABLE 11.6. The Association between Smoking and Chronic Cough

	Diagnosis of chronic cough		
Smoking	Yes	No	Total
Yes	99 (52.73) a	151 (197.27) b	250
No	17 (63.27) c	283 (236.73) d	300
Total	116 ($a + c$)	434 ($b + d$)	550
			Grand total (n)

Note: Expected frequencies are shown in parentheses.

then refers the employees to a medical exam that assesses the presence of lung diseases; chronic cough is included in the review of symptoms. The data are charted in Table 11.6.

The expected frequencies are computed in the same way as in a 2×2 table. (Refer back to Section 11.3 for the formulas.) Note also that the frequencies shown in cells b and d can be determined by subtraction. That is, if you know only the total number of smokers and the number of cases of chronic cough among smokers, you can determine the number of smokers who do not have chronic cough by subtraction $(250 - 99)$.

$$\text{Chi-square} = \frac{(99-52.73)^2}{52.73} + \frac{(17-63.27)^2}{63.27} + \frac{(151-197.27)^2}{197.27} + \frac{(283-236.73)^2}{236.73} = 94.33$$

This is a significant chi-square for $df = 1$ and suggests that the proportions of persons with chronic cough are not equally distributed between smokers and nonsmokers.

11.5   TESTING FOR DIFFERENCES BETWEEN TWO PROPORTIONS

The foregoing chi-square tests also may be considered tests of proportion and may be used as an alternative to the binomial test of proportions (Chapter 10). Tests for differences among groups are based on whether or not the proportions are equal. So a test of independence between gender and smoking is the same as testing that the proportion of male smokers equals the proportion of female smokers. The binomial test is called an exact test of significance, whereas the chi-square test is an approximate test of the comparison of two or more proportions. The chi-square test statistic under the null hypothesis has an approximate chi-square distribution based on asymptotic theory, but the exact probability distribution is not a chi-square. Hence, the significance level based on the table of the chi-square distribution is only an approximation to the true significance level. On the other hand, the binomial distribution is the exact probability of the test statistic and so an exact significance level can be found by referring to the appropriate binomial distribution under the null hypothesis.

11.6   THE SPECIAL CASE OF THE 2 × 2 CONTINGENCY TABLE

Many situations in biomedical research call for the use of a 2 × 2 contingency table
(Table 11.7) in which the researcher might be comparing two levels of a study condition, such as treatment and control, and two levels of an outcome, such as yes/no
or dead/alive. By using algebra, the formula for chi-square has been greatly simplified for easy computation. The calculation formula has many applications in epidemiologic research settings.

In a 2 × 2 table we use an independent chi-square test, where chi-square $= \Sigma(|O -
E| - 1/2)^2/E$. The term "1/2" is called Yates' correction and provides a more precise
estimate of chi-square when there are only two rows and columns.

By algebra, the calculation formula for a 2 × 2 χ^2 is:

$$\chi^2(df = 1) = \frac{(|ad - bc| - N/2)^2 N}{(a + b)(c + d)(a + c)(b + d)}$$

where $df = 1$, χ^2 critical $= 3.84$, and $\alpha = 0.05$.

Now let us apply the calculation formula to a specific example. Data shown in
Table 11.8 reflect the number of male and female smokers between two hypothetical samples of males and females ($n = 54$ and $n = 46$, respectively).

If there is no association between gender and smoking, one would expect that the
deviations between the observed and expected numbers of smokers and nonsmokers in each of the four cells are not statistically significant. If there is an association,
some of the cells will have statistically significant deviations between the observed
and expected frequencies, which would suggest an association between smoking
and gender.

Whether this association is likely or not likely to be due to chance may be evaluated by the chi-square statistic. Using the data in the bivariate 2 × 2 contingency
table (Table 11.8),

$$\chi^2 = \frac{(|21 \times 31 - 15 \times 33| - 100/2)^2\ 100}{(36)\ (64)\ (54)\ (46)} = .196$$

Because the calculated χ^2 does not exceed the critical value (3.84), gender does not
appear to be related to smoking status.

TABLE 11.7. General 2 × 2 Contingency Table

	Outcome		
Study Condition (or factor)	Yes	No	Total
Treatment	a	b	$a + b$
Control	c	d	$c + d$
Total	$a + c$	$b + d$	$a + b + c + d$
			Grand total

TABLE 11.8. Bivariate 2 × 2 Contingency Table

Gender	Smoking Status		
	Yes	No	Row Total
Male	$a = 21$	$b = 33$	$a + b = 54$
Female	$c = 15$	$d = 31$	$c + d = 46$
Column total	$a + c = 36$	$b + d = 64$	Grand total $= 100$

11.7 SIMPSON'S PARADOX IN THE 2 × 2 TABLE

Sometimes, as in a meta-analysis, it may be reasonable to combine results from two or more experiments that produce 2 × 2 contingency tables. We simply cumulate the totals in the individual contingency tables into the corresponding cells for the combined table. An apparent paradox called Simpson's paradox can result, however. In Simpson's paradox, we see a particular association in each table but when we combine the tables the association disappears or is reversed!

To see how this can happen, we take the following fictitious example from Lloyd (1999, pages 153–154). In this example, a new cancer treatment is applied to patients in a particular hospital and the patients are classified as terminal and non-terminal. Before considering the groups separately we naively think that we can evaluate the effectiveness of the treatment by simply comparing its effect on both terminal and nonterminal patients combined. The hospital has records that can be used to compare survival rates over a fixed period of time (say 2 years) for patients on the new treatment and patients taking the standard therapy. The hospital records the results in 2 × 2 tables to see if the new treatment is more effective for each of the groups. This results in the following 2 × 2 tables taken from Lloyd (1999) with permission.

Table for All Patients

Treatment	Survived	Died	Total
New	117	104	221
Old	177	44	221
Total	294	148	442

By examining the table, the result seems clear. In each treatment group, 221 patients got the treatment but 60 more patients survived in the old treatment compared to the new treatment group. This translates into a two-year survival rate of 80.1% for the old treatment group and only 52.9% for the new treatment group. The difference between these two proportions is clearly significant. So the old treatment is superior. Let us slow down a little and investigate more closely what is going on here. Since we can split the data into two tables, one for terminal patients and one for nonterminal patients, it make sense to do this. After all, without treatment terminal patients are likely to have a shorter survival time than nonterminal patients. How do these tables compare and what do they show about the treatments?

Table for Terminal Patients

Treatment	Survived	Died	Total
New	17	101	118
Old	2	36	38
Total	19	137	156

Table for Nonterminal Patients

Treatment	Survived	Died	Total
New	100	3	103
Old	175	8	183
Total	275	11	286

Here we see an entirely different picture! The survival rate is much lower in the table for terminal patients, as we might expect. But the new treatment provides a survival rate of 14.4% compared to a survival rate of only 5.2% for the old treatment. For the nonterminal patients, the new treatment has a 97.1% survival rate compared to a 95.6% rate for the old treatment. In both cases, the new treatment appears to be better (the difference between 97.1% and 95.6% may not be statistically significant).

Simpson's paradox occurs when, as in this example, two tables each show a higher proportion of success (e.g., survival) for the one group (e.g., the new treatment group), but when the data are combined into one table the success rate is higher for the other group (e.g., the old treatment group). Why did this happen? We have a situation in which the survival rates are very different for terminal and nonterminal patients but we did not have uniformity in the number of patients in the terminal group that received the new versus the old treatment. Probably because the new treatment was expected to help the terminal patients, far more terminal patients were given the new treatment compared to the old one (118 received the new treatment and only 38 received the old treatment among the terminal patients. This created a much larger number of nonsurviving patients in the new treatment group than in the old treatment group, even though the percentage of nonsurviving patients was lower. So when the two groups are combined, the new treatment group is penalized in the overall proportion nonsurviving simply because of the much higher number of nonsurviving patients contributed by the terminal group.

So we should not be surprised by the result and the paradox is not a real one. It does not make sense to pool this data when the proportions differ so drastically between the classes of patients. Had randomization been used so that the groups were balanced, we would not see this phenomenon. Simpson's paradox is a warning to think carefully about the data and to avoid combining data into a contingency table when there are known subgroups with markedly different success proportions. In our example, the overall survival rate for terminal patients was only 12.2%, with 19 out of 156 surviving. On the other hand, the survival rate for the nonterminal patients was 96.2%, with 275 out of 286 patients surviving. Although the difference in proportions is very dramatic here, Simpson's paradox can occur with differences that are not as sharp as these. The main ingredient that causes the trouble is the imbalance in sample sizes between the two treatment groups.

11.8   McNEMAR'S TEST FOR CORRELATED PROPORTIONS

In Chapter 9, we discussed the concept of paired observations. An illustration was the paired t test, which is used when two or more measurements are correlated. That is, we might conduct an experiment and collect before and after measurements on each subject. The subject's score on the after measure is in part a function of the status on the before measurement. Other examples in which paired observations occur include studies of twins (who have genetically similar characteristics) and animal experiments that use littermates.

We used the paired t test to examine correlated interval and ratio measurements. McNemar's test is used for categorical data that are correlated, for assessment of equality of proportions when the binary categorical measurements are correlated. When the binary measurements cannot be made on the same subjects, as in the following example, we can still use McNemar's test to advantage if there is a way to pair the subjects so that the results are correlated. Correlation will be discussed in detail in Chapter 12. This can happen, for example, in a case control study where demographic characteristics are used to match subjects.

Here is an example: Suppose that we would like to find out how people stop smoking successfully. In particular, we would like to determine which of two methods is more effective: the nicotine patch or group counseling sessions. So we match 150 subjects who tried to stop by using the nicotine patch with 150 subjects who tried to stop smoking by using group counseling.

Then we proceed as follows. Define 0 as a failure and 1 as a success. The possible pairs are (0, 0), (0, 1), (1, 0), and (1, 1) with the first coordinate representing the nicotine patch subject and the second representing the matched subject who tried group counseling. Let r be the number of cases with (1, 0) (i.e., the first member of the pair being successful on the nicotine patch with the corresponding member of the pair a failure using group counseling) and s the number of cases with (0, 1) (i.e., subjects who fail using the nicotine patch but whose corresponding member of the pair is successful under group counseling). These are called nonconcordant pairs because the subjects in the pair have opposing outcomes. The other pairs (0, 0) (both members of the pair fail) and (1, 1) (both members of the pair succeed) are called concordant pairs because the results are the same for the members of the pair. These are also sometimes called tied pairs because the scores are the same for each member of the pair.

The concordant observations provide information about the degree of positive

TABLE 11.9. Outcomes for Pairs of Subjects that Attempted to Stop Smoking

	Counseling Failure	Counseling Success
Nicotine Patch Failure	$(0, 0)\ n = 143$	$(0, 1)\ s = 48$
Nicotine Patch Success	$(1, 0)\ r = 92$	$(1, 1)\ b = 17$

correlation between the members of the pair but do not provide any information about whether or not the two proportions are equal. If we consider only the tables that have the observed values for $r + s$, the nonconcordant pairs provide all the information we need to test the null hypothesis that the two proportions are equal. This is similar to conditioning on the marginal totals as we did for Fisher's exact test in the 2×2 contingency table that you will encounter in Chapter 14.

Under the null hypothesis, we expect r and s to be about the same. So the expected total for $(1, 0)$ pairs is $(r + s)/2$ and the expected total for $(0, 1)$ is also $(r + s)/2$ under the null hypothesis. We use a chi-square statistic that compares the observed totals r and s to their expected values ($[r + s]/2$ under the null hypothesis). In McNemar's test, we ignore the number of concordant pairs $n + b$, where n is the number of $(0, 0)$ pairs and b is the number of $(1, 1)$ pairs. McNemar's test statistic is $T = (r - [r + s]/2)^2/[r + s]/2 + (s - [r + s]/2)^2/[r + s]/2$. This simplifies to $(r - s)^2/(r + s)$ since $(r - [r + s]/2)^2/[r + s]/2 = ([r - s]/2)^2/[r + s]/2 = (r - s)^2/[2(r + s)]$ and $(s - [r + s]/2)^2/[r + s]/2 = ([s - r]/2)^2/[r + s]/2 = (r - s)^2/[2(r + s)]$ also [see Conover (1999), page 166, for more details on McNemar's test]. The data are shown in Table 11.9. There are 300 matched pairs of subjects. 109 nicotine users were successful $(r + b)$ and 66 counseling users $(s + b)$ were successful. $T = (r - s)^2/(r + s) = (44)^2/140 = 1936/140 = 13.8$ (significant, $p < 0.01$, $df = 1$). Note that n and b are ignored since they do not contribute to determining the difference.

We conclude that the nicotine patch is more commonly used than group counseling among persons who stop smoking. Or put another way, subjects who try to stop smoking are more successful if they use the nicotine patch rather than group counseling.

11.9   RELATIVE RISK AND ODDS RATIOS

The concepts of relative risk and odds ratios are derived from epidemiologic studies. A thorough discussion of them is beyond the scope of this text. We refer the reader to Friis and Sellers (1999) or Lachin (2000) for in-depth coverage of these topics. However, we will review them briefly here, because they are common measures that are germane to any treatment of categorical data.

The relative risk is used in cohort studies, which are a type of prospective study in which persons who have different types of exposure to risk factors for disease are followed prospectively, meaning that disease-free subjects are followed over time and the occurrence of new cases of disease is recorded. The occurrence of new cases of disease (known as incidence) is compared between subjects who have an exposure of

TABLE 11.10. 2 × 2 Table for Assessment of Relative Risk

Factor	Outcome		Total
	Present	Absent	
Yes	a	b	$a + b$
No	c	d	$c + d$

R.R. (relative risk) = $a/(a + b) \div c/(c + d) = a(c + d)/c(a + b)$.

interest and those who do not. Consequently, the subjects must be free from the disease of interest before the exposure occurs, and they must be observed after a period of time to ascertain the effects of exposure. In a cohort study, the measure of association between exposure and disease is known as the relative risk (R.R.).

Relative risk is a number that can vary from very low (approaching 0) to "large." A relative risk of 1 suggests that the risk of an outcome of interest is equally balanced between those exposed and not exposed to the factor. As relative risk increases above 1, the risk factor has a stronger association with the study outcome. Table 11.10 presents the format of a 2 × 2 table for assessment of relative risk; a calculation example is provided in Table 11.11.

Researchers follow a cohort of 300 smokers and a comparison cohort of nonsmokers over a 20-year period. The relative risk of lung cancer associated with smoking is 98/300 ÷ 35/700 = 6.53. These data suggest that the smokers are 6.5 times more likely to develop lung cancer than the nonsmokers. Sometimes the relative risk can be less than 1. This value suggests that the exposure factor is a protective factor. For example, if the incidence of lung cancer had been lower among the smokers, smoking would be a protective factor for lung cancer!

A second type of major epidemiologic study is a case-control study. This study is a type of retrospective study in which cases (those who have a disease of interest) are compared with controls (those who do not have the disease) with respect to exposure history.

For example, we might also study the association between smoking and lung cancer by using the case-control approach. A group of lung cancer patients (the cases) and controls would be assessed for history of smoking. The odds ratio (O.R.) is the measure of association between the factor and outcome in a case-control study. In Table 11.12, we provide a 2 × 2 table for assessment of an odds ratio. The corresponding calculation example is shown in Table 11.13.

TABLE 11.11. Smoking and Lung Cancer Data for a Cohort Study

Smokers	Lung cancer		Total
	Present	Absent	
Yes	98	202	300
No	35	665	700

TABLE 11.12. 2 × 2 Table for Assessment of an Odds Ratio

Factor	Cases	Controls
Yes	a	b
No	c	d
Total	$a + c$	$b + d$

O.R. (odds ratio) = $a/c \div b/d = ad/bc$.

TABLE 11.13. Smoking and Lung Cancer Data for a Case-Control Study

Smokers	Lung Cancer Cases	Controls
Yes	18	15
No	9	12
Total	27	27

O.R. = 12 (18)/9 (15) = 1.6.

In this example, smokers were 1.6 times as likely to develop lung cancer as non-smokers. Note that the odds ratio is a measure of association that is interpreted in a similar way as a relative risk.

Note that throughout the foregoing examples we have calculated only point estimates of relative risk. You might be interested in confidence intervals or hypothesis tests. For example, if we could obtain a 95% confidence interval for relative risk that did not include 1, we would be able to reject the null hypothesis of no difference at the 5% level. This topic is outside the scope of the present text, but the interested reader can find the asymptotic results needed for approximate confidence intervals on relative risk in Lachin (2000), page 24.

11.10 GOODNESS OF FIT TESTS—FITTING HYPOTHESIZED PROBABILITY DISTRIBUTIONS

Goodness of fit tests are tests that compare a parametric distribution to observed data. Tests such as the Kolmogorov–Smirnov test look at how far a parametric cumulative distribution (e.g., normal or negative exponential) deviates from the empirical distribution. There is a chi-square test for goodness of fit. Recall the negative exponential distribution is a distribution with the probability density $f(x) = \lambda \exp(-\lambda x)$ for $x > 0$, where $\lambda > 0$ is known as the rate parameter.

For the chi-square test, we divide the range of possible values for a random variable into connected disjoint intervals. By this we mean that if the random variable can only take on values in the interval [0, 10] then the set of disjoint connected intervals could be [0, 2), [2, 4), [4, 6), [6, 8), and [8, 10]. These intervals are disjoint because they contain no points in common. They are connected because there are no points missing in between the intervals and when they are put together they comprise the entire range of possible values for the random variable.

For each interval, we count the number (or proportion) of observations from the observed data that fall in that interval. We also compute an expected number for the fitted probability distribution. The fitted probability distribution is simply the parametric distribution that uses estimates for the parameters in place of the unknown parameters. For example, a fitted normal distribution would use the sample mean and sample variance in place of the parameters μ and σ^2, respectively. As with the other chi-square tests described in this chapter, we compute the quantities $(O_i - E_i)^2/E_i$ for each interval i and sum them up over all the intervals $i = 1, 2, \ldots, k$. Here E_i is obtained by integrating the fitted probability density function over the ith interval.

Under the null hypothesis that the data come from the parametric distribution, the test statistic has an approximate chi-square distribution with $k - q - 1$ degrees of freedom, where q is the number of parameters estimated from the data to compute the expected values E_i.

So for a normal distribution, we would need to estimate the mean and standard deviation. Consequently, q would be 2 and the degrees of freedom would be $k - 3$. For a negative exponential distribution, we need to estimate only the rate parameter, so $q = 1$ and the degrees of freedom are $k - 2$. Recall that the rate parameter measures how many events we expect per unit time. Generally, we do not know its value a priori but can estimate it after the data have been collected. For a detailed account of goodness of fit tests for both continuous and discrete random variables, see the *Encyclopedia of Statistical Sciences, Volume 3* (1983), pp. 451–461.

The following example, taken from Nelson (1982), represents complete lifetime data for a negative exponential model. The table presents the time to breakdown of insulating fluid at a voltage of 35 kV. In this case, we have 12 observed times, which are shown in Table 11.14.

TABLE 11.14. Seconds to Insulating Fluid Breakdown at 35 kV*

Time (sec)
30
33
41
87
93
98
116
258
461
1180
1350
1500

*Adapted from Nelson, 1982, *p.* 252, Table 2.1.

First, we need to estimate the rate parameter. The best estimate of expected time to failure is the sum of the failure times divided by the number of failures. This estimate is often referred to as the mean time between failures. Using the data in Table 11.14, we calculate the mean time between failures as follows:

$$(30 + 33 + 41 + 87 + 93 + 98 + 116 + 258 + 461 + 1180 + 1350 + 1500)/12$$
$$= 437.25 \text{ seconds}$$

The reciprocal of this quantity is called the failure rate. In our example, it is 0.002287 failures per second.

Now we can determine for any interval the probability of failure in the interval denoted p_i for interval i. Since $S(t) = \exp(-\lambda t)$ is the survival probability for the interval $[0, t]$, we can estimate λ as 0.002287. For any interval, $i = [a_i, b_i]$, and p_i, the probability of failure in interval i, is estimated as $\exp(-0.002287a_i) - \exp(-0.00287b_i)$.

Suppose we have a range of values $[0, \infty]$. Now let us divide $[0, \infty]$ into four disjoint intervals: $[0, 90]$, $[90, 180]$, $[180, 500]$, and $[500, \infty]$. We observe four failures in the first interval, two failures in the second interval, two failures in the third interval, and three in the last interval. For each i, $E_i = np_i$. The resulting computations for this case, where $n = 12$, are given in Table 11.15.

In this example, the chi-square statistic is 2.13. We refer to the chi-square table (Appendix D) for the distribution under the null hypothesis. Since $k = 4$ and $q = 1$, the degrees of freedom are $k - q - 1 = 2$. From Appendix D we see that the p-value is between 0.10 and 0.90. So we cannot reject the null hypothesis of a negative exponential distribution. The data seem to fit the negative exponential distribution reasonably well.

11.11 LIMITATIONS TO CHI-SQUARE AND EXACT ALTERNATIVES

The following are some general caveats regarding use of the chi-square test. These guidelines are based on statisticians' experiences with the test. Many statisticians

TABLE 11.15. Chi-Square Test for Negative Exponential Distribution

Interval	Observed (O)	Expected (E)	$(O - E)^2/E$
[0, 90]	4	$12(1 - \exp[-(0.002287)90]) = 0.186(12) = 2.23$	$(4 - 2.23)^2/2.23 = 1.405$
(90, 180]	3	$12(\exp[-(0.002287)90] - \exp[-(0.002287)180])$ $= (0.834 - 0.597)(12) = (0.237)12 = 2.85$	$(3 - 2.85)^2/2.85 = 0.008$
(180, 500]	2	$12(\exp[-(0.002287)180] - \exp[-(0.002287)500])$ $= (0.597 - 0.319)(12) = (0.278)12 = 3.34$	$(2 - 3.34)^2/3.34 = 0.538$
(500, ∞)	3	$12 (\exp[-(0.002287)500] = 0.319(12) = 3.828$	$(3 - 3.828)^2/3.828 = 0.179$
Total			2.130

have identified the limitations of the chi-square test through the use of simulations. As noted, the test should be used for data in the form of counts, enumerations, or frequencies. A particular cell should not have small frequencies (e.g., $n < 5$), and the grand total N should be greater than 20. The chi-square test is an approximate test, and the approximation can be poor when the cell frequencies are low. In a two-way or N-way table, the subjects being classified should be chosen independently (with the exception of McNemar's test). For example, if one is studying sex differences, one should choose samples of males and females independently.

An example of nonindependent selection would be to choose men and women who are spouses. Similarly, pairs of twins would not qualify as independently selected. In the special case of a 2×2 table, Yates' correction gives an improved estimation of chi-square. Yates' correction is built into the calculation formula as $N/2$ and gives an improved estimate of χ^2 when $df = 1$.

Given that the chi-square test does not involve parameter values directly, it does not have a corresponding confidence interval. Furthermore, it is not easy to calculate the required sample sizes (power testing) for a chi-square test. However, the software package StatXact 5.0, described in Chapter 16, calculates power and sample sizes for the analogous exact tests. .

Among the alternatives for the 2×2 table is Fisher's exact test, which Chapter 14 (section on permutation tests) will cover in detail. We use Fisher's exact test for problems that involve small sizes when expected cell values are smaller than 5. This test is based on specifying that the row and column totals are fixed. Various other exact tests are described in detail in the StatXact users guide.

11.12   EXERCISES

11.1 State in your words definitions of the following terms:
  a. Chi-square
  b. Contingency table (cross-tabulation)
  c. Correlated proportions
  d. Odds ratio
  e. Goodness of fit test
  f. Test for independence of two variables
  g. Homogeneity

11.2 A hospital accrediting agency reported that the survival rate for patients who had coronary bypass surgery in tertiary care centers was 93%. A sample of community hospitals had an average survival rate of 88%. Were the survival rates for the two types of hospitals the same or different?

11.3 Researchers at an academic medical center performed a clinical trial to study the effectiveness of a new medication to lower blood sugar. Diabetic patients were assigned at random to treatment and control conditions. Patients in both groups received counseling regarding exercise and weight loss. Among the

TABLE 11.16. Cross-Tabulation of Lifetime Smoking and Self-Reported Health Status

Self-reported health status	Have you smoked 100 cigarettes in your life?		
	Yes	No	Total
Excellent	142	227	369
Very good/good	368	475	843
Fair/poor	122	155	277
Total	632	857	1,489

Source: Robert Friis, Long Beach Community Health Study (1998 interview wave).

sample of 200 treatment patients, 60% were found to have normal fasting blood glucose levels at follow-up. Among an equal number of controls, only 15% had normal fasting blood glucose levels at follow-up. Demonstrate that the new medication was effective in treating hyperglycemia.

11.4 In a community health survey, individuals were randomly selected for participation in a telephone interview. The study used a cross-sectional design. Table 11.16 shows the results for the cross-tabulation of cigarette smoking and health status. Determine whether the relationship between smoking 100 cigarettes during one's life and self-reported health status is statistically significant at the $\alpha = 0.05$ level.

11.5 In the community health survey described in the previous exercise, respondents' smoking status was classified into three categories (smoker, quitter, never smoker). Table 11.17 shows the results for the cross-tabulation of smoking status and health status. Determine whether the relationship is statistically significant at the $\alpha = 0.05$ level. Compare your results with those obtained in the previous exercise.

11.6 In the same community health survey, the investigators wanted to know whether smoking status varied according to race/ethnicity. Race was measured according to five categories (African American, Asian, Hispanic, Na-

TABLE 11.17. Cross-Tabulation of Smoking Status and Self-Reported Health Status

Self-reported health status	Smoking Status			
	Smoker	Quitter	Never	Total
Excellent	40	100	229	369
Very good/good	172	189	485	846
Fair/poor	61	63	153	277
Total	273	352	867	1,492

Source: Robert Friis, Long Beach Community Health Study (1998 interview wave).

TABLE 11.18. Cross-Tabulation of Race/Ethnicity and Self-Reported Health Status

| Race/Ethnicity | Smoking Status | | | |
	Smoker	Quitter	Never	Total
African American	45	41	123	209
Asian	13	12	53	78
Hispanic	50	75	311	436
Native American	10	5	14	29
European American	144	201	350	695
Total	262	334	851	1, 447

Source: Robert Friis, Long Beach Community Health Study (1998 interview wave).

tive American, European American) and smoking status was classified according to the same categories as in Exercise 11.6. Table 11.18 shows the results for the cross-tabulation of race and health status. Does smoking status vary according to race? Perform the test at the $\alpha = 0.05$ level.

11.7 In the community health survey, the investigators studied the relationship between alcohol drinking status (defined according to four categories) and smoking status (defined according to three categories). Alcohol drinking status was classified according to the categories of current drinker, former drinker, occasional drinker, and never drinker. Table 11.19 shows the resulting cross-tabulation. Inspect the data shown in the table. Do you think that there is an association between alcohol drinking status and smoking status? Confirm your subjective impressions by performing a statistical test at the $\alpha = 0.05$ level.

11.8 A multiphasic health examination was administered to 1000 employees of a pharmaceutical firm. 50% of these employees had elevated diastolic blood pressure and 45% had hypoglycemia. A total of 37% of employees had both elevated diastolic blood pressure and hyperglycemia. Create a 2 × 2 contingency table and fill in all cells of the table. Is the association between hypertension and hyperglycemia statistically significant?

TABLE 11.19. Cross-Tabulation of Smoking Status and Alcohol Drinking Status

| Smoking Status | Alcohol Drinking Status | | | | |
	Current	Former	Occasional	Never	Total
Heavy	56	10	7	8	81
Moderate	78	16	17	6	117
Light	52	10	7	5	74
Total	186	36	31	19	272

Source: Robert Friis, Long Beach Community Health Study (1998 interview wave).

11.13 ADDITIONAL READING

1. Agresti, A. (1990). *Categorical Data Analysis.* Wiley, New York.
2. CYTEL Software Corporation (1998). *StatXact4 for Windows: Statistical Software for Exact Nonparametric Inference User Manual.* CYTEL: Cambridge, Massachusetts.
3. Friis, R. H. and Sellers, T. A. (1999). *Epidemiology for Public Health Practice,* Second Edition. Aspen, Gaithersburg, Maryland.
4. Kotz, S. and Johnson, N. L. (1983). *Encyclopedia of Statistical Sciences, Volume 3,* Faa di Bruno's Formula—Hypothesis Testing. Wiley, New York.
5. Lachin, J.M. (2000). *Biostatistical Methods: The Assessment of Relative Risks.* Wiley, New York.
6. Lloyd, C. J. (1999). *Statistical Analysis of Categorical Data.* Wiley, New York.
7. Nelson, W. (1982). *Applied Life Data Analysis.* Wiley, New York.

CHAPTER 12

Correlation, Linear Regression, and Logistic Regression

> *Biological phenomena in their numerous phases, economic and social, were seen to be only differentiated from the physical by the intensity of their correlations. The idea Galton placed before himself was to represent by a single quantity the degree of relationships, or of partial causality between the different variables of our everchanging universe.*
> —Karl Pearson, *The Life, Letters, and Labours of Francis Galton,*
> Volume IIIA, Chapter XIV, p. 2

The previous chapter presented various chi-square tests for determining whether or not two variables that represented categorical measurements were significantly associated. The question arises about how to determine associations between variables that represent higher levels of measurement. This chapter will cover the Pearson product moment correlation coefficient (Pearson correlation coefficient or Pearson correlation), which is a method for assessing the association between two variables that represent either interval- or ratio-level measurement.

Remember from the previous chapter that examples of interval level measurement are Fahrenheit temperature and I.Q. scores; ratio level measures include blood pressure, serum cholesterol, and many other biomedical research variables that have a true zero point. In comparison to the chi-square test, the correlation coefficient provides additional useful information—namely, the strength of association between the two variables.

We will also see that linear regression and correlation are related because there are formulas that relate the correlation coefficient to the slope parameter of the regression equation.. In contrast to correlation, linear regression is used for predicting status on a second variable (e.g., a dependent variable) when the value of a predictor variable (e.g., an independent variable) is known.

Another technique that provides information about the strength of association between a predictor variable (e.g., a risk factor variable) and an outcome variable (e.g., dead or alive) is logistic regression. In the case of a logistic regression analysis, the outcome is a dichotomy; the predictor can be selected from variables that represent several levels of measurement (such as categorical or ordinal), as we will demonstrate in Section 12.9. For example, a physician may use a patient's total serum cholesterol value and race to predict high or low levels of coronary heart disease risk.

12.1   RELATIONSHIPS BETWEEN TWO VARIABLES

In Figure 12.1, we present examples of several types of relationships between two variables. Note that the horizontal and vertical axes are denoted by the symbols X and Y, respectively.

Both Figures 12.1A and 12.1B represent linear associations, whereas the remaining figures illustrate nonlinear associations. Figures 12.1A and 12.1B portray direct and inverse linear associations, respectively. The remaining figures represent nonlinear associations, which cannot be assessed directly by using a Pearson correlation coefficient. To assess these types of associations, we will need to apply other statistical methods such as those described in Chapter 14 (nonparametric tests). In other cases, we can use data transformations, a topic that will be discussed briefly later in this text.

12.2   USES OF CORRELATION AND REGRESSION

The Pearson correlation coefficient (ρ), is a population parameter that measures the degree of association between two variables. It is a natural parameter for a distribution called the bivariate normal distribution. Briefly, the bivariate normal distribution is a probability distribution for X and Y that has normal distributions for both X and Y and a special form for the density function for the variable pairs. This form allows for positive or negative dependence between X and Y.

The Pearson correlation coefficient is used for assessing the linear (straight line) association between an X and a Y variable, and requires interval or ratio measurement. The symbol for the sample correlation coefficient is r, which is the sample estimate of ρ that can be obtained from a sample of pairs (X, Y) of values for X and Y. The correlation varies from negative one to positive one ($-1 \leq r \leq +1$). A correlation of $+1$ or -1 refers to a perfect positive or negative X, Y relationship, respectively (refer to Figures 12.1A and 12.1B). Data falling exactly on a straight line indicates that $|r| = 1$.

The reader should remember that correlation coefficients merely indicate association between X and Y, and not causation. If $|r| = 1$, then all the sample data fall exactly on a straight line. This one-to-one association observed for the sample data does not necessarily mean that $|\rho| = 1$; but if the number of pairs is large, a high value for r suggests that the correlation between the variable pairs in the population is high.

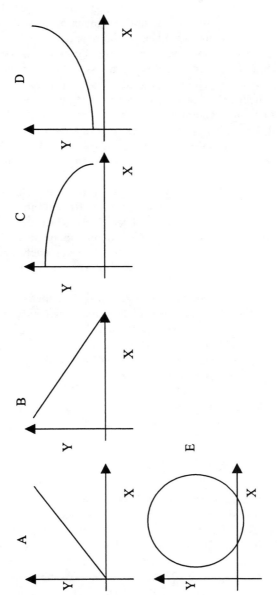

Figure 12.1. Examples of bivariate associations.

Previously, we defined the term "variance" and saw that it is a special parameter of a univariate normal distribution. With respect to correlation and regression, we will be considering the bivariate normal distribution. Just as the univariate normal distribution has mean and variance as natural parameters in the density function, so too is the correlation coefficient a natural parameter of the bivariate normal distribution. This point will be discussed later in this chapter.

Many biomedical examples call for the use of correlation coefficients: A physician might want to know whether there is an association between total serum cholesterol values and triglycerides. A medical school admission committee might want to study whether there is a correlation between grade point averages of graduates and MCAT scores at admission. In psychiatry, interval scales are used to measure stress and personality characteristics such as affective states. For example, researchers have studied the correlation between Center for Epidemiologic Studies Depression (CESD) scores (a measure of depressive symptoms) and stressful life events measures.

Regression analysis is very closely related to linear correlation analysis. In fact, we will learn that the formulae for correlation coefficients and the slope of a regression line are similar and functionally related. Thus far we have dealt with bivariate examples, but linear regression can extend to more than one predictor variable. The linearity requirement in the model is for the regression coefficients and not for the predictor variables. We will provide more information on multiple regression in Section 12.9.

Investigators use regression analysis very widely in the biomedical sciences. As noted previously, the researchers use an independent variable to predict a dependent variable. For example, regression analysis may be used to assess a dose–response relationship for a drug administered to laboratory animals. The drug dose would be considered the independent variable, and the response chosen would be the dependent variable. A dose–response relationship is a type of relationship in which increasing doses of a substance produce increasing biological responses; e.g., the relationship between number of cigarettes consumed and incidence of lung cancer is considered to be a dose–response relationship.

12.3 THE SCATTER DIAGRAM

A scatter diagram is used to portray the relationship between two variables; the relationship occurs in a sample of ordered (X, Y) pairs. One constructs such a diagram by plotting, on Cartesian coordinates, X and Y measurements (X and Y pairs) for each subject. As an example of two highly correlated measures, consider systolic and diastolic blood pressure. Remember that when your blood pressure is measured, you are given two values (e.g., 120/70). Across a sample of subjects, these two values are known to be highly correlated and are said to form a linear (straight line) relationship.

Further, as r decreases, the points on a scatter plot diverge from the line of best fit. The points form a cloud—a scatter cloud—of dots; two measures that are uncorrelated would produce the interior of a circle or an ellipse without tilt. Table 12.1

TABLE 12.1. Systolic and Diastolic Blood Pressure Values for a Sample of 48 Elderly Men

Systolic BP	Diastolic BP	Systolic BP	Diastolic BP	Systolic BP	Diastolic BP	Systolic BP	Diastolic BP
140	78	117	75	145	81	146	83
170	101	141	83	151	83	162	83
141	84	120	76	134	85	158	77
171	92	163	89	178	99	152	86
158	80	155	97	128	73	152	93
175	91	114	76	147	78	106	67
151	78	151	90	146	80	147	79
152	82	136	87	160	91	111	71
138	81	143	84	173	79	149	83
136	80	163	75	143	87	137	77
173	95	143	81	152	69	136	84
143	84	163	94	137	85	132	79

presents blood pressure data collected from a sample of 48 elderly men who participated in a study of cardiovascular health.

In order to produce a scatter diagram, we take a piece of graph paper and draw X and Y axes. The X axis (horizontal axis) is called the abscissa; it is also used to denote the independent variable that we have identified in our analytic model. The Y axis (vertical axis), or ordinate, identifies the dependent, or outcome, variable. We then plot variable pairs on the graph paper.

For example, the first pair of measurements (140, 78) from Table 12.1 comprises a point on the scatter plot. When we plot all of the pairs in the table, the result is the scatter diagram shown in Figure 12.2. For the blood pressure data, the choice of the X or Y axes is arbitrary, for there is no independent or dependent variable.

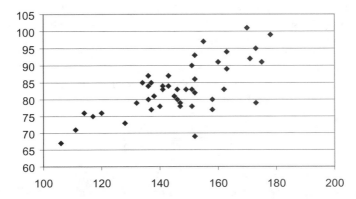

Figure 12.2. Scatter diagram of systolic and diastolic blood pressure (using data from Table 12.1).

12.4 PEARSON'S PRODUCT MOMENT CORRELATION COEFFICIENT AND ITS SAMPLE ESTIMATE

The formulae for a Pearson sample product moment correlation coefficient (also called a Pearson correlation coefficient) are shown in Equations 12.1 and 12.2. The deviation score formula for r is

$$r = \frac{\sum_{i=1}^{n}(X-\bar{X})(Y-\bar{Y})}{\sqrt{\sum_{i=1}^{n}(X-\bar{X})^2 \sum_{i=1}^{n}(Y-\bar{Y})^2}} \tag{12.1}$$

The calculation formula for r is

$$r = \frac{\sum_{i=1}^{n}XY - \dfrac{\left(\sum_{i=1}^{n}X\right)\left(\sum_{i=1}^{n}Y\right)}{n}}{\sqrt{\left[\dfrac{\sum_{i=1}^{n}X^2 - \left(\sum_{i=1}^{n}X\right)^2}{n}\right]\left[\dfrac{\sum_{i=1}^{n}Y^2 - \left(\sum_{i=1}^{n}Y\right)^2}{n}\right]}} \tag{12.2}$$

We will apply these formulae to the small sample of weight and height measurements shown in Table 12.2. The first calculation uses the deviation score formula (i.e., the difference between each observation for a variable and the mean of the variable).

The data needed for the formulae are shown in Table 12.3. When using the calculation formula, we do not need to create difference scores, making the calculations a bit easier to perform with a hand-held calculator.

We would like to emphasize that the Pearson product moment correlation measures the strength of the linear relationship between the variables X and Y. Two variables X and Y can have an exact non-linear functional relationship, implying a form of dependence, and yet have zero correlation. An example would be the function $y = x^2$ for x between -1 and $+1$. Suppose that X is uniformly distributed on $[0, 1]$ and $Y = X_2$ without any error term. For a bivariate distribution, r is an estimate of the correlation (ρ) between X and Y, where

$$\rho = \frac{\mathrm{Cov}(X, Y)}{\sqrt{\mathrm{Var}(X)\mathrm{Var}(Y)}}$$

The covariance between X and Y defined by $\mathrm{Cov}(X, Y)$ is $E[(X-\mu_x)(Y-\mu_y)]$, where μ_x and μ_y are, respectively, the population means for X and Y. We will show that $\mathrm{Cov}(X, Y) = 0$ and, consequently, $\rho = 0$. For those who know calculus, this proof is

TABLE 12.2. Deviation Score Method for Calculating r (Pearson Correlation Coefficient)

ID	Weight (X)	$(X-\bar{X})$	$(X-\bar{X})^2$	Height (Y)	$(Y-\bar{Y})$	$(Y-\bar{Y})^2$	$(X-\bar{X})(Y-\bar{Y})$
1	148	−6.10	37.21	64	1.00	1.00	−6.10
2	172	17.90	320.41	63	0.00	0.00	0.00
3	203	48.90	2391.21	67	4.00	16.00	195.60
4	109	−45.10	2034.01	60	−3.00	9.00	135.30
5	110	−44.10	1944.81	63	0.00	0.00	0.00
6	134	−20.10	404.01	62	−1.00	1.00	20.10
7	195	40.90	1672.81	59	−4.00	16.00	−163.60
8	147	−7.10	50.41	62	−1.00	1.00	7.10
9	153	−1.10	1.21	66	3.00	9.00	−3.30
10	170	15.90	252.81	64	1.00	1.00	15.90
Σ	1541		9108.90	630		54.00	201.00

$$\bar{X} = 1541/10 = 154.10 \qquad\qquad \bar{Y} = 630/10 = 63.00$$

$$r = \frac{\sum_{i=1}^{n}(X_i-\bar{X})(Y_i-\bar{Y})}{\sqrt{\sum_{i=1}^{n}(X_i-\bar{X})^2 \sum_{i=1}^{n}(Y_i-\bar{Y})^2}} \qquad r = \frac{201}{\sqrt{(9108.90)(54)}} \quad r = \frac{201.00}{701.34} = 0.29$$

TABLE 12.3. Calculation Formula Method for Calculating r (Pearson Correlation Coefficient)

ID	Weight (X)	X_2	Height (Y)	Y_2	XY
1	148	21,904	64	4,096	9,472
2	172	29,584	63	3,969	10,836
3	203	41,209	67	4,489	13,601
4	109	11,881	60	3,600	6,540
5	110	12,100	63	3,969	6,930
6	134	17,956	62	3,844	8,308
7	195	38,025	59	3,481	11,505
8	147	21,609	62	3,844	9,114
9	153	23,409	66	4,356	10,098
10	170	28,900	64	4,096	10,880
Σ	1,541	246,577	630	39,744	97,284

$$r = \frac{\sum_{i=1}^{n}X_iY_i - \dfrac{\left(\sum_{i=1}^{n}X_i\right)\left(\sum_{i=1}^{n}Y_i\right)}{n}}{\sqrt{\left[\sum_{i=1}^{n}X_i^2 - \dfrac{\left(\sum_{i=1}^{n}X_i\right)^2}{n}\right]\left[\sum_{i=1}^{n}Y_i^2 - \dfrac{\left(\sum_{i=1}^{n}Y_i\right)^2}{n}\right]}}$$

$$r = \frac{97284 - \dfrac{(1541)(630)}{10}}{\sqrt{\left[246577 - \dfrac{(1541)^2}{10}\right]\left[39744 - \dfrac{(630)^2}{10}\right]}} \qquad r = \frac{201.00}{701.34} = 0.29$$

Display 12.1: Proof of Cov(X, Y) = 0 and $\rho = 0$ for $Y = X^2$

$E(X) = 0$ since $\int_{-1}^{1} x f(x)dx = 0$, also $E(Y) = E(X^2) = \int_{-1}^{1} x^2 f(x)dx = \int_{-1}^{1} x^2(1)dx = \dfrac{x^3}{3}\Big|_{-1}^{+1} = \dfrac{2}{3}$

$\mathrm{Cov}(X, Y) = E\left[(X - 0)\left(Y - \dfrac{2}{3}\right)\right] = E[XY] - \left(\dfrac{2}{3}\right)E[X] = E[XY]$ since $E[XY] = 0$

Now $E[XY] = E[X^3]$ since $Y = X^2$ and $E[X^3] = \int_{-1}^{1} x^3 f(x)dx = \dfrac{x^4}{4}\Big|_{-1}^{+1} = \dfrac{1^4 - (-1)^4}{4} = 0$

---

shown in Display 12.1. However, understanding this proof is not essential to understanding the material in this section.

12.5 TESTING HYPOTHESES ABOUT THE CORRELATION COEFFICIENT

In addition to assessing the strength of association between two variables, we need to know whether their association is statistically significant. The test for the significance of a correlation coefficient is based on a t test. In Section 12.4, we presented r (the sample statistic for correlation) and ρ (the population parameter for the correlation between X and Y in the population).

The test for the significance of a correlation evaluates the null hypothesis (H_0) that $\rho = 0$ in the population. We assume $Y = a + bX + \varepsilon$. Testing $\rho = 0$ is the same as testing $b = 0$. The term ε in the equation is called the noise term or error term. It is also sometimes referred to as the residual term. The assumption required for hypothesis testing is that the noise term has a normal distribution with a mean of zero and unknown variance σ^2 independent of X. The significance test for Pearson's correlation coefficient is

$$t_{df} = \frac{r}{\sqrt{1 - r^2}} \sqrt{n - 2} \tag{12.3}$$

where $df = n - 2$; $n =$ number of pairs.

Referring to the earlier example presented in Table 12.2, we may test whether the previously obtained correlation is significant by using the following procedure:

$$t_{df} = \frac{r}{\sqrt{1 - r^2}} \sqrt{n - 2} \qquad df = 10 - 2 = 8$$

$$t = \frac{0.29}{\sqrt{1 - (0.29)^2}} \sqrt{10 - 2} = \frac{0.29}{\sqrt{1 - (0.0729)}} \sqrt{8} = \frac{0.29}{0.9629}(2.8284) = 0.79$$

where $p =$ n.s., t critical $= 2.306$, 2-tailed.

12.6 CORRELATION MATRIX

A correlation matrix presents correlation coefficients among a group of variables. An investigator portrays all possible bivariate combinations of a set of variables in order to ascertain patterns of interesting associations for further study. Table 12.4 illustrates a matrix of correlations among seven risk factor variables for coronary heart disease among a sample of older men. Note that the upper and lower diagonals of the grid are bisected by diagonal cells in which all of the values are 1.000, meaning that these cells show the variables correlated with themselves. The upper and lower parts of the diagonal are equivalent. The significance of the correlations are indicated with one asterisk or two asterisks for a correlation that is significant at the $p < 0.05$ or $p < 0.01$ levels, respectively. A correlation matrix can aid in data reduction (identifying the most important variables in a data set) or descriptive analyses (describing interesting patterns that may be present in the data set).

12.7 REGRESSION ANALYSIS AND LEAST SQUARES INFERENCE REGARDING THE SLOPE AND INTERCEPT OF A REGRESSION LINE

We will first consider methods for regression analysis and then relate the concept of regression analysis to testing hypotheses about the significance of a regression line.

TABLE 12.4. Matrix of Pearson Correlations among Coronary Heart Disease Risk Factors, Men Aged 57–97 Years ($n = 70$)

	Age in years	Weight in pounds	Height in inches	Diastolic blood pressure	Systolic blood pressure	Cholesterol level	Blood sugar
Age in years	1.000	−0.021	−0.033	0.104	0.276*	−0.063	−0.039
Weight in pounds	−0.021	1.000	0.250*	0.212	0.025	−0.030	−0.136
Height in inches	−0.033	0.250*	1.000	0.119	−0.083	−0.111	0.057
Diastolic blood pressure	0.104	0.212	0.119	1.000	0.671**	0.182	0.111
Systolic blood pressure	0.276*	0.025	−0.083	0.671**	1.000	0.060	0.046
Cholesterol level	−0.063	−0.030	−0.111	0.182	0.060	1.000	0.006
Blood sugar	−0.039	−0.136	0.057	0.111	0.046	0.006	1.000

*Correlation is significant at the 0.05 level (2-tailed).
**Correlation is significant at the 0.01 level (2-tailed).
Note: The correlation of a variable with itself is always 1.0 and has no particular value but is included as the diagonal elements of the correlation matrix.

The method of least squares provides the underpinnings for regression analysis. In order to illustrate regression analysis, we present the simplified scatter plot of six observations in Figure 12.3.

The figure shows a line of best linear fit, which is the only straight line that minimizes the sum of squared deviations from each point to the regression line. The deviations are formed by subtending a line that is parallel to the Y axis from each point to the regression line. Remember that each point in the scatter plot is formed from measurement pairs (x, y values) that correspond to the abscissa and ordinate. Let Y correspond to a point on the line of best fit that corresponds to a particular y measurement. Then $Y - \hat{Y}$ = the deviations of each observed ordinate from Y, and

$$\sum (Y - \hat{Y})^2 \xrightarrow{\text{min}}$$

From algebra, we know that the general form of an equation for a straight line is: $Y = a + bX$, where a = the intercept (point where the line crosses the ordinate) and b = the slope of the line. The general form of the equation $Y = a + bX$ assumes Cartesian coordinates and the data points do not deviate from a straight line. In regression analysis, we need to find the line of best fit through a scatterplot of (X, Y) measurements. Thus, the straight-line equation is modified somewhat to allow for error between observed and predicted values for Y. The model for the regression equation is $Y = a + bX + e$, where e denotes an error (or residual) term that is estimated by $Y - \hat{Y}$ and $\Sigma(Y - \hat{Y})^2 = \Sigma e^2$. The prediction equation for $\hat{Y}$ is $\hat{Y} = a + bX$.

The term $\hat{Y}$ is called the expected value of Y for X. $\hat{Y}$ is also called the conditional mean. The prediction equation $\hat{Y} = a + bX$ is called the estimated regression equation for Y on X. From the equation for a straight line, we will be able to estimate (or predict) a value for Y if we are given a value for X. If we had the slope and intercept for Figure 12.2, we could predict systolic blood pressure if we knew only a subject's diastolic blood pressure. The slope (b) tells us how steeply the line inclines; for example, a flat line has a slope equal to 0.

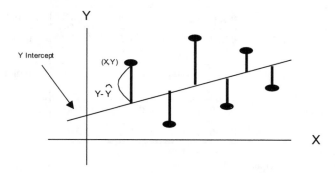

Figure 12.3. Scatter plot of six observations.

Substituting for Y in the sums of squares about the regression line gives $\Sigma(Y - \hat{Y})^2$ $= \Sigma(Y - a - bX)^2$. We will not carry out the proof. However, solving for b, it can be demonstrated that the slope is

$$b = \frac{\sum_{i=1}^{n}(X_i - \overline{X})(Y_i - \overline{Y})}{\sum_{i=1}^{n}(X_i - \overline{X})^2} \tag{12.4}$$

Note the similarity between this formula and the deviation score formula for r shown in Section 12.4. The equation for a correlation coefficient is

$$r = \frac{\sum_{i=1}^{n}(X_i - \overline{X})(Y_i - \overline{Y})}{\sqrt{\sum_{i=1}^{n}(X_i - \overline{X})^2 \sum_{i=1}^{n}(Y_i - \overline{Y})^2}}$$

This equation contains the term $\Sigma_{i=1}^{n}(Y_i - \overline{Y})^2$ in the denominator whereas the formula for the regression equation does not. Using the formula for sample variance, we may define

$$S_y^2 = \sum_{i=1}^{n}\frac{(Y_i - \overline{Y})^2}{n - 1}$$

and

$$S_y^2 = \sum_{i=1}^{n}\frac{(X_i - \overline{X})^2}{n - 1}$$

The terms s_y and s_x are simply the square roots of these respective terms. Alternatively, $b = (S_y/S_x)r$. The formulas for estimated y and the y-intercept are:

estimated $y(\hat{Y})$: $\hat{Y} = a + b\overline{X}$ intercept (a): $a = \overline{X} - b\overline{X}$

In some instances, it may be easier to use the calculation formula for a slope, as shown in Equation 12.5:

$$b = \frac{\sum_{i=1}^{n}X_iY_i - \dfrac{\sum_{i=1}^{n}X_i \sum_{i=1}^{n}Y_i}{n}}{\sum_{i=1}^{n}X_i^2 - \dfrac{\left(\sum_{i=1}^{n}Y_i\right)^2}{n}} \tag{12.5}$$

In the following examples, we will demonstrate sample calculations using both the deviation and calculation formulas. From Table 12.2 (deviation score method):

$$\sum(X-\overline{X})(Y-\overline{Y}) = 201 \qquad \sum(X-\overline{X})^2 = 9108.90$$

$$b = \frac{201}{9108.90} = 0.0221$$

From Table 12.3 (calculation formula method):

$$\Sigma XY = 97{,}284 \quad \Sigma X \Sigma Y = (1541)(630) \qquad n = 10 \ \Sigma X_2 = 246{,}577$$

$$b = \frac{97{,}284 - \dfrac{(1541)(630)}{10}}{246{,}577 - \dfrac{(1541)^2}{10}} \qquad b = 0.0221$$

Thus, both formulas yield exactly the same values for the slope. Solving for the y-intercept (a), $a = Y - b\overline{X} = 63 - (0.0221)(154.10) = 59.5944$.

The regression equation becomes $\hat{Y} = 59.5944 + 0.0221x$ or, alternatively, height $= 59.5944 + 0.0221$ weight. For a weight of 110 pounds we would expect height $= 59.5944 + 0.0221(110) = 62.02$ inches.

We may also make statistical inferences about the specific height estimate that we have obtained. This process will require several additional calculations, including finding differences between observed and predicted values for Y, which are shown in Table 12.5.

We may use the information in Table 12.5 to determine the standard error of the estimate of a regression coefficient, which is used for calculation of a confidence interval about an estimated value of $Y(\hat{Y})$. Here the problem is to derive a confi-

TABLE 12.5. Calculations for Inferences about Predicted Y and Slope

	Weight (X)	$X-\overline{X}$	$(X-\overline{X})^2$	Height (Y)	Predicted Height ($\hat{Y}$)	$Y-\hat{Y}$	$(Y-\hat{Y})^2$
	148	−6.1	37.21	64	62.8652	1.1348	1.287771
	172	17.9	320.41	63	63.3956	−0.3956	0.156499
	203	48.9	2391.21	67	64.0807	2.9193	8.522312
	109	−45.1	2034.01	60	62.0033	−2.0033	4.013211
	110	−44.1	1944.81	63	62.0254	0.9746	0.949845
	134	−20.1	404.01	62	62.5558	−0.5558	0.308914
	195	40.9	1672.81	59	63.9039	−4.9039	24.04824
	147	−7.1	50.41	62	62.8431	−0.8431	0.710818
	153	−1.1	1.21	66	62.9757	3.0243	9.14639
	170	15.9	252.81	64	63.3514	0.6486	0.420682
Total	1541		9108.9				49.56468

dence interval about a single point estimate that we have made for Y. The calculations involve the sum of squares for error (SSE), the standard error of the estimate ($s_{y.x}$), and the standard error of the expected Y for a given value of x [$SE(\hat{Y})$]. The respective formulas for the confidence interval about $\hat{Y}$ are shown in Equation 12.6:

$$SSE = \Sigma(Y - \hat{Y})^2 \qquad \text{sum of squares for error}$$

$$S_{y.x} = \sqrt{\frac{SSE}{n-2}} \qquad \text{standard error of the estimate} \qquad (12.6)$$

$$SE(\hat{Y}) = S_{y.x}\sqrt{\frac{1}{n} + \frac{(x - \bar{X})^2}{\Sigma(Xi - \bar{X})^2}} \qquad \text{standard error of } \hat{Y} \text{ for a given value of } x$$

$\hat{Y} \pm (t_{df_{n-2}})[SE(\hat{Y})]$ is the confidence interval about $\hat{Y}$; e.g., t critical is $100(1 - \alpha/2)$ percentile of Student's t distribution with $n - 2$ degrees of freedom.

The sum of squares for error $SSE = \Sigma(Y - \hat{Y})^2 = 49.56468$ (from Table 12.5). The standard error of the estimate refers to the sample standard deviation associated with the deviations about the regression line and is denoted by $s_{y.x}$:

$$S_{y.x} = \sqrt{\frac{SSE}{n-2}}$$

From Table 12.5

$$S_{y.x} = \sqrt{\frac{49.56468}{8}} = 2.7286$$

The value $S_{y.x}$ becomes useful for computing a confidence interval about a predicted value of Y. Previously, we determined that the regression equation for predicting height from weight was height = $59.5944 + 0.0221$ weight. For a weight of 110 pounds we predicted a height of 62.02 inches. We would like to be able to compute a confidence interval for this estimate. First we calculate the standard error of the expected Y for a given value of [$SE(\hat{Y})$]:

$$SE(\hat{Y}) = S_{y.x}\sqrt{\frac{1}{n} + \frac{(x - \bar{X})^2}{\Sigma(Xi - \bar{X})^2}} = 2.7286\sqrt{\frac{1}{10} + \frac{110}{9108.9} - (154.1)^2} = 0.5599$$

The 95% confidence interval is

$$\hat{Y} \pm (t_{df_{n-2}})[SE(\hat{Y})] \quad 95\% \text{ CI } [62.02 \pm 2.306(0.5599)] = [63.31 \leftrightarrow 60.73]$$

We would also like to be able to determine whether the population slope (β) of the regression line is statistically significant. If the slope is statistically significant, there is a linear relationship between X and Y. Conversely, if the slope is not statistically significant, we do not have enough evidence to conclude that even a weak linear relationship exists between X and Y. We will test the following null hypothesis: H_o: $\beta = 0$. Let b = estimated population slope for X and Y. The formula for estimating the significance of a slope parameter β is shown in Equation 12.7.

$$t = \frac{b - \beta}{SE(b)} = \frac{b}{SE(b)} \quad \text{test statistic for the significance of } \beta$$

(12.7)

$$SE(b) = \frac{S_{y.x}}{\sqrt{\Sigma(X_i - \bar{X})^2}} \quad \text{standard error of the slope estimate } [SE(b)]$$

The standard error of the slope estimate $[SE(b)]$ is (note: refer to Table 12.5 and the foregoing sections for the values shown in the formula)

$$SE(b) = \frac{2.7286}{\sqrt{9108.9}} = 0.02859 \qquad t = \frac{0.0221}{0.02859} = 0.77 \qquad p = \text{n.s.}$$

In agreement with the results for the significance of the correlation coefficient, these results suggest that the relationship between height and weight is not statistically significant These two tests (i.e., for the significance of r and significance of b) are actually mathematically equivalent.

This t statistic also can be used to obtain a confidence interval for the slope, namely $[b - t_{1-\alpha/2}\, SE(b), b + t_{1-\alpha/2}\, SE(b)]$, where the critical value for t is the $100(1 - \alpha/2)$ percentile for Student's t distribution with $n - 2$ degrees of freedom. This interval is a $100(1 - \alpha)\%$ confidence interval for β.

Sometimes we have knowledge to indicate that the intercept is zero. In such cases, it makes sense to restrict the solution to the value $a = 0$ and arrive at the least squares estimate for b with this added restriction. The formula changes but is easily calculated and there exist computer algorithms to handle the zero intercept case.

When the error terms are assumed to have a normal distribution with a mean of 0 and a common variance σ^2, the least squares solution also has the property of maximizing the likelihood. The least squares estimates also have the property of being the minmum variance unbiased estimates of the regression parameters [see Draper and Smith (1998) page 137]. This result is called the Gauss–Markov theorem [see Draper and Smith (1998) page 136].

12.8 SENSITIVITY TO OUTLIERS, OUTLIER REJECTION, AND ROBUST REGRESSION

Outliers refer to unusual or extreme values within a data set. We might expect many biochemical parameters and human characteristics to be normally distributed, with the majority of cases falling between ± 2 standard deviations. Nevertheless, in a large data set, it is possible for extreme values to occur. These extreme values may be caused by actual rare events or by measurement, coding, or data entry errors. We can visualize outliers in a scatter diagram, as shown in Figure 12.4.

The least squares method of regression calculates "b" (the regression slope) and "a" (the intercept) by minimizing the sum of squares $[\Sigma(Y - \hat{Y})^2]$ about the regres-

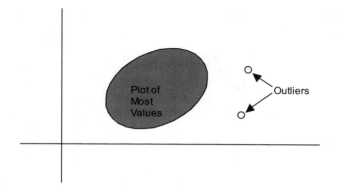

Figure 12.4. Scatter diagram with outliers.

sion line. Outliers cause distortions in the estimates obtained by the least squares method. Robust regression techniques are used to detect outliers and minimize their influence in regression analyses.

Even a few outliers may impact both the intercept and the slope of a regression line. This strong impact of outliers comes about because the penalty for a deviation from the line of best fit is the square of the residual. Consequently, the slope and intercept need to be placed so as to give smaller deviations to these outliers than to many of the more "normal" observations.

The influence of outliers also depends on their location in the space defined by the distribution of measurements for X (the independent variable). Observations for very low or very high values of X are called leverage points and have large effects on the slope of the line (even when they are not outliers). An alternative to least squares regression is robust regression, which is less sensitive to outliers than is the least squares model. An example of robust regression is median regression, a type of quantile regression, which is also called a minimum absolute deviation model.

A very dramatic example of a major outlier was the count of votes for Patrick Buchanan in Florida's Palm Beach County in the now famous 2000 presidential election. Many people believe that Buchanan garnered a large share of the votes that were intended for Gore. This result could have happened because of the confusing nature of the so-called butterfly ballot.

In any case, an inspection of two scatter plots (one for vote totals by county for Buchanan versus Bush, Figure 12.5, and one for vote totals by county for Buchanan versus Gore, Figure 12.6) reveals a consistent pattern that enables one to predict the number of votes for Buchanan based on the number of votes for Bush or Gore. This prediction model would work well in every county except Palm Beach, where the votes for Buchanan greatly exceeded expectations. Palm Beach was a very obvious outlier. Let us look at the available data published over the Internet.

Table 12.6 shows the counties and the number of votes that Bush, Gore, and Buchanan received in each county. The number of votes varied largely by the size of the county; however, from a scatter plot you can see a reasonable linear relation-

TABLE 12.6. 2000 Presidential Vote by County in Florida

County	Gore	Bush	Buchanan
Alachua	47,300	34,062	262
Baker	2,392	5,610	73
Bay	18,850	38,637	248
Bradford	3,072	5,413	65
Brevard	97,318	115,185	570
Broward	386,518	177,279	789
Calhoun	2,155	2,873	90
Charlotte	29,641	35,419	182
Citrus	25,501	29,744	270
Clay	14,630	41,745	186
Collier	29,905	60,426	122
Columbia	7,047	10,964	89
Dade	328,702	289,456	561
De Soto	3,322	4,256	36
Dixie	1,825	2,698	29
Duval	107,680	152,082	650
Escambia	40,958	73,029	504
Flagler	13,891	12,608	83
Franklin	2,042	2,448	33
Gadsden	9,565	4,750	39
Gilchrist	1,910	3,300	29
Glades	1,420	1,840	9
Gulf	2,389	3,546	71
Hamilton	1,718	2,153	24
Hardee	2,341	3,764	30
Hendry	3,239	4,743	22
Hernando	32,644	30,646	242
Highlands	14,152	20,196	99
Hillsborough	169,529	180,713	845
Holmes	2,154	4,985	76
Indian River	19,769	28,627	105
Jackson	6,868	9,138	102
Jefferson	3,038	2,481	29
Lafayette	788	1,669	10
Lake	36,555	49,965	289
Lee	73,530	106,123	306
Leon	61,425	39,053	282
Levy	5,403	6,860	67
Liberty	1,011	1,316	39
Madison	3,011	3,038	29
Manatee	49,169	57,948	272
Marion	44,648	55,135	563
Martin	26,619	33,864	108
Monroe	16,483	16,059	47
Nassau	6,952	16,404	90
Okaloosa	16,924	52,043	267

TABLE 12.6. *Continued*

County	Gore	Bush	Buchanan
Okeechobee	4,588	5,058	43
Orange	140,115	134,476	446
Osceola	28,177	26,216	145
Palm Beach	268,945	152,846	3,407
Pasco	69,550	68,581	570
Pinellas	200,212	184,884	1,010
Polk	74,977	90,101	538
Putnam	12,091	13,439	147
Santa Rosa	12,795	36,248	311
Sarasota	72,854	83,100	305
Seminole	58,888	75,293	194
St. Johns	19,482	39,497	229
St. Lucie	41,559	34,705	124
Sumter	9,634	12,126	114
Suwannee	4,084	8,014	108
Taylor	2,647	4,051	27
Union	1,399	2,326	26
Volusia	97,063	82,214	396
Wakulla	3,835	4,511	46
Walton	5,637	12,176	120
Washington	2,796	4,983	88

ship between; for instance, the total number of votes for Bush and the total number for Buchanan. One could form a regression equation to predict the total number of votes for Buchanan given that the total number of votes for Bush is known. Palm Beach County stands out as a major exception to the pattern. In this case, we have an outlier that is very informative about the problem of the butterfly ballots.

Palm Beach County had by far the largest number of votes for Buchanan (3407 votes). The county that had the next largest number of votes was Pinellas County, with only 1010 votes for Buchanan. Although Palm Beach is a large county, Broward and Dade are larger; yet, Buchanan gained only 789 and 561 votes, respectively, in the latter two counties.

Figure 12.5 shows a scatterplot of the votes for Bush versus the votes for Buchanan. From this figure, it is apparent that Palm Beach County is an outlier.

Next, in Figure 12.6 we see the same pattern we saw in Figure 12.5 when comparing votes for Gore to votes for Buchanan, and in Figure 12.7, votes for Nader to votes for Buchanan. In each scatter plot, the number of votes for any candidate is proportional to the size of each county, with the exception of Palm Beach County. We will see that the votes for Nader correlate a little better with the votes for Buchanan than do the votes for Bush or for Gore; and the votes for Bush correlate somewhat better with the votes for Buchanan than do the votes for Gore. If we exclude Palm Beach County from the scatter plot and fit a regression function with or

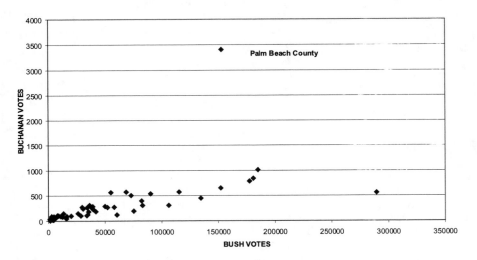

Figure 12.5. Florida presidential vote (all counties).

without an intercept term, we can use this regression function to predict the votes for Buchanan.

For example, Figures 12.8 and Figures 12.9 show the regression equations with and without intercepts, respectively, for predicting votes for Buchanan as a function of votes for Nader based on all counties except Palm Beach. We then use these equations to predict the Palm Beach outcome; then we compare our results to the

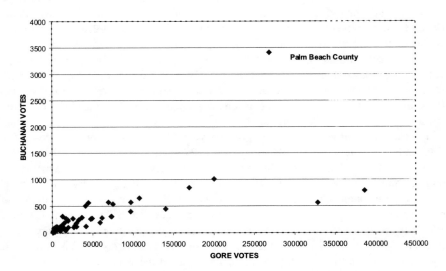

Figure 12.6. Florida presidential votes (all counties).

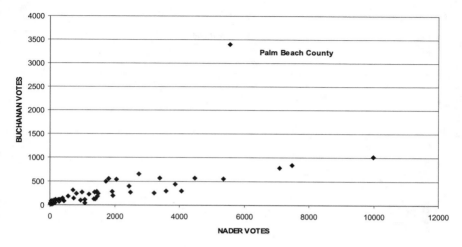

Figure 12.7. Florida presidential votes (all counties).

3407 votes that actually were counted in Palm Beach County as votes for Buchanan.

Since Nader received 5564 votes in Palm Beach County, we derive, using the equation in Figure 12.8, the prediction of Y for Buchanan: $\hat{Y} = 0.1028(5564) + 68.93 = 640.9092$. Or, if we use the zero intercept formula, we have $\hat{Y} = 0.1194 (5564) = 664.3416$.

Similar predictions for the votes for Buchanan using the votes for Bush as the

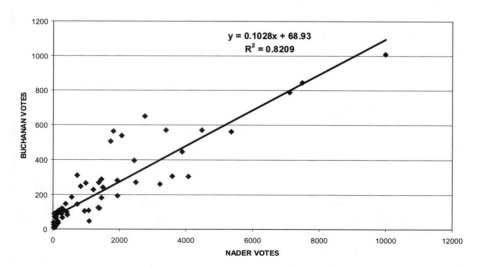

Figure 12.8. Florida presidential vote (Palm Beach county omitted).

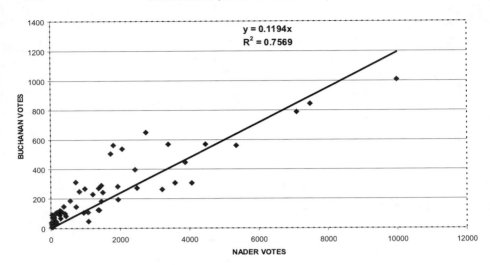

Figure 12.9. Florida presidential vote (Palm Beach county omitted).

covariate X give the equations $\hat{Y} = 0.0035\ X + 65.51 = 600.471$ and $\hat{Y} = 0.004\ X = 611.384$ (zero intercept formula), since Bush reaped 152,846 votes in Palm Beach County. Votes for Gore also could be used to predict the votes for Buchanan, although the correlation is lower ($r = 0.7940$ for the equation with intercept, and $r = 0.6704$ for the equation without the intercept).

Using the votes for Gore, the regression equations are $\hat{Y} = 0.0025\ X + 109.24$ and $\hat{Y} = 0.0032\ X$, respectively, for the fit with and without the intercept. Gore's 268,945 votes in Palm Beach County lead to predictions of 781.6025 and 1075.78 using the intercept and nonintercept equations, respectively.

In all cases, the predictions of votes for Buchanan ranged from around 600 votes to approximately 1076 votes—far less than the 3407 votes that Buchanan actually received. This discrepancy between the number of predicted and actual votes leads to a very plausible argument that at least 2000 of the votes awarded to Buchanan could have been intended for Gore.

An increase in the number of votes for Gore would eliminate the outlier with respect to the number of votes cast for Buchanan that were detected for Palm Beach County. This hypothetical increase would be responsive to the complaints of many voters who said they were confused by the butterfly ballot. A study of the ballot shows that the punch hole for Buchanan could be confused with Gore's but not with that of any other candidate. A better prediction of the vote for Buchanan could be obtained by multiple regression. We will review the data again in Section 12.9.

The undo influence of outliers on regression equations is one of the problems that can be resolved by using robust regression techniques. Many texts on regression models are available that cover robust regression and/or the regression diagnostics that can be used to determine when the assumptions for least squares regression do not apply. We will not go into the details of these topics; however, in

Section 12.12 (Additional Reading), we provide the interested reader with several good texts. These texts include Chatterjee and Hadi (1988); Chatterjee, Price, and Hadi (1999); Ryan (1997); Montgomery, and Peck (1992); Myers (1990); Draper, and Smith (1998); Cook (1998); Belsley, Kuh, and Welsch (1980); Rousseeuw and Leroy (1987); Bloomfield and Steiger (1983); Staudte and Sheather (1990); Cook and Weisberg (1982); and Weisberg (1985).

Some of the aforementioned texts cover diagnostic statistics that are useful for detecting multicollinearity (a problem that occurs when two or more predictor variables in the regression equation have a strong linear interrelationship). Of course, multicollinearity is not a problem when one deals only with a single predictor. When relationships among independent and dependent variables seem to be nonlinear, transformation methods sometimes are employed. For these methods, the least squares regression model is fitted to the data after the transformation [see Atkinson (1985) or Carroll and Ruppert (1988)].

As is true of regression equations, outliers can adversely affect estimates of the correlation coefficient. Nonparametric alternatives to the Pearson product moment correlation exist and can be used in such instances. One such alternative, called Spearman's rho, is covered in Section 14.7.

12.9   GALTON AND REGRESSION TOWARD THE MEAN

Francis Galton (1822–1911), an anthropologist and adherent of the scientific beliefs of his cousin Charles Darwin, studied the heritability of such human characteristics as physical traits (height and weight) and mental attributes (personality dimensions and mental capabilities). Believing that human characteristics could be inherited, he was a supporter of the eugenics movement, which sought to improve human beings through selective mating.

Given his interest in how human traits are passed from one generation to the next, he embarked in 1884 on a testing program at the South Kensington Museum in London, England. At his laboratory in the museum, he collected data from fathers and sons on a range of physical and sensory characteristics. He observed among his study group that characteristics such as height and weight tended to be inherited. However, when he examined the children of extremely tall parents and those of extremely short parents, he found that although the children were tall or short, they were closer to the population average than were their parents. Fathers who were taller than the average father tended to have sons who were taller than average. However, the average height of these taller than average sons tended to be lower than the average height of their fathers. Also, shorter than average fathers tended to have shorter than average sons; but these sons tended to be taller on average than their fathers.

Galton also conducted experiments to investigate the size of sweet pea plants produced by small and large pea seeds and observed the same phenomenon for a successive generation to be closer to the average than was the previous generation. This finding replicated the conclusion that he had reached in his studies of humans.

Galton coined the term "regression," which refers to returning toward the average. The term "linear regression" got its name because of Galton's discovery of this phenomenon of regression toward the mean. For more specific information on this topic, see Draper and Smith (1998), page 45.

Returning to the relationship that Galton discovered between the height at adulthood of a father and his son, we will examine more closely the phenomenon of regression toward the mean. Galton was one of the first investigators to create a scatter plot in which on one axis he plotted heights of fathers and on the other, heights of sons. Each single data point consisted of height measurements of one father–son pair. There was clearly a high positive correlation between the heights of fathers and the heights of their sons. He soon realized that this association was a mathematical consequence of correlation between the variables rather than a consequence of heredity.

The paper in which Galton discussed his findings was entitled "Regression toward mediocrity in hereditary stature." His general observations were as follows: Galton estimated a child's height as

$$\hat{Y} = \overline{Y} + \frac{2(X - \overline{X})}{3}$$

where $\hat{Y}$ is the predicted or estimated child's height, $\overline{Y}$ is the average height of the children, X is the parent's height for that child, and $\overline{X}$ is the average height of all parents. Apparently, the choice of X was a weighted average of the mother's and father's heights.

From the equation you can see that if the parent has a height above the mean for parents, the child also is expected to have a greater than average height among the children, but the increase $\hat{Y} = \overline{Y}$ is only 2/3 of the predicted increase of the parent over the average for the parents. However, the interpretation that the children's heights tend to move toward mediocrity (i.e., the average) over time is a fallacy sometimes referred to as the regression fallacy.

In terms of the bivariate normal distribution, if Y represents the son's height and X the parent's height, and the joint distribution has mean μ_x for X, mean μ_y for Y, standard deviation σ_x for X, standard deviation σ_y for Y, and correlation ρ_{xy} between X and Y, then $E(Y - \mu_y | X = x) = \rho_{xy}\, \sigma_y\, (x - \mu_x)/\sigma_x$.

If we assume $\sigma_x = \sigma_y$, the equation simplifies to $\rho_{xy}(x - \mu_x)$. The simplified equation shows mathematically how the phenomenon of regression occurs, since $0 < \rho_{xy} < 1$. All of the deviations of X about the mean must be reduced by the multiplier ρ_{xy}, which is usually less than 1. But the interpretation of a progression toward mediocrity is incorrect. We see that our interpretation is correct if we switch the roles of X and Y and ask what is the expected value of the parent's height (X) given the son's height (Y), we find mathematically that $E(X - \mu_x | Y = y) = \rho_{xy}\, \sigma_x(y - \mu_y)/\sigma_y$, where μ_y is the overall mean for the population of the sons. In the case when $\sigma_x = \sigma_y$, the equation simplifies to $\rho_{xy}(y - \mu_y)$. So when y is greater than μ_y, the expected value of X moves closer to its overall mean (μ_x) than Y does to its overall mean (μ_y).

Therefore, on the one hand we are saying that tall sons tend to be shorter than their tall fathers, whereas on the other hand we say that tall fathers tend to be shorter than their tall sons. The prediction for heights of sons based on heights of fathers indicates a progression toward mediocrity; the prediction of heights of fathers based on heights of sons indicates a progression away from mediocrity. The fallacy lies in the interpretation of a progression. The sons of tall fathers appear to be shorter because we are looking at (or conditioning on) only the tall fathers. On the other hand, when we look at the fathers of tall sons we are looking at a different group because we are conditioning on the tall sons. Some short fathers will have tall sons and some tall fathers will have short sons. So we err when we equate these conditioning sets. The mathematics is correct but our thinking is wrong. We will revisit this fallacy again with students' math scores.

When trends in the actual heights of populations are followed over several generations, it appears that average height is increasing over time. Implicit in the regression model is the contradictory conclusion that the average height of the population should remain stable over time. Despite the predictions of the regression model, we still observe the regression toward the mean phenomenon with each generation of fathers and sons.

Here is one more illustration to reinforce the idea that interchanging the predictor and outcome variables may result in different conclusions. Michael Chernick's son Nicholas is in the math enrichment program at Churchville Elementary School in Churchville, Pennsylvania. The class consists of fifth and sixth graders, who take a challenging test called the Math Olympiad test. The test consists of five problems, with one point given for each correct answer and no partial credit given. The possible scores on any exam are 0, 1, 2, 3, 4, and 5. In order to track students' progress, teachers administer the exam several times during the school year. As a project for the American Statistical Association poster competition, Chernick decided to look at the regression toward the mean phenomenon when comparing the scores on one exam with the scores on the next exam.

Chernick chose to compare 33 students who took both the second and third exams. Although the data are not normally distributed and are very discrete, the linear model provides an acceptable approximation; using these data, we can demonstrate the regression toward the mean phenomenon. Table 12.7 shows the individual student's scores and the average scores for the sample for each test.

Figure 12.10 shows a scatter plot of the data along with the fitted least squares regression line, its equation, and the square of the correlation.

The term R^2 (Pearson correlation coefficient squared) when multiplied by 100 refers to the percentage of variance that an independent variable (X) accounts for in the dependent variable (Y). To find the Pearson correlation coefficient estimate of the relationship between scores for exam # 2 and exam # 3, we need to find the square root of R^2, which is shown in the figure as 0.3901; thus, the Pearson correlation coefficient is 0.6246. Of the total variance in the scores, almost 40% of the variance in the exam # 3 score is explained by the exam # 2 score. The variance in exam scores is probably attributable to individual differences among students. The

TABLE 12.7. Math Olympiad Scores

Student Number	Exam # 2 Score	Exam # 3 Score
1	5	4
2	4	4
3	3	1
4	1	3
5	4	4
6	1	1
7	2	3
8	2	2
9	4	4
10	4	3
11	3	3
12	5	5
13	0	1
14	3	1
15	3	3
16	3	2
17	3	2
18	1	3
19	3	2
20	2	3
21	3	2
22	0	2
23	3	2
24	3	2
25	3	2
26	3	2
27	2	0
28	1	2
29	0	1
30	2	2
31	1	1
32	0	1
33	1	2
Average score:	2.363	2.272

average scores for exam # 2 and exam # 3 are 2.363 and 2.272, respectively (refer to Table 12.7).

In Table 12.8, we use the regression equation shown in Figure 12.10 to predict the individual exam # 3 scores based on the exam # 2 scores. We also can observe the regression toward the mean phenomenon by noting that for scores of 0, 1, and 2 (all below the average of 2.272 for exam # 3), the predicted values for Y are higher than the actual scores, but for scores of 3, 4, and 5 (all above the mean of 2.272), the predicted values for Y are lower than the actual scores. Hence, all predicted scores

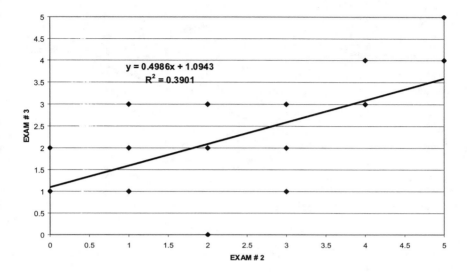

Figure 12.10. Linear regression of olympiad scores of advanced students predicting exam # 3 from exam # 2.

($\hat{Y}$s) for exam # 3 are closer to the overall class mean for exam # 3 than are the actual exam # 2 scores.

Note that a property of the least squares estimate is that if we use $x = 2.363$, the mean for the x's, then we get an estimate of $y = 2.272$, the mean of the y's. So if a student had a score that was exactly equal to the mean for exam # 2, we would predict that the mean of the exam # 3 scores would be that student's score for exam # 3. Of course, this hypothetical example cannot happen because the actual scores can be only integers between 0 and 5.

Although the average scores on exam # 3 are slightly lower than the average scores on exam # 2. the difference between them is not statistically significant, according to a paired t test ($t = 0.463$, $df = 32$).

TABLE 12.8. Regression toward the Mean Based on Predicting Exam #3 Scores from Exam # 2 Scores

	Exam # 2 Score	Prediction for Exam # 3
Scores	0	1.0943
Below	1	1.5929
Mean	2	2.0915
Scores	3	2.5901
Above	4	3.0887
Mean	5	3.5873

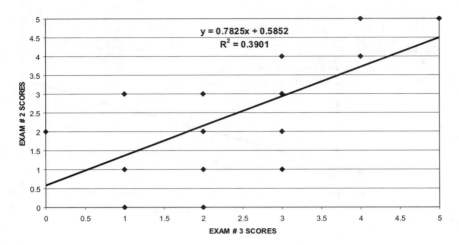

Figure 12.11. Linear regression of olympiad scores predicting exam # 2 from exam # 3, advanced students (tests reversed).

To demonstrate that it is flawed thinking to surmise that the exam # 3 scores tend to become more mediocre than the exam # 2 scores, we can turn the regression around and use the exam # 3 scores to predict the exam # 2 scores. Figure 12.11 exhibits this reversed prediction equation.

Of course, we see that the R^2 value remains the same (and also the Pearson correlation coefficient); however, we obtain a new regression line from which we can demonstrate the regression toward the mean phenomenon displayed in Table 12.9.

Since the average score on exam # 2 is 2.363, the scores 0, 1, and 2 are again below the class mean for exam # 2 and the scores 3, 4, and 5 are above the class mean for exam # 2. Among students who have exam # 3 scores below the mean, the prediction is for their scores on exam # 2 to increase toward the mean score for exam # 2. The corresponding prediction among students who have exam # 3 scores above the mean is that their scores on exam # 2 will decrease. In this case, the degree of shift between actual and predicted scores is less than in the previous case in which

TABLE 12.9. Regression toward the Mean Based on Predicting Exam # 2 Scores from Exam # 3 Scores

	Exam # 3 Score	Prediction for Exam # 2
Scores	0	0.585
Below	1	1.368
Mean	2	2.150
Scores	3	2.933
Above	4	3.715
Mean	5	4.498

exam # 2 scores were used to predict exam # 3 scores. Again, according to an important property of least squares estimates, if we use the exam # 3 mean of 2.272 for x, we will obtain the exam # 2 mean of 2.363 for y (which is exactly the same value for the mean of exam # 2 shown in Table 12.7).

Now let's examine the fallacy of our thinking regarding the trend in exam scores toward mediocrity. The predicted scores for exam # 3 are closer to the mean score for exam # 3 than are the actual scores on exam # 2. We thought that both the lower predicted and observed scores on exam # 3 meant a trend toward mediocrity. But the predicted scores for exam # 2 based on scores on exam # 3 are also closer to the mean of the actual scores on exam # 2 than are the actual scores on exam # 3. This finding indicates a trend away from mediocrity in moving in time from scores on exam # 2 to scores on exam # 3. But this is a contradiction because we observed the opposite of what we thought we would find. The flaw in our thinking that led to this contradiction is the mistaken belief that the regression toward the mean phenomenon implies a trend over time.

The fifth and sixth grade students were able to understand that the better students tended to receive the higher grades and the weaker students the lower grades. But chance also could play a role in a student's performance on a particular test. So students who received a 5 on an exam were probably smarter than the other students and also should be expected to do well on the next exam. However, because the maximum possible score was 5, by chance some students who scored 5 on one exam might receive a score of 4 or lower on the next exam, thus lowering the expected score below 5.

Similarly, a student who earns a score of 0 on a particular exam is probably one of the weaker students. As it is impossible to earn a score of less than 0, a student who scores 0 on the first exam has a chance of earning a score of 1 or higher on the next exam, raising the expected score above 0. So the regression to the mean phenomenon is real, but it does not mean that the class as a group is changing. In fact, the class average could stay the same and the regression toward the mean phenomenon could still be seen.

12.10 MULTIPLE REGRESSION

The only difference between multiple linear regression and simple linear regression is that the former introduces two or more predictor variables into the prediction model, whereas the latter introduces only one. Although we often use a model of $Y = \alpha + \beta X$ for the form of the regression function that relates the predictor (independent) variable X to the outcome or response (dependent) variable Y, we could also use a model such as $Y = \alpha + \beta X^2$ or $Y = \alpha + \beta \ln X$ (where ln refers to the log function). The function is linear in the regression parameters α and β.

In addition to the linearity requirement for the regression model, the other requirement for regression theory to work is that the observed values of Y differ from the regression function by an independent random quantity, or noise term (error variance term). The noise term has a mean of zero and variance of σ^2. In addition,

σ^2 does not depend on X. Under these assumptions the method of least squares provides estimates a and b for α and β, respectively, which have desirable statistical properties (i.e., minimum variance among unbiased estimators).

If the noise term also has a normal distribution, then its maximum likelihood estimator can be obtained. The resulting estimation is known as the Gauss–Markov theorem, the derivation of which is beyond the scope of the present text. The interested reader can consult Draper and Smith (1998), page 136, and Jaske (1994).

As with simple linear regression, the Gauss–Markov theorem applies to multiple linear regression. For a simple linear regression, we introduced the concept of a noise, or error, term. The prediction equation for multiple linear regression also contains an error term. Let us assume a normally distributed additive error term with variance that is independent of the predictor variables. The least squares estimates for the regression coefficients used in the multiple linear regression model exist; under certain conditions, they are unique and are the same as the maximum likelihood estimates [Draper and Smith (1998) page 137].

However, the use of matrix algebra is required to express the least squared estimates. In practice, when there are two or more possible variables to include in a regression equation, one new issue arises regarding the particular subset of variables that should go into the final regression equation. A second issue concerns the problem of multicollinearity, i.e., the predictor variables are so highly intercorrelated that they produce instability problems.

In addition, one must assess the correlation between the best fitting linear combination of predictor variables and the response variable instead of just a simple correlation between the predictor variable and the response variable. The square of the correlation between the set of predictor variables and the response variable is called R^2, the multiple correlation coefficient. The term R^2 is interpreted as the percentage of the variance in the response variable that can be explained by the regression function. We will not study multiple regression in any detail but will provide an example to guide you through calculations and their interpretation.

The term "multicollinearity" refers to a situation in which there is a strong, close to linear relationship among two or more predictor variables. For example, a predictor variable X_1 may be approximately equal to $2X_2 + 5X_3$ where X_2 and X_3 are two other variables that we think relate to our response variable Y.

To understand the concept of linear combinations, let us assume that we include all three variables $(X_1 + X_2 + X_3)$ in a regression model and that their relationship is exact. Suppose that the response variable $Y = 0.3\,X_1 + 0.7\,X_2 + 2.1\,X_3 + \varepsilon$, where ε is normally distributed with mean 0 and variance 1.

Since $X_1 = 2X_2 + 5X_3$, we can substitute the right-hand side of this equation into the expression for Y. After substitution we have $Y = 0.3(2\,X_2 + 5X_3) + 0.7X_2 + 2.1X_3 + \varepsilon = 1.3X_2 + 3.6X_3 + \varepsilon$. So when one of the predictors can be expressed as a linear function of the other, the regression coefficients associated with the predictor variables do not remain the same. We provided examples of two such expressions: $Y = 0.3X_1 + 0.7X_2 + 2.1X_3 + \varepsilon$ and $Y = 0.0X_1 + 1.3X_2 + 3.6X_3 + \varepsilon$. There are an infinite number of possible choices for the regression coefficients, depending on the linear combinations of the predictors.

In most practical situations, an exact linear relationship will not exist; even a relationship that is close to linear will cause problems. Although there will be (unfortunately) a unique least squares solution, it will be unstable. By unstable we mean that very small changes in the observed values of Y and the X's can produce drastic changes in the regression coefficients. This instability makes the coefficients impossible to interpret.

There are solutions to the problem that is caused by a close linear relationship among predictors and the outcome variable. The first solution is to select only a subset of the variables, avoiding predictor variables that are highly interrelated (i.e., multicollinear). Stepwise regression is a procedure that can help overcome multicollinearity, as is ridge regression. The topic of ridge regression is beyond the scope of the present text; the interested reader can consult Draper and Smith (1998), Chapter 17. The problem of multicollinearity is also called "ill-conditioning"; issues related to the detection and treatment of regression models that are ill-conditioned can be found in Chapter 16 of Draper and Smith (1998). Another approach to multicollinearity involves transforming the set of X's to a new set of variables that are "orthogonal." Orthogonality, used in linear algebra, is a technique that will make the X's uncorrelated; hence, the transformed variables will be well-conditioned (stable) variables.

Stepwise regression is one of many techniques commonly found in statistical software packages for multiple linear regression. The following account illustrates how a typical software package performs a stepwise regression analysis. In stepwise regression we start with a subset of the X variables that we are considering for inclusion in a prediction model. At each step we apply a statistical test (often an F test) to determine if the model with the new variable included explains a significantly greater percentage of the variation in Y than the previous model that excluded the variable.

If the test is significant, we add the variable to the model and go to the next step of examining other variables to add or drop. At any stage, we may also decide to drop a variable if the model with the variable left out produces nearly the same percentage of variation explained as the model with the variable entered. The user specifies critical values for F called the "F to enter" and the "F to drop" (or uses the default critical values provided by a software program).

Taking into account the critical values and a list of X variables, the program proceeds to enter and remove variables until none meets the criteria for addition or deletion. A variable that enters the regression equation at one stage may still be removed at another stage, because the F test depends on the set of variables currently in the model at a particular iteration.

For example, a variable X may enter the regression equation because it has a great deal of explanatory power relative to the current set under consideration. However, variable X may be strongly related to other variables (e.g., U, V, and Z) that enter later. Once these other variables are added, the variable X could provide little additional explanatory information than that contained in variables U, V, and Z. Hence, X is deleted from the regression equation.

In addition to multicollinearity problems, the inclusion of too many variables in the equation can lead to an equation that fits the data very well but does not do nearly as well as equations with fewer variables when predicting future values of Y based on known values of x. This problem is called overfitting. Stepwise regression is useful because it reduces the number of variables in the regression, helping with overfitting and multicollinearity problems. However, stepwise regression is not an optimal subset selection approach; even if the F to enter criterion is the same as the F to leave criterion, the resulting final set of variables can differ from one another depending on the variables that the user specifies for the starting set.

Two alternative approaches to stepwise regression are forward selection and backward elimination. Forward selection starts with no variables in the equation and adds them one at a time based solely on an F to enter criterion. Backward elimination starts with all the variables in the equation and drops variables one at a time based solely on an F to drop criterion. Generally, statisticians consider stepwise regression to be better than either forward selection or backward elimination. Stepwise regression is preferred to the other two techniques because it tends to test more subsets of variables and generally settles on a better choice than either forward selection or backward elimination. Sometimes, the three approaches will lead to the same subset of variables, but often they will not.

To illustrate multiple regression, we will consider the example of predicting votes for Buchanan in Palm Beach County based on the number of votes for Nader, Gore, and Bush (refer back to Section 12.7). For all counties except Palm Beach, we fit the model $Y = \alpha + \beta_1 X_1 + \beta_2 X_2 + \beta_3 X_3 + \varepsilon$, where X_1 represents votes for Nader, X_2 votes for Bush, and X_3 votes for Gore; ε is a random noise term with mean 0 and variance σ^2 that is independent of X_1, X_2, and X_3; and α, β_1, β_2, and β_3 are the regression parameters. We will entertain this model and others with one of the predictor variables left out. To do this we will use the SAS procedure REG and will show you the SAS code and output. You will need a statistical computer package to solve most multiple regression problems. Multiple regression, which can be found in most of the common statistical packages, is one of the most widely used applied statistical techniques.

The following three regression models were considered:

1. A model including votes for Nader, Bush, and Gore to predict votes for Buchanan
2. A model using only votes for Nader and Bush to predict votes for Buchanan
3. A model using votes for Nader and Bush and an nteraction term defined as the product of the votes for Nader and the votes for Bush

The coefficient for votes for Gore in model (1) was not statistically significant, so model (2) is probably better than (1) for prediction. Model (3) provided a slightly better fit than model (2), and under model (3) all the coefficients were statistically significant. The SAS code (presented in italics) used to obtain the results is as follows:

data florida:
  input county $ gore bush buchanan nader;
  cards;

alachua 47300 34062 262 3215
baker 2392 5610 73 53
bay 18850 38637 248 828

.

.

.

walton 5637 12176 120 265
washngtn 2796 4983 88 93
;
data florid2;
  set florida;
  if county = 'palmbch' then delete;
  nbinter = nader*bush;
run;

proc reg;
model buchanan = nader bush gore;
run;

proc reg;
model buchanan = nader bush;
run;
proc reg;
model buchanan = nader bush nbinter;
run;

The data statement at the beginning creates an SAS data set "florida" with "county" as a character variable and "gore bush buchanan and nader" as numeric variables. The input statement identifies the variable names and their formats ($ is the symbol for a character variable). The statement "cards" indicates that the input is to be read from the lines of code that follow in the program.

On each line, a character variable of 8 characters or less (e.g., alachua) first appears; this character variable is followed by four numbers indicating the values for the numeric variables gore, bush, buchanan, and nader, in that order. The process is continued until all 67 lines of counties are read. Note that, for simplicity, we show only the input for the first three lines and the last two lines, indicating with three dots that the other 62 counties fall in between. This simple way to read data is suitable for small datasets; usually, it is preferable to store data on files and have SAS read the data file.

The next data step creates a modified data set, florid2, for use in the regression modeling. Consequently, we remove Palm Beach County (i.e., the county variable with the value 'palmbch'). We also want to construct an interaction term for the third model. The interaction between the votes for Nader and the votes for Bush is modeled by the product nader*bush. We call this new variable nbinter.

Now we are ready to run the regressions. Although we could use three model statements in a single regression procedure, instead we performed the regression as three separate procedures. The model statement specifies the dependent variable on the left side of the equation. On the right side of the equation is the list of predictor variables. For the first regression we have the variables nader, bush, and gore; for the second just the variables nader and bush. The third regression specifies nader, bush, and their interaction term nbinter.

The output (presented in bold face) appears as follows:

Model: MODEL1 (using votes for Nader, Bush, and Gore to predict votes for Buchanan)
Dependent Variable: BUCHANAN

Analysis of Variance

Source	DF	Sum of Squares	Mean Square	F Value	Prob>F
Model	3	2777684.5165	925894.82882	114.601	0.0001
Error	62	500914.34717	8079.26366		
C Total	65	3278598.8636			

Root MSE	89.88472	R-square	0.8472	
Dep Mean	211.04545	Adj R-sq	0.8398	
C. V.	42.59022			

Parameter Estimates

Variable	DF	Parameter Estimate	Standard Error	T for H0: Parameter = 0	Prob>|T|
INTERCEP	1	54.757978	14.29169893	3.831	0.0003
NADER	1	0.077460	0.01255278	6.171	0.0001
BUSH	1	0.001795	0.00056335	3.186	0.0023
GORE	1	−0.000641	0.00040706	−1.574	0.1205

Model: MODEL2 (using votes for Nader and Bush to predict votes for Buchanan)
Dependent Variable: BUCHANAN

Analysis of Variance

Source	DF	Sum of Squares	Mean Square	F Value	Prob>F
Model	2	2757655.9253	1378827.9626	166.748	0.0001
Error	63	520942.93834	8268.93553		
C Total	65	3278598.8636			

Root MSE	90.93369	R-square	0.8411	
Dep Mean	211.04545	Adj R-sq	0.8361	
C. V.	43.08725			

Parameter Estimates

Variable	DF	Parameter Estimate	Standard Error	T for H0: Parameter = 0	Prob>|T|
INTERCEP	1	60.155214	14.03642389	4.286	0.0001
NADER	1	0.072387	0.01227393	5.898	0.0001
BUSH	1	0.001220	0.00043382	2.812	0.0066

Model: MODEL3 (using votes for Nader and Bush plus an interaction term, Nader*Bush)
Dependent Variable: BUCHANAN

Analysis of Variance

Source	DF	Sum of Squares	Mean Square	F Value	Prob>F
Model	3	2811645.8041	937215.26803	124.439	0.0001
Error	62	466953.05955	7531.50096		
C Total	65	3278598.8636			

Root MSE	86.78422	R-square	0.8576
Dep Mean	211.04545	Adj R-sq	0.8507
C. V.	41.12110		

Parameter Estimates

Variable	DF	Parameter Estimate	Standard Error	T for H0: Parameter = 0	Prob>|T|
INTERCEP	1	36.353406	16.7731503	2.261	0.0273
NADER	1	0.098017	0.01512781	6.479	0.0001
BUSH	1	0.001798	0.00046703	3.850	0.0003
NBINTER	1	−0.000000232	0.00000009	−2.677	0.0095

For each model, the value of R^2 describes the percentage of the variance in the votes for Buchanan that is explained by the predictor variables. By taking into account the joint influence of the significant predictor variables in the model, the adjusted R^2 provides a better measure of goodness of fit than do the individual predictors. Both models (1) and (2) have very similar R^2 and adjusted R^2 values. Model (3) has slightly higher R^2 and adjusted R^2 values than does either model (1) or model (2).

The F test for each model shows a p-value less than 0.0001 (the column labeled Prob>F), indicating that at least one of the regression parameters is different from zero. The individual t test on the coefficients suggests the coefficients that are different from zero. However, we must be careful about the interpretation of these results, due to multiple testing of coefficients.

Regarding model (3), since Bush received 152,846 votes and Nader 5564, the equation predicts that Buchanan should have 659.236 votes. Model (1) uses the 268,945 votes for Gore (in addition to those for Nader and Bush) to predict 587.710 votes for Buchanan. Model (2) predicts the vote total for Buchanan to be 649.389. Model (3) is probably the best model, for it predicts that the votes for Buchanan will be less than 660. So again we see that any reasonable model would predict that Buchanan would receive 1000 or fewer votes, far less than the 3407 he actually received!

12.11   LOGISTIC REGRESSION

Logistic regression is a method for predicting binary outcomes on the basis of one or more predictor variables (covariates). The goal of logistic regression is the same as the goal of ordinary multiple linear regression; we attempt to construct a model to best describe the relationship between a response variable and one or more independent explanatory variables (also called predictor variables or covariates). Just as in ordinary linear regression, the form of the model is linear with respect to the regression parameters (coefficients). The only difference that distinguishes logistic regression from ordinary linear regression is the fact that in logistic regression the response variable is binary (also called dichotomous), whereas in ordinary linear regression it is continuous.

A dichotomous response variable requires that we use a methodology that is very different from the one employed in ordinary linear regression. Hosmer and Lemeshow (2000) wrote a text devoted entirely to the methodology and many important applications of handling dichotomous response variables in logistic regression equations. The same authors cover the difficult but very important practical problem of model building where a "best" subset of possible predictor variables is to be selected based on data. For more information, consult Hosmer and Lemeshow (2000).

In this section, we will present a simple example along with its solution. Given that the response variable Y is binary, we will describe it as a random variable that takes on either the value 0 or the value 1. In a simple logistic regression equation with one predictor variable, X, we denote by $\pi(x)$ the probability that the response variable Y equals 1 given that $X = x$. Since Y takes on only the values 0 and 1, this probability $\pi(x)$ also is equal to $E(Y|X = x)$ since $E(Y|X = x) = 0 \, P(Y = 0|X = x) + 1 \, P(Y = 1|X = x) = P(Y = 1|X = x) = \pi(x)$.

Just as in simple linear regression, the regression function for logistic regression is the expected value of the response variable, given that the predictor variable $X = x$. As in ordinary linear regression we express this function by a linear relationship of the coefficients applied to the predictor variables. The linear relationship is specified after making a transformation. If X is continuous, in general X can take on all values in the range $(-\infty, +\infty)$. However, Y is a dichotomy and can be only 0 or 1. The expectation for Y, given $X = x$, is that $\pi(x)$ can belong only to $[0, 1]$. A linear combination such as $\alpha + \beta x$ can be in $(-\infty, +\infty)$ for continuous variables. So we consider the logit transformation, namely $g(x) = \ln[\pi(x)/(1 - \pi(x))]$. Here the transformation $w(x) = [\pi(x)/(1 - \pi(x))]$ can take a value from $[0, 1]$ to $[0, +\infty)$ and ln (the logarithm to the base e) takes $w(x)$ to $(-\infty, +\infty)$. So this logit transformation puts $g(x)$ in the same interval as $\alpha + \beta x$ for arbitrary values of α and β.

The logistic regression model is then expressed simply as $g(x) = \alpha + \beta x$ where g is the logit transform of π. Another way to express this relationship is on a probability scale by reversing (taking the inverse) the transformations, which gives $\pi(x) = \exp(\alpha + \beta x)/[1 + \exp(\alpha + \beta x)]$, where exp is the exponential function. This is because the exponential is the inverse of the function ln. That means that $\exp(\ln(x)) = x$. So $\exp[g(x)] = \exp(\alpha + \beta x) = \exp\{\ln[\pi(x)/(1 - \pi(x))]\} = \pi(x)/1 - \pi(x)$. We then solve $\exp(\alpha + \beta x) = \pi(x)/1 - \pi(x)$ for $\pi(x)$ and get $\pi(x) = \exp(\alpha + \beta x)[1 - \pi(x)] = \exp(\alpha + \beta x) - \exp(\alpha + \beta x)\pi(x)$. After moving $\exp(\alpha + \beta x) \, \pi(x)$ to the other side of the equation, we have $\pi(x) + \exp(\alpha + \beta x)\pi(x) = \exp(\alpha + \beta x)$ or $\pi(x)[1 + \exp(\alpha + \beta x)] = \exp(\alpha + \beta x)$. Dividing both sides of the equation by $1 + \exp(\alpha + \beta x)$ at last gives us $\pi(x) = \exp(\alpha + \beta x)/[1 + \exp(\alpha + \beta x)]$.

The aim of logistic regression is to find estimates of the parameters α and β that best fit an available set of data. In ordinary linear regression, we based this estimation on the assumption that the conditional distribution of Y given $X = x$ was normal. Here we cannot make that assumption, as Y is binary and the error term for Y given $X = x$ takes on one of only two values, $-\pi(x)$ when $Y = 0$ and $1 - \pi(x)$ when $Y = 1$ with probabilities $1 - \pi(x)$ and $\pi(x)$, respectively. The error term has mean zero and variance $[1 - \pi(x)]\pi(x)$. Thus, the error term is just a Bernoulli random variable shifted down by $\pi(x)$.

The least squares solution was used in ordinary linear regression under the usual assumption of constant variance. In the case of ordinary linear regression, we were told that the maximum likelihood solution was the same as the least squares solution [Draper and Smith (1998), page 137, and discussed in Sections 12.8 and 12.10 above]. Because the distribution of error terms is much different for logistic regression than for ordinary linear regression, the least squares solution no longer applies; we can follow the principle of maximizing the likelihood to obtain a sensible solution. Given a set of data (y_i, x_i) where $i = 1, 2, \ldots, n$ and the y_i are the observed responses and can have a value of either 0 or 1, and the x_i are the corresponding covariate values, we define the likelihood function as follows:

$$L(x_1, y_1, x_2, y_2, \ldots, x_n, y_n) = \pi(x_1)^{y_1}[1 - \pi(x_1)]^{(1-y_1)}$$
$$\pi(x_2)^{y_2}[1 - \pi(x_2)]^{(1-y_2)}\pi(x_3)^{y_3}[1 - \pi(x_3)]^{(1-y_3)}, \ldots, \pi(x_n)^{y_n}[1 - \pi(x_n)]^{(1-y_n)} \quad (12.1)$$

This formula specifies that if $y_i = 0$, then the probability that $y_i = 0$ is $1 - \pi(x_i)$; whereas, if $y_i = 1$, then the probability of $y_i = 1$ is $\pi(x_i)$. The expression $\pi(x_i)^{y_i}[1 - \pi(x_i)]^{(1-y_i)}$ provides a compact way of expressing the probabilities for $y_i = 0$ or $y_i = 1$ for each i regardless of the value of y. These terms shown on the right side of the equal sign of Equation 12.8 are multiplied in the likelihood equation because the observed data are assumed to be independent. To find the maximum values of the likelihood we solve for α and β by simply computing their partial derivatives and setting them equal to zero. This computation leads to the likelihood equations $\Sigma[y_i - \pi(x_i)] = 0$ and $\Sigma x_i[y_i - \pi(x_i)] = 0$ which we solve simultaneously for α and β. Recall that in the likelihood equations $\pi(x_i) = \exp(\alpha + \beta x_i)/[1 + \exp(\alpha + \beta x_i)]$, so the parameters α and β enter the likelihood equations through the terms with $\pi(x_i)$.

Generalized linear models are linear models for a function $g(x)$. The function g is called the link function. Logistic regression is a special case where the logit function is the link function. See Hosmer and Lemeshow (2000) and McCullagh and Nelder (1989) for more details.

Iterative numerical algorithms for generalized linear models are required to solve maximum likelihood equations. Software packages for generalized linear models provide solutions to the complex equations required for logistic regression analysis. These programs allow you to do the same things we did with ordinary simple linear regression—namely, to test hypotheses about the coefficients (e.g., whether or not they are zero) or to construct confidence intervals for the coefficients. In many applications, we are interested only in the predicted values $\pi(x)$ for given values of x.

Table 12.10 reproduces data from Campbell and Machin (1999) regarding hemoglobin levels among menopausal and nonmenopausal women. We use these data in order to illustrate logistic regression analysis.

Campbell and Machin used the data presented in Table 12.10 to construct a logistic regression model, which addressed the risk of anemia among women who were younger than 30. Female patients who had hemoglobin levels below 12 g/dl were categorized as anemic. The present authors (Chernick and Friis) dichotomized the subjects into anemic and nonanemic in order to examine the relationship of age (under and over 30 years of age) to anemia. (Refer to Table 12.11.)

We note from the data that two out of the five women under 30 years of age were anemic, while only two out of 15 women over 30 were anemic. None of the women who were experiencing menopause was anemic. Due to blood and hemoglobin loss during menstruation, younger, nonmenopausal women (in comparison to menopausal women) were hypothesized to be at higher risk for anemia.

In fitting a logistic regression model for anemia as a function of the dichotomized age variable, Campbell and Machin found that the estimate of the regression parameter β was 1.4663 with a standard error of 1.1875. The Wald test, analogous to the t test for the significance of a regression coefficient in ordinary linear regression, is used in logistic regression. It also evaluates whether the logistic

TABLE 12.10. Hemoglobin Level (Hb), Packed Cell Volume (PCV), Age, and Menopausal Status for 20 Women*

Subject Number	Hb (g/dl)	PCV (%)	Age (yrs)	Menopause (0 = No, 1 = Yes)
1	11.1	35	20	0
2	10.7	45	22	0
3	12.4	47	25	0
4	14.0	50	28	0
5	13.1	31	28	0
6	10.5	30	31	0
7	9.6	25	32	0
8	12.5	33	35	0
9	13.5	35	38	0
10	13.9	40	40	0
11	15.1	45	45	1
12	13.9	47	49	0
13	16.2	49	54	1
14	16.3	42	55	1
15	16.8	40	57	1
16	17.1	50	60	1
17	16.6	46	62	1
18	16.9	55	63	1
19	15.7	42	65	1
20	16.5	46	67	1

*Adapted from Campbell and Machin (1999), page 95, Table 7.1.

TABLE 12.11. Women Reclassified by Age Group and Anemia (Using Data from Table 12.10)

Subject Number	Anemic (0 = No, 1 = Yes)	Age (0 = under 30, 1 = 30 or over)
1	1	0
2	1	0
3	0	0
4	0	0
5	0	0
6	1	1
7	1	1
8	0	1
9	0	1
10	0	1
11	0	1
12	0	1
13	0	1
14	0	1
15	0	1
16	0	1
17	0	1
18	0	1
19	0	1
20	0	1

regression coefficient is significantly different from 0. The value of the Wald statistic was 1.5246 for these data ($p = 0.2169$, n.s.).

With such a small sample size ($n = 20$) and the dichotomization used, one cannot find a statistically significant relationship between younger age and anemia. We can also examine the exponential of the parameter estimate. This exponential is the estimated odds ratio (OR), defined elsewhere in this book. The OR turns out to be 4.33, but the confidence interval is very wide and contains 0.

Had we performed the logistic regression using the actual age instead of the dichotomous values, we would have obtained a coefficient of -0.2077 with a standard error of 0.1223 for the regression parameter, indicating a decreasing risk of anemia with increasing age. In this case, the Wald statistic is 2.8837 ($p = 0.0895$), indicating that the downward trend is statistically significant at the 10% level even for this relatively small sample.

12.12   EXERCISES

12.1   Give in your own words definitions of the following terms that pertain to bivariate regression and correlation:

    a. Correlation versus association
    b. Correlation coefficient
    c. Regression
    d. Scatter diagram
    e. Slope (b)

12.2 Research papers in medical journals often cite variables that are correlated with one another.
    a. Using a health-related example, indicate what investigators mean when they say that variables are correlated.
    b. Give examples of variables in the medical field that are likely to be correlated. Can you give examples of variables that are positively correlated and variables that are negatively correlated?
    c. What are some examples of medical variables that are not correlated? Provide a rationale for the lack of correlation among these variables.
    d. Give an example of two variables that are strongly related but have a correlation of zero (as measured by a Pearson correlation coefficient).

12.3 List the criteria that need to be met in order to apply correctly the formula for the Pearson correlation coefficient.

12.4 In a study of coronary heart disease risk factors, an occupational health physician collected blood samples and other data on 1000 employees in an industrial company. The correlations (all significant at the 0.05 level or higher) between variable pairs are shown in Table 12.12. By checking the appropriate box, indicate whether the correlation denoted by r_1 is lower than, equal to, or higher than the correlation denoted by r_2.

12.5 Some epidemiologic studies have reported a negative association between moderate consumption of red wine and coronary heart disease mortality. To what extent does this correlation represent a causal association? Can you identify any alternative arguments regarding the interpretation that

TABLE 12.12. Correlations between Variable Pairs in a Risk Factor Study*

Variable Pair	r_1	Variable Pair	r_2	$r_1 < r_2$	$r_1 = r_2$	$r_1 > r_2$
LDL chol/HDL chol	0.87	HDL chol/SUA	0.49			
HDL chol/glucose	0.01	Trigl/glucose	−0.09			
Glucose/Hba$_1$c	0.76	Glucose/SUA	−0.76			
Trigl/glucose	−0.09	Glucose/SUA	−0.76			
HDL chol/SUA	0.49	Glucose/SUA	−0.76			

*Abbreviations: chol = cholesterol; SUA = serum uric acid; Trigl = triglycerides; Hba1c = glycosolated hemoglobin.

consumption of red wine causes a reduction in coronary heart disease mortality?

12.6   A psychiatric epidemiology study collected information on the anxiety and depression levels of 11 subjects. The results of the investigation are presented in Table 12.13. Perform the following calculations:
a. Scatter diagram
b. Pearson correlation coefficient
c. Test the significance of the correlation coefficient at $\alpha = 0.05$ and $\alpha = 0.01$.

12.7   Refer to Table 12.1 in Section 12.3. Calculate r between systolic and diastolic blood pressure. Calculate the regression equation between systolic and diastolic blood pressure. Is the relationship statistically significant at the 0.05 level?

12.8   Refer to Table 12.14:
a. Create a scatter diagram of the relationships between age (X) and cholesterol (Y), age (X) and blood sugar (Y), and cholesterol (X) and blood sugar (Y).
b. Calculate the correlation coefficients (r) between age and cholesterol, age and blood sugar, and cholesterol and blood sugar. Evaluate the significance of the associations at the 0.05 level.
c. Determine the linear regression equations between age (X) and cholesterol (Y), age (X) and blood sugar (Y), and cholesterol (X) and blood sugar (Y). For age 93, what are the estimated cholesterol and blood pressure values? What is the 95% confidence interval about these values? Are the slopes obtained for the regression equations statistically significant (at the 0.05 level)? Do these results agree with the significance of the correlations?

TABLE 12.13. Anxiety and Depression Scores of 11 Subjects

Subject ID	Anxiety Score	Depression Score
1	24	14
2	9	5
3	25	16
4	26	17
5	35	22
6	17	8
7	49	37
8	39	41
9	8	6
10	34	28
11	28	33

TABLE 12.14 : Age, Cholesterol Level, and Blood Sugar Level of Elderly Men

Age		Cholesterol		Blood Sugar	
76	80	275	360	125	139
76	80	245	238	127	137
76	80	245	267	138	131
76	63	237	295	129	160
93	63	263	245	151	147
91	63	251	305	138	139
91	64	195	276	137	148
97	76	260	275	129	175
72	76	245	259	138	151
72	76	268	245	139	147
72	76	254	226	150	126
72	57	282	247	159	129

12.9   An experiment was conducted to study the effect on sleeping time of increasing the dosage of a certain barbiturate. Three readings were made at each of three dose levels:

Sleeping Time (Hrs) Y	Dosage (μM/kg) X
4	3
6	3
5	3
9	10
8	10
7	10
13	15
11	15
9	15
$\Sigma Y = 72$	$\Sigma X = 84$
$\Sigma Y^2 = 642$	$\Sigma X^2 = 1002$
$\Sigma XY = 780$	

a. Plot the scatter diagram.
b. Determine the regression line relating dosage (X) to sleeping time (Y).
c. Place a 95% confidence interval on the slope parameter β.
d. Test at the 0.05 level the hypothesis of no linear relationship between the two variables.
e. What is the predicted sleeping time for a dose of 12 μM/kg?

12.10   In the text, a correlation matrix was described. Using your own words, explain what is meant by a correlation matrix. What values appear along the diagonal of a correlation? How do we account for these values?

12.11   An investigator studying the effects of stress on blood pressure subjected mine monkeys to increasing levels of electric shock as they attempted to obtain food from a feeder. At the end of a 2-minute stress period, blood pressure was measured. (Initially, the blood pressure readings of the nine monkeys were essentially the same).

Blood Pressure Y	Shock Intensity X
125	30
130	30
120	30
150	50
145	50
160	50
175	70
180	70
180	70

Some helpful intermediate calculations: $\Sigma X = 450$, $\Sigma Y = 1365$, $\Sigma X^2 = 24900$, $\Sigma Y^2 = 211475$, $(\Sigma X)^2 = 202500$, $(\Sigma Y)^2 = 1863225$, $\Sigma X Y = 71450$, and $(\Sigma X)(\Sigma Y) = 614250$. Using this information,
  a. Plot the scatter diagram.
  b. Determine the regression line relating blood pressure to intensity of shock.
  c. Place a 95% confidence interval on the slope parameter β.
  d. Test the null hypothesis of no linear relationship between blood pressure and shock intensity (stress level). (Use $\alpha = 0.01$.)
  e. For a shock intensity level of 60, what is the predicted blood pressure?

12.12   Provide the following information regarding outliers.
  a. What is the definition of an outlier?
  b. Are outliers indicators of errors in the data?
  c. Can outliers sometimes be errors?
  d. Give an example of outliers that represent erroneous data.
  e. Give an example of outliers that are not errors.

12.13   What is logistic regression? How is it different from ordinary linear regression? How is it similar to ordinary linear regression?

12.14 In a study on the elimination of a certain drug in man, the following data were recorded:

Time in Hours X	Drug Concentration (μg/ml) Y
0.5	0.42
0.5	0.45
1.0	0.35
1.0	0.33
2.0	0.25
2.0	0.22
3.0	0.20
3.0	0.20
4.0	0.15
4.0	0.17

Intermediate calculations show $\Sigma X = 21$, $\Sigma Y = 2.74$, $\Sigma X^2 = 60.5$, $\Sigma Y^2 = 0.8526$, and $\Sigma X Y = 4.535$.

a. Plot the scatter diagram.

b. Determine the regression line relating time (X) to concentration of drug (Y).

c. Determine a 99% confidence interval for the slope parameter β.

d. Test the null hypothesis of no relationship between the variables at $\alpha = 0.01$.

e. Is (d) the same as testing that the slope is zero?

f. Is (d) the same as testing that the correlation is zero?

g. What is the predicted drug concentration after two hours?

12.15 What is the difference between a simple and a multiple regression equation?

12.16 Give an example of a multiple regression problem and identify the terms in the equation.

12.17 How does the multiple correlation coefficient R^2 for the sample help us interpret a multiple regression problem?

12.18 A regression problem with five predictor variables results in an R^2 value of 0.75. Interpret the finding.

12.19 When one of the five predictor variables in the preceding example is eliminated from the analysis, the value of R^2 drops from 0.75 to 0.71. What does this tell us about the variable that was dropped?

12.20 What is multicollinearity? Why does it occur in multiple regression problems?

12.21 What is stepwise regression? Why is it used?

12.22 Discuss the regression toward the mean phenomenon. Give a simple real-life example.

12.23 Give an example of a logistic regression problem. How is logistic regression different from multiple linear regression?

12.24 When a regression model is nonlinear or the error terms are not normally distributed, the standard hypothesis testing methods and confidence intervals do not apply. However, it is possible to solve the problem by bootstrapping. How might you bootstrap the data in a regression model? [Hint: There are two ways that have been tried. Consider the equation $Y = \alpha + \beta_1 X_1 + \beta_2 X_2 + \beta_3 X_3 + \beta_4 X_4 + \varepsilon$ and think about using the vector (Y, X_1, X_2, X_3, X_4). Alternatively, to help you apply the bootstrap, what do you know about the properties of ε and its relationship to the estimated residuals $e = Y - (a + b_1 X_1 + b_2 X_2 + b_3 X_3 + b_4 X_4)$, where a, b_1, b_2, b_3, and b_4 are the least squares estimates of the parameters α, β_1, β_2, β_3, and β_4, respectively.] Refer to Table 12.1 in Section 12.3. Calculate r between systolic and diastolic blood pressure. Calculate the regression equation between systolic and diastolic blood pressure. Is the relationship statistically significant at the 0.05 level?

12.13 ADDITIONAL READING

1. Atkinson, A. C. (1985). *Plots, Transformations, and Regression.* Oxford University Press, New York.
2. Belsley, D. A., Kuh, E. and Welsch, R. E. (1980). *Regression Diagnostics.* Wiley, New York.
3. Bloomfield, P. and Steiger, W. (1983). *Least Absolute Deviations.* Birkhauser, Boston.
4. Campbell, M. J. and Machin, D. (1999). *Medical Statistics: A Commonsense Approach,* Third Edition. Wiley, Chichester, England.
5. Carroll, R. J. and Ruppert, D. (1988). *Transformation and Weighting in Regression.* Chapman and Hall, New York.
6. Chatterjee, S. and Hadi, A. S. (1988). *Sensitivity Analysis in Linear Regression.* Wiley, New York.
7. Chatterjee, S., Price, B. and Hadi, A. S. (1999). *Regression Analysis by Example,* Third Edition. Wiley, New York.
8. Cook, R. D. (1998). *Regression Graphics.* Wiley, New York.
9. Cook, R. D. and Weisberg, S. (1982). *Residuals and Influence in Regression.* Chapman and Hall, London.
10. Draper, N. R. and Smith, H. (1998). *Applied Regression Analysis,* Third Edition. Wiley, New York.
11. Hosmer, D. W. and Lemeshow, S. (2000). *Applied Logistic Regression,* Second Edition. Wiley, New York.

12. Jaske, D. R. (1994). Illustrating the Gauss–Markov Theorem. *The American Statistician* **48,** 237–238.

13. McCullagh, P. and Nelder, J. A. (1989). *Generalized Linear Models,* Second Edition. Chapman and Hall, London.

14. Montgomery, D. C. and Peck, E. A. (1992). *Introduction to Linear Regression Analysis.* Second Edition. Wiley, New York.

15. Myers, R. H. (1990). *Classical and Modern Regression with Applications,* Second Edition. PWS-Kent, North Scituate, Massachusetts.

16. Rousseeuw, P. J. and Leroy, A. M. (1987). *Robust Regression and Outlier Detection.* Wiley, New York.

17. Ryan, T. P. (1997). *Modern Regression Methods.* Wiley, New York.

18. Staudte, R. G. and Sheather, S. J. (1990). *Robust Estimation and Testing.* Wiley, New York.

19. Weisberg, S. (1985). *Applied Linear Regression,* Second Edition. Wiley, New York.

CHAPTER 13

One-Way Analysis of Variance

Statistical methods of analysis are intended to aid the interpreta-
tion of data that are subject to appreciable haphazard variability.
—Sir David R. Cox and David V. Hinkley, *Theoretical Statistics*, p. 1

The analysis of variance is a comparison of different populations in studies that have several treatments or conditions. For example, we may want to compare mean scores from three or more populations that represent three or more study conditions. Remember that we used the Z test or t test to compare two populations, as in comparing an experimental group with a control group. The analysis of variance will enable us to extend the comparison to more than two groups.

In this text, we will consider only the one-way analysis of variance (ANOVA). Typically, ANOVA is used to compare population means (μ's) that represent interval- or ratio-level measurement. In the one-way analysis of variance, there is a single factor (such as classification according to treatment group) that differentiates the groups.

Other types of analyses of variance are also important in statistics. ANOVA may be extended to two-way, three-way, and N-way designs. To illustrate, the two-way analysis would examine the effects of two variables, such as treatment group and age group, on an outcome variable. The N-way ANOVAs are used in experimental studies that have multiple factorial designs. However, the problem of assessing the associations of several variables with an outcome variable becomes daunting.

One common use of the two-way analysis of variance is the randomized block design. In this design, one factor could be the treatment and the other would be the blocks. Blocks refer to homogeneous groupings of subsets of subjects; for example, subsets defined by race or other demographic characteristics. These characteristics, when uncontrolled, may increase the size of the error variance. In the randomized block design, we look for treatment effects and block effects, both of which are called the main effects. There is also the possibility of considering interaction effects between the treatments and the blocks. Interaction means that certain combinations of treatments and blocks may have greater or smaller impact on the outcome than do than the sum of their main effects. As is true of regression, the

Introductory Biostatistics for the Health Sciences, by Michael R. Chernick
and Robert H. Friis. ISBN 0-471-41137-X. Copyright © 2003 Wiley-Interscience.

analysis of variance, which represents an important area in applied statistics, is the subject of entire books.

Scheffe (1959) wrote the classic theoretical text on analysis of variance. Fisher and McDonald (1978) authored a more recent text, which provides an advanced treatment of fixed effects designs (as opposed to random effects). Other, less advanced, treatments can be found in Hocking (1985), Dunn and Clark (1974), and Miller (1986).

In statistical computer packages, the analysis of variance can be treated as a regression problem with dummy variables. A dummy variable is a type of dichotomous variable created by recoding the classifications of a categorical variable. For example, a single category of race (e.g., African American) would be coded as present (1) or absent (0). In the case of a regression problem, we may regard an ANOVA as a type of linear model. Such a linear model (called the general linear model) can employ a mix of categorical and continuous variables to describe a relationship between them and a response variable. You may often see this type of analysis referred to as analysis of covariance. All these models have the decomposition of variance of the response Y into proportions explained by the predictor variables. This is the so-called ANOVA that we will describe in this chapter.

In Chapter 12 we discussed R^2, which is a ratio of the part of the variance in the response variable Y that is explained by the regression equation divided by the total variance of the response variable Y. In the ANOVA table (refer to Appendix A), we will see the case of an F test in which at least one of the means of a response variable is different from the other means. There is a direct mathematical relationship between this F statistic and R^2.

In Chapter 12, we emphasized simple linear regression and correlation and briefly touched on multiple regression by giving one example. Analogously, multiway analysis of variance is similar to multiple linear regression, in that there are two or more categorical variables in the model to explain the response Y. We will not go into the details here; the interested reader can consult some of the texts listed in Section 13.7.

13.1   THE PURPOSE OF ONE-WAY ANALYSIS OF VARIANCE

The purpose of the one-way analysis of variance (ANOVA) is to determine whether three or more groups have the same mean (i.e., H_0: $\mu_1 = \mu_2 = \mu_3, \ldots, \mu_k$). It is a generalization of the t test to three or more groups. But the difference is that for a one-sided t test, when you reject the null hypothesis of equality of means, the alternative tells you which one of the two means is greater ($\mu > \mu_0$, $\mu < \mu_0$, or $\mu_1 > \mu_2$, $\mu_1 < \mu_2$). With the analysis of variance, the corresponding test is an F test. It tells you that the means are different but not necessarily which one is larger than the others. As a result, if we want to identify specific differences we need to carry out additional tests, as described in Section 13.5.

The analysis of variance is based on a linear model that says that the response for group j, denoted X_j, satisfies Equation 13.1 for a one-way ANOVA:

$$X_{ij} = \mu_j + \varepsilon_{ij} \tag{13.1}$$

where i is the ith observation from the jth group $j = 1, 2, \ldots, k$; j is the group label and we have $k \geq 3$ groups; μ_j is the mean for group j; and ε_{ij} is an independent error term assumed to have a normal distribution with mean 0 and variance σ^2 independent of j.

The test statistic is the ratio of estimates of two sources of variation called the within-group variance and the between-group variance. If the treatment makes a difference, then we expect that the between-group variance will exceed the within-group variance. These variances or sums of squares when normalized have independent chi-square distributions with n_w and n_b degrees of freedom, respectively, when the modeling assumptions in Equation 13.1 hold and the null hypothesis is true. The sums of squares divided by their degrees of freedom are called mean squares.

The ratio of these mean squares is the test statistic for the analysis of variance. When the means are equal, this ratio has an F distribution with n_b degrees of freedom in the numerator and n_w degrees of freedom in the denominator. It is this F distribution that we refer to in order to determine whether or not to reject the null hypothesis. We also can compute a p-value from this F distribution as we have done with other tests. The F distribution is more complicated than the t distribution because it has two degrees of freedom parameters instead of just one.

13.2   DECOMPOSING THE VARIANCE AND ITS MEANING

Cochran's theorem is the basis for the sums of squares having independent chi-square distributions when Equation 13.1 holds [see Rao (1997), page 4]. It can be deduced from Cochran's theorem in the case of the one-way ANOVA that $\Sigma(X_{ij} - \overline{X})^2 = \Sigma(X_{ij} - X_i)^2 + \Sigma(X_i - \overline{X})^2$, where the following holds:

X_{ij} is normally distributed with mean μ_i

The variance is σ^2

X_{ij} is the jth observation from the ith group

X_i. is the average of all observations in the ith group

X is the average over all the observations in all groups

Let Q, Q_1, and Q_2 refer to total sum of squares, within-groups sum of squares, and between-groups sum of squares, respectively. We have that $Q = Q_1 + Q_2$ $Q = \Sigma(X_{ij} - \overline{X})^2$ normalized has a chi-square distribution with $n_w + n_b - 1$ degrees of freedom; $Q_1 = \Sigma(X_{ij} - X_i)^2$ has a chi-square distribution with n_w degrees of freedom; and $Q_2 = \Sigma(X_i - \overline{X})^2$ has a chi-square distribution with $n_b - 1$ degrees of freedom. Q_2 is independent of $\Sigma(X_{ij} - X_i)^2$. The symbol n_b is the number of groups and n_w is the number of degrees of freedom for error. The total sample size equals $n - n_b$. For Q_2 to have a chi-square distribution when appropriately normalized, we need the null hypothesis that all μ_i are equal to be true. The F distribution is obtained by taking $[Q_2/(n_b - 1)]/[Q_1/n_w]$. When the alternative holds, the normalized Q_2 has what is called a noncentral chi-square distribution, and the ratio tends to be centered above 1. The distribution of $[Q_2/(n_b - 1)]/[Q_1/n_w]$ is then called a noncentral F distribution.

The mathematical relationship between this F statistic and the sample multiple correlation coefficient R^2 (discussed in Chapter 12) is as follows: $R^2 = (n_b - 1)F/\{(n_b - 1)F + n_w\}$ or $F = \{R^2/(n_b - 1)\}/\{(1 - R^2)/n_w\}$

13.3 NECESSARY ASSUMPTIONS

The assumptions for the one-way analysis of variances are:

1. $X_{ij} = \mu_j + \varepsilon_{ij}$, where i is the ith observation from the jth group, $j = 1, 2, \ldots, k$; k is the group label for $k \geq 3$ group; μ_j is the mean for group j; and ε_{ij} is an independent error term.
2. The ε_{ij} has a normal distribution with mean 0 and variance σ^2 independent of j.
3. Under the null hypothesis, $\mu_j = \mu$ for all j.

To express this in nonmathematical terms, all observations in the jth group are independent and normally distributed with the same mean and variance. However, two different groups can have different means but must have the same variance. Under the null hypothesis, all groups must also have the same mean.

The sensitivity of the analysis to violations of these assumptions has been well studied; see Miller (1986) for a discussion. When these assumptions are violated, we can use a nonparametric alternative called the Kruskal–Wallis test (refer to Section 14.6.)

13.4 *F* DISTRIBUTION AND APPLICATIONS

The F distribution will be used to evaluate the significance of the association between an independent variable and an outcome variable in an ANOVA. The F distribution is defined as the distribution of $(Z/n_1)/(W/n_2)$, where Z has a chi-square distribution with n_1 degrees of freedom, W has a chi-square distribution with n_2 degrees of freedom, and Z and W are statistically independent. In the one-way analysis of variance, $Z = Q_2/\sigma^2$, $W = Q_1/\sigma^2$, $n_1 = n_w$, and $n_2 = n_b - 1$; so the ratio $[Q_2/(n_b - 1)]/[Q_1/n_w]$ has the central F distribution with $n_b - 1$ numerator degrees of freedom and n_w denominator degrees of freedom under the null hypothesis. Note that the common variance σ^2 appears in both the numerator and denominator and hence cancels out of the ratio.

The probability density function for this F distribution has been derived and is described in statistical texts [see page 246 in Mood, Graybill, and Boes (1974)].

TABLE 13.1. General One-Way ANOVA Table

Source of Variation	Sum of Squares	Degrees of Freedom (df)	Mean Square	F ratio
Between	SS_b	$n_b - 1$	$MS_b = SS_b/(n_b - 1)$	$F = MS_b/MS_w$
Within	SS_w	n_w	$MS_w = SS_w/n_w$	—
Total	SS_t	$n_b + n_w - 1 = n - 1$	—	—

The F distribution depends on the two degrees of freedom parameters n_1 and n_2, called, respectively, the numerator and denominator degrees of freedom. We include tables of the central F distribution based on degree of freedom parameters in Appendix A. A sample ANOVA is presented in Table 13.1.

Although we do not cover the two-way analysis of variance, Table 13.2 shows the typical two-way ANOVA table that should help you see how the ANOVA table generalizes to N-way ANOVAs. Note that as more factors appear, we have more than one F test. This appearance of multiple F tests is analogous to the several F and/or t tests in regression that are used to determine the significance of the regression coefficients. ANOVA Table 13.2 is not the most general table. A treatment by block effect also can be considered in the model; in this case, the table would have another row for the interaction term.

We will illustrate the one-way analysis of variance with a numerical example. Table 13.3 shows some hypothetical data for the weight gain of pigs fed with three different brands of cereal. A total of 12 pigs are randomly assigned (4 each) to the three cereal brands.

To generate the ANOVA table, we must calculate SS_b and SS_w. As a first step in obtaining SS_w, we calculate the means for each brand. $\overline{X}_A = (1 + 2 + 2 + 1)/4 = 1.5$. $\overline{X}_B = (7 + 8 + 9 + 8)/4 = 8$. $\overline{X}_C = (12 + 14 + 16 + 18)/4 = 15$. The grand mean is $X = (1.5 + 8 + 15)/3 = 8.167$. Now $SS_W = Q_1 = (1 - 1.5)^2 + (2 - 1.5)^2 + (2 - 1.5)^2 + (1 - 1.5)^2 + (7 - 8)^2 + (8 - 8)^2 + (9 - 8)^2 + (8 - 8)^2 + (12 - 15)^2 + (14 - 15)^2 + (16 - 15)^2 + (18 - 15)^2 = 0.25 + 0.25 + 0.25 + 0.25 + 1 + 0 + 1 + 0 + 9 + 1 + 1 + 9 = 23$. Note that SS_w represents the sum of squared deviations of the individual observations from their group means.

Now let us compute SS_b. We can calculate this directly or calculate SS_t and get SS_b by the equation $SS_b = SS_t - SS_w$. Since SS_t is a little easier to compute, let us do

TABLE 13.2. Typical Two-Way ANOVA Table

Source of Variation	Sum of Squares	Degrees of Freedom (df)	Mean Square	F Ratio
Treatment	SS_{tr}	$n_{tr} - 1$	$MS_{tr} = SS_{tr}/(n_{tr} - 1)$	$F = MS_{tr}/MS_r$
Blocks	SS_{bl}	$n_{bl} - 1$	$MS_{bl} = SS_{bl}/(n_{bl} - 1)$	$F = MS_{bl}/MS_r$
Residual	SS_r	$(n_{tr} - 1)(n_{bl} - 1)$	$MS_r = SS_r/[(n_{tr} - 1)(n_{bl} - 1)]$	—
Total	SS_t	$n_{tr} n_{bl} - 1$	—	—

TABLE 13.3. Weight Gain for 12 Pigs Fed with Three Brands of Cereal

Brand A (Gain in oz)	Brand B (Gain in oz)	Brand C (Gain in oz)
1	7	12
2	8	14
2	9	16
1	8	18

it by the subtraction method first. We need to get the overall or "grand" mean—the weighted average of the group means weighted by their respective sample sizes. In this case, since all three groups have 4 pigs each, the result is the same as taking the arithmetic average of the three group averages. So $\overline{X}_g = (1.5 + 8 + 15)/3 = 8.1667$. For SS_t, we do the same computations as for SS_w except that instead of subtracting the group means, we subtract the grand mean before taking the square. So for SS_t we have $SS_t = Q = (1 - 8.1667)^2 + (2 - 8.1667)^2 + (2 - 8.1667)^2 + (1 - 8.1667)^2 + (7 - 8.1667)^2 + (8 - 8.1667)^2 + (9 - 8.1667)^2 + (8 - 8.1667)^2 + (12 - 8.1667)^2 + (14 - 8.1667)^2 + (16 - 8.1667)^2 + (18 - 8.1667)^2 = 51.3616 + 38.0282 + 38.0282 + 51.3616 + 2.7789 + 0.0278 + 0.6944 + 0.0278 + 14.6942 + 34.0274 + 61.3606 + 96.6938 = 391.0845$.

So by subtraction, $SS_b = 391.0845 - 23.0 = 368.0845$. Now we can fill in the ANOVA table. Table 13.4 is the ANOVA table of the form of Table 13.1 as applied to these data.

An F statistic of 72.00 is highly significant. Compare it to values in the F distribution table with 2 degrees of freedom in the numerator and 9 degrees of freedom in the denominator (Appendix A). The critical values are 4.26 at the 5% level and 8.02 at the 1% level. So we see that the p-value is considerably less than 0.01.

SS_b can be calculated directly. The formula is $n_{ob}\{(\overline{X}_A - \overline{X})^2 + (\overline{X}_B - \overline{X})^2 + (\overline{X}_C - \overline{X})^2\} = 4\{(1.5 - 8.167)^2 + (8 - 8.167)^2 + (15 - 8.167)^2\} = 4\{44.444 + 0.0279 + 46.690\} = 364.647$. This formula applies to balanced designs where n_{ob} is the common number of observations in each group. The difference between the results obtained from the two methods for calculating SS_b (364.667 versus 364.647) is due to rounding errors. Using SAS software and applying the GLM procedure to these data, we found that $SS_b = 364.667$. So most of the rounding error was in our calculation of SS_t in the first approach.

TABLE 13.4. One-Way ANOVA Table for Pig Feeding Experiment

Source of Variation	Sum of Squares	Degrees of Freedom (df)	Mean Square	F Ratio
Between	368.0845	2	$MS_b = 368.0845/2 = 184.0423$	$F = 184.0423/2.556 = 72.00$
Within	23	9	$MS_w = 23/9 = 2.556$	—
Total	385.0845	11	—	—

13.5 MULTIPLE COMPARISONS

13.5.1 General Discussion

The result of rejecting the null hypothesis in the analysis of variance is to conclude that there is a difference among the means. However, if we have three or more populations, then how exactly do these means differ? Sometimes researchers consider the precise nature of the differences among these means to be an important scientific issue. Alternatives to the analysis of variance, called ranking and selection procedures, address this issue directly. As the alternative methods are beyond the scope of the present text, we refer the interested reader to Gibbons, Olkin, and Sobel (1977) for an explanation of the ranking and selection methodology.

In the framework of the analysis of variance, the traditional approach is to do the F test first. If the null hypothesis is rejected, we can then look at several hypotheses that compare the pair-wise differences of the means or other linear combinations of the means that might be of interest. For example, we may be interested in $\mu_1 - \mu_2$ and $\mu_3 - \mu_4$. A less obvious contrast might be $\mu_1 - 2\mu_2 + \mu_3$. Any such linear combination of means can be considered, although in most practical situations mean differences are considered and are tested against the null hypothesis prove that they are zero. Since many hypotheses are being tested simultaneously, the methodology must take this fact into account. Such methodology is sometimes called simultaneous inference (for example, see Miller, 1981) or multiple comparisons [see Hochberg and Tamhane (1987) or Hsu (1996)]. Resampling approaches, including bootstrapping, have also been successfully employed to accomplish this task [see Westfall and Young (1993)].

13.5.2 Tukey's Honest Significant Difference (HSD) Test

In order to find out which means are significantly different from one another, we are at first tempted to look at the various t tests that compare the differences of the individual means. For k groups there are $k(k-1)/2$ such comparisons. Even for $k = 4$, there are six comparisons.

The original t tests might have been constructed to test the hypotheses at the 5% significance level. The threshold C for such a test is determined by the t distribution so that if T is the test statistic, then $P(|T| > C) = 0.05$ The constant C is found from the table of the t distribution and depends on the degrees of freedom. But this condition is set for just one such test.

If we do six such tests and set the thresholds to satisfy $P(|T| > C) = 0.05$ for each test statistic, the probability that at least one of the test statistics will exceed the threshold is much higher than 0.05. The methods of Scheffe, Tukey, and Dunnett, among others, are designed to guard against this. See Miller (1981) for coverage of all these methods. For these methods, we choose a threshold or thresholds so that the probability that any one of the thresholds is exceeded is no greater than 0.05. See Hsu (1996), Chapter 5, pp. 119–174, to see all such procedures.

In our example, when the test statistic exceeds the threshold, the result amounts to declaring a significant difference between a particular pair of group means. The family-wise error rate is (by definition) the probability that any such declaration would be incorrect. In doing multiple comparisons, we usually want to control this family-wise error rate at a level of 0.05 (or 0.10).

When we use Tukey's honest significant difference test, our test statistic has exactly the same form as that of a t test. Our confidence interval for the mean difference has the same form as a confidence interval using the t distribution. The only difference in the confidence interval between the HSD test and the t test is that the choice of the constant C is larger than what we would choose for a single t test.

In the application, we assume that the k groups each have equivalent sample sizes, n. This is called a balanced design. To calculate the confidence interval we need a table of constants derived by Tukey (reprinted in Appendix B). We simply compare the difference between the two sample means to the Tukey HSD for one-way ANOVA, which is determined by Equation 13.2:

$$HSD = q(\alpha, k, N-k)\sqrt{MSw/n} \qquad (13.2)$$

where k = the number of groups, n = the number of samples per group, N is the total number of samples, MSw is the within group mean square, and α is the significance level or family-wise error rate. The constant $q(\alpha, k, N-k)$ is found in Tukey's tables.

Note the use of the term q in the equation. The quantity q is sometimes called the studentized range. A table for the studentized range for values of $\alpha = 0.01, 0.05,$ and 0.10 is given in Appendix B.

13.6　EXERCISES

13.1　Complete the following ANOVA table:

Source of Variation	Sum of Squares	Degrees of Freedom	Mean Square	F Ratio
Between	300			
Within	550	15		
Total		21		

13.2　Complete the following ANOVA table:

Source of Variation	Sum of Squares	Degrees of Freedom	Mean Square	F Ratio
Between	200	10		
Within				
Total	500	15		

13.3   Why does one use a Tukey's HSD rather than a *t* test when comparing mean differences in ANOVA?

13.4   Samples were taken of individuals with each blood type to see if the average white blood cell count differed among types. Ten individuals in each group were sampled. The results are given in the table below:

Average White Blood Cell Count by Blood Type

	A	B	AB	O	Grand Totals
	5,000	7,000	7,200	5,550	
	5,550	7,500	7,770	6,570	
	6,000	8,500	8,600	7,620	
	6,500	5,000	6,000	5,900	
	8,000	6,100	5,950	7,100	
	7,700	7,200	7,540	6,980	
	10,000	9,900	11,000	8,750	
	6,100	6,400	6,200	7,700	
	7,200	7,300	7,000	8,100	
	5,500	5,800	6,100	4,900	
	9,000	8,950	7,800	5,800	
Σx	76,550	79,650	81,160	74,970	312,330 (grand total)
$\bar{x}$	7655.0	7965.0	8116.0	7497.0	7808.25 (grand mean)

Source: Modification to Exercise 10.9, page 171, Kuzma and Bohnenblust (2001).

a. State the null hypothesis.
b. Construct an ANOVA table.

13.5   Using the data from the example in Exercise 13.4 and the ANOVA table from that exercise, determine the *p*-value for the test (use the *F* statistic and the appropriate degrees of freedom based on the within and between sum of squares). Is there a statistically significant difference in the white blood cell counts among the groups?

13.6   Five individuals were selected at random from three communities, and their ages were recorded in the table below. The investigator was interested in determining whether these communities differed in mean age.

Ages of Individuals ($n = 5$ in Each Group) in Three Communities

	Community A	Community B	Community C	Grand Totals
	12	26	35	
	27	40	53	
	18	18	43	
	30	25	33	
	16	39	44	
Σx	103	148	208	459 (grand total)
$\bar{x}$	20.6	29.6	41.6	30.6 (grand mean)

Source: Modification to Exercise 10.10, page 172, Kuzma and Bohnenblust (2001).

a. State the null hypothesis.
b. Construct an ANOVA table.

13.7 Using the data from the example in Exercise 13.6 and the ANOVA table from that exercise, determine the p-value for the test (use the F statistic and the appropriate degrees of freedom based on the within and between sum of squares). Is there a statistically significant difference in the ages among the groups?

13.8 Researchers studied the association between birth mothers' smoking habits and the birth weights of their babies. Group 1 consisted of nonsmokers. Group 2 comprised smokers who smoked less than one pack of cigarettes per day. Group 3 smoked more than one but fewer than two packs per day. Group 4 smoked more than two packs per day.

Birth Weights of Infants ($n = 11$ in Each Group)
by Mother's Smoking Status

Subject Number	Group 1 (birthweight in grams)	Subject Number	Group 2 (birthweight in grams)	Subject Number	Group 3 (birthweight in grams)	Subject Number	Group 4 (birthweight in grams)
1	3510	12	3444	23	2608	34	2232
2	3174	13	3111	24	2555	35	2331
3	3580	14	2890	25	3100	36	2200
4	3232	15	3002	26	1775	37	2121
5	3884	16	2995	27	2985	38	2001
6	3982	17	3101	28	2479	39	1566
7	4055	18	3400	29	2901	40	1676
8	3459	19	3764	30	2778	41	1783
9	3998	20	2997	31	2099	42	2002
10	3852	21	3031	32	2500	43	2118
11	3421	22	3120	33	2322	44	1882

Source: Modification of data in Exercise 10.14, page 173, Kuzma and Bohnenblust (2001).

Use the above table to construct an ANOVA table for the test of no mean differences in birth weight among the groups. What is the p-value for this test? What do you conclude about the effect of smoking on birth weight?

13.9 Four brands of cereal are compared to see if they produce significant weight gain in rats. Four groups of seven rats each were given a diet of the respective cereal brand. At the end of the experimental period, the rats were weighed and the weight was compared to the weight just prior to the start of the cereal diet. Determine whether each brand has a statistically significant effect on the amount of weight gain. The data are provided in the table below.

Rat Weight by Brand of Cereal

Brand A (weight gain in oz)	Brand B (weight gain in oz)	Brand C (weight gain in oz)	Brand D (weight gain in oz)
9	5	2	3
7	4	1	8
8	6	1	5
8	4	2	9
7	5	2	2
8	7	3	7
8	3	2	8

Source: Modification of Exercise 10.13, page 173, Kuzma and Bohnenblust (2001).

13.10 A botanist wants to determine the effect of microscopic worms on seedling growth. He prepares 16 identical planting pots and then introduces four sets of worm populations into them. There are four groups of pots with four pots in each group. The worm population group sizes are 0 (introduced into the first group of four pots), 500 (introduced into the second group of four pots), 1000 (introduced into the third group of four pots), and 4000 (introduced into the fourth group of four pots). Two weeks after planting, he measures the seedling growth in centimeters. The results are given in the table below.

Seedling Growth in Centimeters by Worm Population Group

Group 1 (0 worms)	Group 2 (500 worms)	Group 3 (1000 worms)	Group 4 (4000 worms)
10.7	11.1	5.7	4.7
9.0	11.1	5.1	3.2
13.4	8.9	7.2	6.5
9.2	11.4	4.8	5.3

Source: Adapted from Exercise 9.16, pages 584–585, Moore (1995).

a. State the null hypothesis and determine the ANOVA table.
b. What is the result of the F test?
c. Apply Tukey's HSD test to see which means differ if the ANOVA was significant at the 5% level.

13.11 Analysis of variance may be used in an industrial setting. For example, managers of a soda-bottling company suspected that four filling machines were not filling the soda cans in a uniform way. An experiment on four machines doing five runs each gave the data in the following table.

Liquid Weight of Machine-Filled Cans in Ounces

Machine A	Machine B	Machine C	Machine D
12.05	11.98	12.04	12.00
12.07	12.05	12.03	11.97
12.04	12.06	12.03	11.98
12.04	12.02	12.00	11.99
11.99	11.99	11.96	11.96

Based on the analysis of variance, is there a difference in the average number of ounces filled by the four machines? Apply Tukey's HSD test to compare the mean differences if the overall ANOVA test is significant at the 5% level.

13.12 The following table shows the home run production of five of baseball's greatest sluggers over a period of 10 years. Each has hit at least 56 home runs in a season and all but Griffey have had seasons with 60 or more. Sosa, Bonds, and Griffey are still active, McGwire has retired, and Ruth is deceased, so this time period constitutes the final 10 years of McGwire's and Ruth's respective careers.

Home Run Production for Five Great Sluggers

	Ruth	McGwire	Sosa	Bonds	Griffey
	25	42	15	34	27
	47	9	10	46	45
	60	9	8	37	40
	54	39	33	33	17
	46	52	25	42	49
	49	58	36	40	56
	46	70	66	37	56
	41	65	63	34	48
	34	32	50	49	40
	22	29	64	73	22
Total	424	405	370	425	400
Average	42.4	40.5	37.0	42.5	40.0

a. Construct an ANOVA table to test whether or not there are statistically significant differences in the home run production of these sluggers over the ten-year period.
b. If the F test indicates significant differences at the 0.05 significance level, apply Tukey's HSD to see if there is a slugger who stands out with the lowest average. Is there a slugger with an average significantly higher than the rest? Is Bonds at 42.5 significantly higher than Sosa at 37.0?

13.7 ADDITIONAL READING

1. Dunn, O. J. and Clark, V. A. (1974). *Applied Statistics: Analysis of Variance and Regression.* Wiley, New York.
2. Fisher, L. and McDonald, J. (1978). *Fixed Effects Analysis of Variance.* Academic Press, New York.
3. Gibbons, J. D., Olkin, I., and Sobel, M. (1977). *Selecting and Ordering Populations: A New Statistical Methodology.* Wiley, New York.
4. Hochberg, Y. and Tamhane, A. C. (1987). *Multiple Comparison Procedures.* Wiley, New York.
5. Hocking, R. R. (1985). *The Analysis of Linear Models.* Brooks/Cole, Monterey, California.
6. Hsu, J. C. (1996). *Multiple Comparisons: Theory and Methods.* Chapman and Hall, London.
7. Kuzma, J. W. and Bohnenblust, S. E. (2001). *Basic Statistics for the Health Sciences,* Fourth Edition. Mayfield, Mountain View, California.
8. Miller, Jr., R. G. (1981). *Simultaneous Statistical Inference,* Second Edition. Springer-Verlag, New York.
9. Miller, Jr., R. G. (1986). *Beyond ANOVA: Basics of Applied Statistics.* Wiley, New York.
10. Mood, A. M., Graybill, F. A., and Boes, D. C. (1974). *Introduction to the Theory of Statistics,* Third Edition. McGraw-Hill, New York.
11. Moore, D. S. (1995). *The Basic Practice of Statistics.* W. H. Freeman, New York.
12. Rao, P. S. R. S. (1997). *Variance Components Estimation: Mixed Models, Methodologies and Applications.* Chapman and Hall, London.
13. Scheffe, H. (1959). *The Analysis of Variance.* Wiley, New York.
14. Westfall, P. H. and Young, S. S. (1993). *Resampling-Based Mutiple Testing: Examples and Methods for p-Value Adjustment.* Wiley, New York.

CHAPTER 14

Nonparametric Methods

A precise and universally acceptable definition of the term "non-parametric" is not presently available.
—John E. Walsh, *Handbook of Nonparametric Statistics, Volume 1,* Chapter 1, p. 2

14.1 ADVANTAGES AND DISADVANTAGES OF NONPARAMETRIC VERSUS PARAMETRIC METHODS

With the exception of the bootstrap, the techniques covered in the first 13 chapters are all parametric techniques. By parametric we mean that they are based on probability models for the data that involve only a few unknown values, called parameters, which refer to measurable characteristics of populations. Usually, the parametric model that we have used has been the normal distribution; the unknown parameters that we attempt to estimate are the population mean μ and the population variance σ^2.

However, many tests (e.g., the F test to determine equal variances), and estimating methods (e.g., the least squares solution to linear regression problems) are sensitive to parametric modeling assumptions. These procedures can be shown in theory to be optimal when the parametric model is correct, but inaccurate or misleading when the model does not hold, even approximately.

Procedures that are not sensitive to the parametric distribution assumptions are called robust. Student's t test for differences between two means when the populations are assumed to have the same variance is robust, because the sample means in the numerator of the test statistic are approximately normal by the central limit theorem.

With nonparametric techniques, the distribution of the test statistic under the null hypothesis has a sampling distribution for the observed data that does not depend on any unknown parameters. Consequently, these tests do not require an assumption of a parametric family. As an example, the sign test for the paired difference between two population medians has a test statistic, T, which equals the number of positive differences between pairs. T has a binomial distribution with parameters n = sample size and $p = 1/2$ under the null hypothesis that the medians are equal. Note that this sampling distribution for the test statistic is completely known under the null hypothesis since the sample size is given and $p = 1/2$. There are no unknown parameters that need to be estimated from the data. The sign test is explained in Section 14.5.

The lack of dependence on parametric assumptions is the advantage of nonparametric tests over parametric ones. Nonparametric tests preserve the significance level of the test regardless of the distribution of the data in the parent population.

When a parametric family is appropriate, the price one pays for a distribution-free test is a loss in power in comparison to the parametric test. Also, in generating the test statistic for a nonparametric procedure, we may throw out useful information. For example, the most common popular tests covered in this chapter are rank tests, which keep only the ranks of the observations and not their numerical values.

In the next section, we will show you how to rank the data in rank tests. Examples of these tests are the Wilcoxon rank-sum test, the Wilcoxon signed-rank test, and the Kruskal–Wallis test. Conover (1999) has written an excellent text on the applications of nonparametric methods.

14.2   PROCEDURES FOR RANKING DATA

Ranking data becomes useful when we are dealing with inferences about two or more populations and believe that parametric assumptions such as the normality of their distributions do not apply. Suppose, for example, that we have two samples from two distinct populations. Our null hypothesis is that the two populations are identical. You may think of this as stating that they have the same medians. We are not checking for differences in means because the mean may not even exist for these populations. Table 14.1 shows how to rank data from two populations.

Let us denote the sample from the first population with n_1 observations $x_1, x_2, x_3,$ $\ldots, x_{n1}$. The second sample consists of n_2 observations. For the purpose of the analysis, we will pool the data from the two samples. We will label the observations from the second sample $x_{n_1+1}, x_{n_1+2}, x_{n_1+3}, \ldots, x_{n_1+n_2}$. Now, to rank the data, we order the observations from smallest to largest and denote the ordered observations as y's. If x_5 is the smallest observation, x_5 becomes y_1, and if x_3 is the next smallest, x_3 becomes y_2, and so forth. We continue in this way until all the x's are assigned to all the y's.

TABLE 14.1. Terminology for Ranking Data from Two Independent Samples

First Sample (x_i)	Second Sample (x_{i+1})
$x_1, x_2, x_3, \ldots, x_{n_1}$	$x_{n_1+1}, x_{n_1+2}, x_{n_1+3}, \ldots, x_{n_1+n_2}$
Ordered Observations (y_i)	
$y_1, y_2, y_3, \ldots, y_{n_1}, y_{n_1+1}, \ldots, y_{n_1+n_2}$	

In Table 14.2, we present hypothetical data to illustrate ranking. The y's refer to the ranked observations from the first and second samples. We have two groups, control and treatment, x_c and x_t, respectively.

To illustrate the procedures described in the previous paragraph, suppose a researcher conducted a study to determine whether physical therapy increased the weight lifting ability of elderly male patients. As the researcher believed that the data were not normally distributed, a nonparametric test was applied. The data under the unsorted scores column represent the values as they were collected directly from the subjects. Then the two data sets were combined and sorted in ascending order. Each score was then assigned a rank, which is shown in parentheses. (Refer to the columns labeled "sorted scores.") The term ΣR means that we should sum the ranks in a particular column; the symbols T and T' refer to the sum of the ranks in the control and treatment groups, respectively. In this example, $T = 25$ and $T' = 30$. We do not need to keep track of both of these statistics because the sum of all the ranks is $T + T'$ and is known to be $n(n + 1)/2$, where n is the sum of the sample sizes in the two groups, in this case $n = 2(5) = 10$, and so the sum of the ranks is $10(11)/2 = 55$. In summing all the ranks we are just adding up the integers from 1 to 10 in our example.

A possible ambiguity can occur when some data points share the same value. In that case, the ordering among the tied values can be done by any system (e.g., choose the lowest indexed x first). Rather than assigning them separate ranks in arbitrary order, sometimes we prefer to give all the tied observations the same rank. That rank would be the average rank among the tied observations. If, for example, the 3rd, 4th, 5th, and 6th smallest values were all tied, they would all get the rank of 4.5 [i.e., $(3 + 4 + 5 + 6)/4$]. Now that the x's have been rearranged from the smallest to the largest values (the arrangement is sometimes called the rank order), the rank

TABLE 14.2. **Left Leg Lifting Test Data among Elderly Male Patients Who Are Receiving Physical Therapy; Maximum Weight (Unsorted, Sorted, and Ranked) For Treatment and Control Groups**

Unsorted scores		Sorted scores (ranks shown in parentheses)	
Control Group (x_c)	Treatment Group (x_t)	Control Group (y_c)	Treatment Group (y_t)
25	26		16 (1)
66	85	18 (2)	
34	48	25 (3)	
18	68		26 (4)
57	16	34 (5)	
			48 (6)
$n_1 = 5$	$n_2 = 5$	57 (7)	
		66 (8)	
			68 (9)
			85 (10)
		$T = \Sigma R = 25$	$T' = \Sigma R = 30$

transformation is made by replacing the value of the observation with its y subscript. This subscript is called the rank of the observation. Refer to Table 14.1 for an example. You can see that the lowest rank is y_1. If x_5 is the smallest observation, its rank would be 1. If x_3 and x_9 are tied, they both would be assigned to y_2 and y_3 and have a rank of 2.5.

If the two distributions of the parent populations are the same, then the ranks will be well mixed among the populations (i.e., both groups should have a similar number of high and low ranks in their respective samples). However, if the alternative is true (that the population distributions are different) and the median or center of one distribution is very different from the other, the group with the smaller median should tend to have more lower ranks than the group with the higher median. A test statistic based on the ranks of one group should be able to detect this difference. In Section 14.3, we will consider an example: the Wilcoxon rank-sum test.

14.3 WILCOXON RANK-SUM TEST (THE MANN–WHITNEY TEST)

A nonparametric analog to the unpaired t test, the Wilcoxon rank-sum test is used to compare central tendency, i.e., the locations of two independent samples selected from two populations. Conover (1999) is an important reference for this test. The data must be taken from a continuous scale and represent at least ordinal measurement. The Wilcoxon test statistic is calculated by taking the sum of the ranks of n_1 observations from group one. There are also n_2 observations in group two, but only group one is needed to perform the test. The sum of all the ranks $(T + T')$ is $(n_1 + n_2)(n_1 + n_2 + 1)/2$. Referring to Table 14.2: $(5 + 5)(5 + 5 + 1)/2 = 55$. You can verify this sum by checking Table 14.2. Since $n_1/(n_1 + n_2)$ is the probability that a randomly selected observation is from group one, multiplying these two numbers together gives the expected rank sum for group one. This value is $(n_1)(n_1 + n_2 + 1)/2 = (5)(11)/2 = 27.5$. We will use the rank sum for group one as the test statistic. The distribution of the rank sum can be found in tables for small to moderate values of n_1 and n_2. For $n_1 = 5$ and $n_2 = 5$, the critical value is 18. A rank sum that is less than 18 or greater than $55 - 18 = 37$ is significant ($p < 0.05$, two-tailed test). Thus, in our example, since $T = 25$ the difference between the treatment and control groups is not statistically significant.

Here is a second example that uses small sample sizes. Recall in Section 8.7 the table for pig blood loss data to compare the treatment and the control groups. In Section 9.9, we used these data to demonstrate the two-sample t test when both of the variances for the parent population are assumed to be unknown and equal. Note that if the variances are equal, we are only entertaining the possibility of a difference in the center or median of the distribution. Because these data did not fit well to the normal distribution, we might perform a Wilcoxon rank-sum test to determine whether we can detect differences between the medians of the two populations. Table 14.3 shows the data and the pooled ranks.

The ranks in Table 14.3 are obtained as follows. First we list all the data irrespective of control group or treatment group assignment: 786, 375, 4446, 2886,

TABLE 14.3. Pig Blood Loss Data (ml)

Control Group Pigs (pooled rank)	Treatment Group Pigs (pooled rank)
786 (9)	543 (5)
375 (1)	666 (7)
4446 (19)	455 (3)
2886 (16)	823 (11)
478 (4)	1716 (14)
587 (6)	797 (10)
434 (2)	2828 (15)
4764 (20)	1251 (13)
3281 (17)	702 (8)
3837 (18)	1078 (12)
Sample mean $(X_c) = 2187.40$	Sample mean $(X_t) = 1085.90$
Sample s.d. $(s_c) = 1824.27$	Sample s.d. $(s_t) = 717.12$

478, 587, 434, 4764, 3281, 3837, 543, 666, 455, 823, 1716, 797, 2828, 1251, 702, 1078. Next we rearrange these values from smallest to largest: 375, 434, 455, 478, 543, 587, 666, 702, 786, 797, 823, 1078, 1251, 1716, 2828, 2886, 3281, 3837, 4446, 4764.

The ranks are then given as follows: $375 \rightarrow 1, 434 \rightarrow 2, 455 \rightarrow 3, 478 \rightarrow 4, 543 \rightarrow 5, 587 \rightarrow 6, 666 \rightarrow 7, 702 \rightarrow 8, 786 \rightarrow 9, 797 \rightarrow 10, 823 \rightarrow 11, 1078 \rightarrow 12, 1251 \rightarrow 13, 1716 \rightarrow 14, 2828 \rightarrow 15, 2886 \rightarrow 16, 3281 \rightarrow 17, 3837 \rightarrow 18, 4446 \rightarrow 19, 4764 \rightarrow 20$. These ranks are then associated with observations in each group; the ranks are given next to the numbers in Table 14.3. The test statistic T is then the sum of the ranks in the control group, namely, $9 + 1 + 19 + 16 + 4 + 6 + 2 + 20 + 17 + 18 = 112$. The sum of the ranks for the treatment group T' is $5 + 7 + 3 + 11 + 14 + 10 + 15 + 13 + 8 + 12 = 98$. The higher rank sum for the control group is consistent with the tendency for greater blood loss in the control group. Note that $n_1 = n_2 = 10$ and $n_1 + n_2 = 20$. The sum of all the ranks $(T + T') = 1 + 2 + 3 + \ldots, 20 = 210$. $T + T' = (n_1 + n_2)(n_1 + n_2 + 1)/2 = (20)(21)/2 = 210$. We also know that $T = 112$. Alternatively, we can calculate $T' = 210 - T = 210 - 112 = 98$.

Consulting tables for the Mann–Whitney (Wilcoxon) test statistic, we see that the 10th percentile critical value is 88 and the 90th percentile critical value is 122. We observed that $T = 112$ and $T' = 98$. The two-sided p-value of the observed statistic must be greater than 0.20. When the null hypothesis is true, the probability is 0.80 that the rank sum statistics fall between 88 and 122. Both T and T' fall within the range of 98 on the low side and 112 on the high side. So the difference in the rank sums is not statistically significant at $\alpha = 0.20$.

Recall that in Chapter 9 (using the same data as in this example), we found a one-sided p-value of less than 0.05 when applying the t test; i.e., the results were significant. Why did the t test give a different answer from the Wilcoxon test, and which test should we believe? First of all, two dubious assumptions were made in applying the t test: the first was that the two distributions were normal and the second was that they both had the same variance. Histograms for the two samples would probably convince you that the distributions are not normal. Also, the sample standard deviation for the control group is approximately 2½ times as large as for the treatment group, indicating that the variances are not equal. Because we are on shaky ground with the parametric assumptions, we should trust the nonparametric analysis and conclude that there is insufficient information to detect a difference between the two populations. The nonsignificant results for the Wilcoxon test do not mean that the central tendencies of the two groups are the same. Tests such as the Wilcoxon rank-sum test are not very powerful at detecting differences in means (or medians) when the variances of the two samples differ greatly, as is true of this case. As the sample size is only 10 for each group, we may wish that we had collected data on more pigs so that a difference in the blood loss distributions could have been detected.

Most of the time, we will be using the normal approximation for the Wilcoxon rank-sum test. Consequently, we have not included tables of critical values for this test for use with small sample sizes. For large values (n_1 or n_2 greater than 20) a normal approximation can be used. As before, we will use the sum of the ranks from the first sample. The test statistic for the sum of the ranks for the control group is denoted as T. To use the normal approximation when there are many ties, take

$$Z = \frac{T - \dfrac{n_1(n_1 + n_2 + 1)}{2}}{S}$$

where S is the standard deviation for T and $n_1(n_1 + n_2 + 1)/2$ is the expected value of the rank sum under the null hypothesis. S is the square root of S^2, where

$$S^2 = \frac{n_1 n_2 \Sigma R_i^2}{(n_1 + n_2)(n_1 + n_2 - 1)} - \frac{n_1 n_2 (n_1 + n_2 + 1)^2}{4(n_1 + n_2 - 1)}$$

Here ΣR_i^2 is the sum of the squares of the ranks for all the data. This result is given in Conover (1999), page 273, using slightly different notation.

When there are no ties, Conover (1999) recommends a simpler approximation, namely,

$$Z' = \frac{T - \dfrac{n_1(n_1 + n_2 + 1)}{2}}{\sqrt{\dfrac{n_1 n_2 (n_1 + n_2 + 1)}{12}}}$$

To summarize, Equation 14.1 describes the normal approximation for the Wilcoxon rank-sum test for comparing two independent samples (no ties) that can be used when n_1 and n_2 are large enough. Let T be the sum of the ranks for the pooled observations from one of the groups (samples). Then

$$Z' = \frac{T - \dfrac{n_1(n_1 + n_2 + 1)}{2}}{\sqrt{\dfrac{n_1 n_2 (n_1 + n_2 + 1)}{12}}} \tag{14.1}$$

where T is the sum of the ranks in one of the groups (e.g., control group) and n_1 and n_2 are, respectively, the sample sizes for samples from population 1 and population 2.

In the event of ties, the following normal approximation Wilcoxon rank-sum test for comparing two independent samples (ties) should be used when n_1 and n_2 are large enough (i.e., greater than 20). Let T be the sum of the ranks for the pooled observations from one of the groups (samples). Then

$$Z = \frac{T - \dfrac{n_1(n_1 + n_2 + 1)}{2}}{S} \tag{14.2}$$

where T is the sum of the ranks from one of the groups (e.g., control group); n_1 and n_2 are, respectively, the sample sizes for sample 1 and sample 2; and

$$S^2 = \frac{n_1 n_2 \Sigma R_i^2}{n_1 + n_2(n_1 + n_2 - 1)} - \frac{n_1 n_2 (n_1 + n_2 + 1)^2}{4(n_1 + n_2 - 1)}$$

where $\Sigma_{i=1}^{N} R_i^2$ is the sum of the squares of the ranks for all the data ($N = n_1 + n_2$).

In the next two sections, we will look at the nonparametric analogs to the paired t test. They are the Wilcoxon signed-rank test (in Section 14.4) and the simpler but less powerful sign test (in Section 14.5).

14.4   WILCOXON SIGNED-RANK TEST

Remember that a paired t test involved taking the difference between two paired observations, i.e., $d_i = X_{i_{t_1}} - X_{i_{t_2}}$. The Wilcoxon signed-rank test is a nonparametric rank test that is analogous to the paired t test but is applicable when the differences (d_i) between the two groups are not approximately normally distributed. The procedure of the Wilcoxon signed-rank test involves first computing the paired differences, as with the t test. The absolute values of the differences are then computed and the data ranked based on these absolute differences. After the ranks are determined, the observations are split into two distinct groups that separate the ones that have negative differences from the ones that have positive differences. The rank sums are then computed for the positive differences, with the test statistic denoted as T^+. This test statistic is then compared to the tables for the signed-rank test; the tables are based on the distribution of this statistic when the central tendencies of the two populations are the same. Alternatively, we could have computed the sum of the negative ranks and denoted it by T^-.

If the two populations are the same, the paired differences will be symmetric about zero and therefore will have about the same number of positive and negative differences, and the magnitude of these differences will not depend on the sign (i.e., whether or not they are in the positive difference group). Assume that we find the differences between paired observations by subtracting the values for the second observation from the values for the first observation (as shown in Table 14.4). If the proportion of positive differences is high, it suggests that population one has a higher median than population two. A low proportion of positive differences indicates that population one has a lower median than population two. In the event that a particular paired difference is identical (i.e., 0), that observation is omitted from the calculation, and we proceed as if the number of pairs is one less than the original number.

Recall from Chapter 9 the two cities data that we used to illustrate the paired t test. We will use these data to demonstrate how the signed-rank test works. (See Table 14.4.)

The fact that all the ranks are positive is a strong indicator that Washington was warmer than New York. This finding replicates the very highly significant difference that was found using the paired t test.

The absolute value of the difference determines the ranks. The smallest absolute value gets rank 1, the next rank 2, and so on until we reach the largest with rank 12. However, in the example in Table 14.4 there is a tie for the lowest, with four cases having the value 2. When ties occur, all tied observations get the average of the tied ranks. So the average of ranks 1, 2, 3, and 4 is 10/4 = 2.5. Similarly the observed absolute difference of 3 is tied in two cases and hence the average of the ranks 5 and 6 gives a rank of 5.5 to each of those tied observations.

The sum of the positive ranks is 78, and the sum of the negative ranks is 0. Since n is small (12), we refer to the tables for the signed-rank test statistic. Recall that the

TABLE 14.4. Daily Temperatures, Washington versus New York

Day	Washington Mean Temperature (°F)	New York Mean Temperature (°F)	Paired Difference #1–#2	Absolute Difference	Rank (sign)
1 (January 15)	31	28	3	3	5.5 (+)
2 (February 15)	35	33	2	2	2.5 (+)
3 (March 15)	40	37	3	3	5.5 (+)
4 (April 15)	52	45	7	7	12 (+)
5 (May 15)	70	68	2	2	2.5 (+)
6 (June 15)	76	74	2	2	2.5 (+)
7 (July 15)	93	89	4	4	7.5 (+)
8 (August 15)	90	85	5	5	10 (+)
9 (September 15)	74	69	5	5	10 (+)
10 (October 15)	55	51	4	4	7.5 (+)
11 (November 15)	32	27	5	5	10 (+)
12 (December 15)	26	24	2	2	2.5 (+)

sum of the positive ranks is denoted by T^+. Referring to Appendix C, we find that for $n = 12$ and $p = 0.005$, the critical value is 8. This outcome means that the probability of observing a value less than 8 is 0.005. Similarly, from the tables the probability of observing a value greater than 70 is 0.005. This is based on symmetry since the probability of the positive ranks being less than 8 under the null hypothesis is the same as the probability of being greater than $78 - 8 = 70$. Since we observed a signed-rank score of 78, we know that the one-sided p-value is less than 0.005. So we conclude that there is a difference between the two populations in the mean temperature.

A normal approximation can be used for large n. Conover (1999) recommends that n be at least 50.

Let

$$Z = \frac{T^+ - \dfrac{n(n + 1)}{4}}{\sqrt{\dfrac{n(n + 1)(2n + 1)}{24}}}$$

Then Z has approximately a standard normal distribution. So the standard normal tables (Appendix E) may be used after calculating Z in order to obtain an approximate p-value for large n.

Another normal approximation that is simpler than the foregoing approximation is based on the statistic $T = T^+ - T^-$. The statistic T has a mean of zero under the null hypothesis. So there is no expected value to subtract. For T (in the case when there are no ties) we define the standard normal approximation as

$$Z = \frac{T}{\sqrt{\dfrac{n(n + 1)(2n + 1)}{6}}}$$

In the event of ties, we use $Z = T/\sqrt{\Sigma R_i^2}$, where R_i is the absolute rank of the ith observation (both positive and negative ranks are included in this sum).

The temperature data (refer to Table 14.4) are highly unusual because of the extreme differences between the two cities; same-day pairing for each month of the year is used to remove the seasonal effect. As a second example of pairing, we will look at how twins score on a psychological test for aggressiveness (refer to Table 14.5). The data are from Conover (1999). The research question being addressed is whether first-born twins are more aggressive than second-born twins.

The value of n is 11 because we discard one pair of observations for which the difference is 0. Here we see that the sum of the ranks for a sample size of 11 is 66 ($1 + 2 + 3 + \ldots + 11$). From the paired difference column, we see that the sum of the positive ranks is 41.5 and the sum of the negative ranks is 24.5. From the table for the signed-rank test with $n = 11$ (Appendix C), we see that the critical value at the one-sided 5% significance level is 55. Given that the sum of the positive ranks is 41.5, we cannot reject the null hypothesis because the p-value is greater than 0.05. Therefore, first-born twins do not tend to be more aggressive than second-born twins.

TABLE 14.5. Aggressiveness Scores for 12 Sets of Identical Twins

Twin Set	Twin #1 (First Born) Aggressiveness	Twin #2 (Second Born) Aggressiveness	Paired Difference	Absolute Difference	Rank (sign)
1	86	88	−2	2	3(−)
2	71	77	−6	6	7 (−)
3	77	76	1	1	1.5 (+)
4	68	64	4	4	4 (+)
5	91	96	−5	5	5.5 (−)
6	72	72	0	0	—
7	77	65	12	12	10 (+)
8	91	90	1	1	1.5 (+)
9	70	65	5	5	5.5 (+)
10	71	80	−9	9	9 (−)
11	88	81	7	7	8 (+)
12	87	72	15	15	11 (+)

Source: adapted from Conover (1999), page 355, Example 1, with permission.

The normal approximations for the signed-rank test, recommended when n is 50 or more, are summarized in Equations 14.3 (no ties) and 14.4 (ties). A normal approximation to the Wilcoxon signed-rank test for comparing two dependent samples (no ties) is

$$Z = \frac{T}{\sqrt{\dfrac{n(n + 1)(2n + 1)}{6}}} \qquad (14.3)$$

where $T = T^+ - T^-$ is the sum of the ranks, and n is the common sample size for both population 1 and population 2. A normal approximation to the wilcoxon signed-rank test for comparing two independent samples (ties) is

$$Z = \frac{T}{\sqrt{\sum\limits_{i=1}^{n} R_i^2}} \qquad (14.4)$$

where $T^+ - T^-$ is the sum of the ranks, $\sum_{i=1}^{n} R_i^2$ is the sum of the squares of the absolute ranks, and n is the common sample size for both population 1 and population 2.

14.5   SIGN TEST

The sign test is very much like the signed-rank test, only simpler. Again we compute the paired differences, but instead of determining the ranks of the absolute differences we just keep track of the number of positive (or negative differences). The sign of paired differences will have a binomial distribution with parameter p. If we define p (the binomial success parameter) to be the probability of a positive sign, and we eliminate cases with zero for the paired difference, then the parameter p will be equal to 0.5 under the null hypothesis. So the sign test is simply a test that a binomial parameter $p = 0.5$, versus either a one-sided or two-sided alternative. Let us look at the two examples from the previous section to illustrate the sign test. First we will consider the temperature data for the two cities and then the example of aggressiveness among twins.

Referring to Table 14.6, we see that the number of successes is 12, meaning that for every month the temperature was higher in Washington than in New York. The p-value for the test is defined as the probability of as extreme or a more extreme outcome than the observed one under the null hypothesis. We see that the p-value is $(1/2)^{12} = 0.000244$. Remember from Chapter 5 that this probability is equivalent to the probability of 12 consecutive heads in a coin toss experiment with a fair coin. From this information, we can see that the significance of the test is less than $p = 0.05$ or $p = 0.001$, indicating that the differences are highly significant. In general, the sign test is not as powerful as the signed-rank test because it disregards the information in the rank of the difference. Yet, in Table 14.6, the evidence is very strong that the p-value is small, even for the sign test. Now let us apply the sign test to the twin data (Table 14.7).

In this case, the p-value is the probability of getting 7 or more successes (shown in Table 14.7 as 7 positive differences) in 11 trials when the binomial probability of success is $p = 0.50$. The probability of observing 7 or more successes in 11 trials when $p = 0.50$ is found to be 0.2744. So a p-value of 0.2744 indicates that the observed number of successes easily could have happened by chance. Therefore, we cannot reject the null hypothesis.

TABLE 14.6. Daily Temperatures for Two Cities

Day	Washington Mean Temperature (°F)	New York Mean Temperature (°F)	Paired Difference #1 – #2	Sign
1 (January 15)	31	28	3	+
2 (February 15)	35	33	2	+
3 (March 15)	40	37	3	+
4 (April 15)	52	45	7	+
5 (May 15)	70	68	2	+
6 (June 15)	76	74	2	+
7 (July 15)	93	89	4	+
8 (August 15)	90	85	5	+
9 (September 15)	74	69	5	+
10 (October 15)	55	51	4	+
11 (November 15)	32	27	5	+
12 (December 15)	26	24	2	+

TABLE 14.7.   Aggressiveness Scores for 12 Sets of Identical Twins

Twin Set	Twin #1 (First Born) Aggressiveness	Twin #2 (Second Born) Aggressiveness	Paired Difference	Rank (sign)
1	86	88	-2	−
2	71	77	-6	−
3	77	76	1	+
4	68	64	4	+
5	91	96	-5	−
6	72	72	0	—
7	77	65	12	+
8	91	90	1	+
9	70	65	5	+
10	71	80	-9	−
11	88	81	7	+
12	87	72	15	+

14.6   KRUSKAL–WALLIS TEST: ONE-WAY ANOVA BY RANKS

The Kruskal–Wallis test is a nonparametric analog to the one-way analysis of variance discussed in Chapter 13. It is a simple generalization of the Wilcoxon rank-sum test. The problem is to identify whether or not three or more populations (independent samples) have the same distribution (or central tendency). We test the null hypothesis (H_0) that the distributions of the parent populations are the same against the alternative (H_1) that the distributions are different. The rationale for the test involves pooling all of the data and then applying a rank transformation. If the null hypothesis is true, each group should have rank sums that are similar. If at least one group has a higher (or lower) median than the others, it should have a higher (or lower) rank sum. Table 14.8 provides an example of data layout for several samples (e.g., k samples), following the model for the Kruskal–Wallis test.

To describe the test procedure, we need to use some mathematical notation. Let X_{ij} represent the jth observation from the ith population. We assume that there are $k \geq 3$ populations and for population i we have n_i observations. $N =$ the total number

TABLE 14.8.   Data Layout for Kruskal–Wallis Test

Observation	Sample 1	Sample 2	. . .	Sample k
1	$X_{1,1}$	$X_{2,1}$		$X_{k,1}$
2	$X_{1,2}$	$X_{2,2}$		$X_{k,2}$
. . .	. . .	. . .		. . .
n_k	X_{1,n_1}	X_{2,n_2}		X_{k,n_1}

Source: adapted from Conover, 1999, page 288.

of observations. Let $N = \Sigma_{i=1}^{k} n_i$ and for each i let R_i be the sum of the ranks for the observations in the ith population. That is, $R_i = \Sigma_{j=1}^{n_i} R(X_{ij})$ for each i, where $i = 1, 2, \ldots, k$). The test statistic is defined as

$$T = \frac{1}{S^2}\left(\sum_{i=1}^{k} \frac{R_i^2}{n_1} - \frac{N(N+1)^2}{4}\right)$$

where

$$S^2 = \frac{1}{N-1}\left(\sum_{i=1}^{k}\sum_{j=1}^{n_1} R(X_{ij})^2 - N\frac{(N+1)^2}{4}\right)$$

In the absence of ties, S^2 simplifies to $N(N+1)/12$, and T is defined by the following equation for a chi-square approximation to the Kruskal–Wallis rank test for comparing three or more independent samples (no ties) is

$$T = \frac{12}{N(N+1)}\sum_{i=1}^{k} \frac{R_i^2}{n_1} - 3(N+1) \tag{14.5}$$

where n_i is the sample size for the ith population and N is the total sample size.

This test statistic has a distribution with a chi-square approximation when there are no ties. Under the null hypothesis that the distributions are the same, the test statistic's distribution has been tabulated for small values of N. The tables of critical values for T are not included in this text. When N is large, an approximate chi-square distribution can be used. In fact, the test statistic T has approximately a chi-square distribution with $k-1$ degrees of freedom, where k again refers to the number of samples. The approximate test has been shown to work well even when N is not very large. See Conover (1999) for details and references.

Equation 14.6 gives the chi-square approximation to the Kruskal–Wallis rank test for comparing three or more independent samples in the event of ties:

$$T = \frac{1}{S^2}\left(\sum_{i=1}^{k} \frac{R_i^2}{n_1} - \frac{N(N+1)^2}{4}\right) \tag{14.6}$$

where

$$R_i = \sum_{j=1}^{n_1} R(X_{ij})$$

$$S^2 = \frac{1}{N-1}\left(\sum_{i=1}^{k}\sum_{j=1}^{n_1} R(X_{ij})^2 - N\frac{(N+1)^2}{4}\right)$$

n_i is the sample size for the ith population
N is the total sample size

The SAS procedure NPAR1WAY can be used to perform the Kruskal–Wallis test. That procedure also allows you to compare the results to the F test used for a one-way ANOVA.

To illustrate the Kruskal–Wallis test, we take an example from Conover (1999). In this example, three instructors are compared to determine whether they are similar or different in their grading practices. (See Table 14.9.). This example demonstrates a special case in which there are many ties, which occur because the ordinal data have a restricted range.

Table 14.9 provides the rankings for these data. As is usual with grades, f is the lowest rank, then D, then C, then B, and finally A. From the pooled total we see that the number of Fs given by the three instructors is 9. As a result, each of the 9 students gets an average rank of $5 = (9 + 1)/2$. The respective counts and rankings for the remaining grades are D (19, rank 19), C (34, rank 46.5), B (27, rank 76), and A (20, rank 99.5). The ranking of 19 for Ds is based on the fact that there are 9 Fs and 19 Ds. So the rank for Ds is $9 + (19 + 1)/2 = 9 + 10 = 19$. The rank for Cs comes from 28 Ds and Fs along with 34 Cs for $28 + (34 + 1)/2 = 28 + 17.5 = 45.5$. For Bs we get the rank from 62 Cs, Ds and Fs along with 27 Bs for $62 + (27 + 1)/2 = 62 + 14 = 76$. Finally, the rank for the As is obtained by taking the 89 Bs, Cs, Ds and Fs along with 20 As for $89 + (20 + 1)/2 = 89 + 10.5 = 99.5$. Conover (1999) chooses to rank the As with the lowest rank and the Fs with the highest rank. We chose to give As the highest rank and Fs the lowest. For purposes of the analysis, assigning the highest rank to A or f does not affect the outcome of the test. Our choice was made because we like to think of high ranks corresponding to high grades. For each cell in Table 14.9, we multiply the number shown in the cell by the rank for that row (e.g., $4 \times 99.5 = 398$. Table 14.10 shows the resulting values; for example, the value in cell one is 398. Then we apply the formulas in Equation 14.6. Based on the formula for S^2, we see that $S^2 = \{(5)^2 \ 9 + (19)^2 \ 19 + (45.5)^2 \ 34 + (76)^2 \ 27 + (99.5)^2 \ 20 - 109 \ (110)^2/4\}/108 = 941.708$ and $T = \{(2359.5)^2/43 + (2023.5)^2/38 + (1612)^2/28 - 109(110)^2/4\}/S^2 = 0.321$. These results for T and S^2 are identical to Conover's, even though we ranked the grades in the opposite way. Based on the approximate chi-square with 2 degrees of freedom distribution for T, the critical value for $\alpha = 0.05$ is 5.991. Because our calculated $T = 0.321$, the association between instructors and grades assigned is not statistically significant.

TABLE 14.9. Grade Counts for Students by Instructor

	Instructor				
Grade	1	2	3	Row Totals	Rank
A	4	10	6	20	99.5
B	14	6	7	27	76
C	17	9	8	34	45.5
D	6	7	6	19	19
F	2	6	1	9	5
Total # of students	43	38	28	109	

Source: adapted from Conover, 1999, page 293, example 2, with permission.

TABLE 14.10. Ranks for Grade Counts for Students by Instructor

Grade	Instructor 1	Instructor 2	Instructor 3	Row Totals
A	398	995	597	1990
B	1064	456	532	2052
C	773.5	409.5	364	1547
D	114	133	114	361
F	10	30	5	45
Rank sums by instructor	2359.5	2023.5	1612	5995

14.7 SPEARMAN'S RANK-ORDER CORRELATION COEFFICIENT

In Section 12.4, we introduced the Pearson product moment correlation between two random variables X and Y. Recall that the Pearson correlation coefficient is a measure of the degree of the linear relationship between X and Y. Statistical significance tests for a nonzero correlation were derived when X and Y can be assumed to have a bivariate normal distribution. We also saw that if X and Y are functionally related in a nonlinear way, the absolute value of the correlation would be less than 1. For example, a nonlinear functional relationship might be $Y = X_2$. In this case, if we looked at values in the range on X between zero and 1, we would find a positive correlation that is less than 1. Looking at the interval between -1 and zero, we would find a negative correlation between zero and -1.

Now we will measure correlation in a more general way that satisfies two conditions. (1) X and Y are allowed to have any joint distribution and not necessarily the bivariate normal distribution. (2) The correlation between X and Y will have the property that as X increases Y increases (or decreases), then the correlation measure will be $+1$ (or -1). In this case if $Y = \ln(X)$ for $X > 1$ or $Y = X^2$ for $X > 0$, then the correlation between Y and X will be $+1$ since Y never decreases as X increases over the range of permissible values. Similarly, if $Y = \exp(-X)$ for $X > 0$, then Y and X will have correlation equal to -1. Statisticians have derived nonparametric measures of correlation that exhibit the foregoing two properties. Two examples are Spearman's rho (ρ_{sp}), attributed to Spearman (1904), and Kendall's tau (τ), introduced in Kendall (1938). Both of these measures have been shown to satisfy conditions (1) and (2) above.

In this text, we will discuss only Spearman's rho, which is very commonly used and easy to describe. Rho is derived as follows:

1. Separately rank the measurements (X_i, Y_i) for the Xs and Ys in increasing order.
2. Replace the pair (X_i, Y_i) for each i with its rank pair (i.e., if X_i has rank 4 and Y_i rank 7, the transformation replaces the pair with the rank pair (4, 7)).
3. Apply the formula for Pearson's product moment correlation to the rank pairs instead of to the original pairs. The result is Spearman's rho.

Spearman's rho enjoys the property that all of its values lie between −1 and 1. This result obtains because rho is the Pearson correlation formula applied to ranks. If Y is a monotonically increasing function of X (i.e., as X increases, Y increases), then the rank of X_i will match the rank of Y_i. This relationship means that the ranked pairs will be $(1, 1), (2, 2), (3, 3), \ldots, (n, n)$.

A scatter plot would show these points falling perfectly on a 45° line in a plane. Recall that for Pearson's correlation formula, a perfect linear relationship with a positive slope gives a correlation coefficient of 1. So if Y is a monotonically increasing function of X, the Spearman correlation coefficient (rho) between X and Y is 1. Similarly, one can argue that if Y is a monotonically decreasing function of X, the rank pairs will be $(1, n), (2, n-1), (3, n-2), \ldots, (n-1, 2), (n, 1)$. The smallest value of X corresponds to the largest value of Y. Consider the example $Y = \exp(-X)$ with values at $X = 1, 1.5, 2, 2.5,$ and 3. The number of pairs is $n = 5$ and these pairs are $[X, \exp(-X)]$, which equal $(1, 0.368), (1.5, 0.223),$ $(2, 0.135), (2.5, 0.082),$ and $(3, 0.050)$ where we have rounded $\exp(-X)$ to three decimal places. Note that the ranks for the Xs are 1 for 1, 2 for 1.5, 3 for 2, 4 for 2.5, and 5 for 3. The corresponding Ys have ranks 5 for 0.368, 4 for 0.223, 3 for 0.135, 2 for 0.082, and 1 for 0.050. So the pairs are $(1, 5), (2, 4), (3, 3), (4, 2)$ and $(5, 1)$. A scatter plot of such pairs would show that these rank pairs fall perfectly on a line with a slope of −1. Hence, the Spearman correlation coefficient in this case is −1.

The computational formula for Spearman's rank correlation rho with ties is given by Equation 14.7:

$$\rho_{sp} = \frac{\sum_{i=1}^{n} R(X_i)R(Y_i) - n\left(\frac{n+1}{2}\right)^2}{\left[\sum_{i=1}^{n} R(X_i)^2 - n\left(\frac{n+1}{2}\right)^2\right]^{1/2}\left[\sum_{i=1}^{n} R(Y_i)^2 - n\left(\frac{n+1}{2}\right)^2\right]^{1/2}} \qquad (14.7)$$

where n is the number of ranked pairs, $R(X_i)$ is the rank of X_i, and $R(Y_i)$ is the rank of Y_i.

When there are no ties, the formula in Equation 14.7 simplifies to Equation 14.8:

$$\rho_{sp} = 1 - \frac{6T}{n(n^2 - 1)}$$

where $T = \sum_{i=1}^{n}[R(X_i) - R(Y_i)]^2$, n is the number of ranked pairs, $R(X_i)$ is the rank of X_i, and $R(Y_i)$ is the rank of Y_i.

To illustrate the use of the foregoing equations, we will compute the Spearman rank correlation coefficient between temperatures paired by date and for the twins' aggressiveness scores paired by birth order of the siblings. Table 14.11 illustrates the computation for the temperatures.. Since there are no ties in rank, we can use Equation 14.8. The term in the last column of Table 14.11 is the ith term in the sum $(\Sigma[R(X_i) - R(Y_i)]^2)$.

TABLE 14.11. Daily Temperature Comparison for Two Cities

Day	Washington Mean Temperature (°F) (rank)	New York Mean Temperature (°F) (rank)	Rank Pair	Term $[R(X_i) - R(Y_i)]^2$
1 (January 15)	31 (2)	28 (3)	(2, 3)	1
2 (February 15)	35 (4)	33 (4)	(4, 4)	0
3 (March 15)	40 (5)	37 (5)	(5, 5)	0
4 (April 15)	52 (6)	45 (6)	(6, 6)	0
5 (May 15)	70 (8)	68 (8)	(8, 8)	0
6 (June 15)	76 (10)	74 (10)	(10, 10)	0
7 (July 15)	93 (12)	89 (12)	(12, 12)	0
8 (August 15)	90 (11)	85 (11)	(11, 11)	0
9 (September 15)	74 (9)	69 (9)	(9,9)	0
10 (October 15)	55 (7)	51 (7)	(7, 7)	0
11 (November 15)	32 (3)	27 (2)	(3, 2)	1
12 (December 15)	26 (1)	24 (1)	(1, 1)	0
T	—	—	—	2
$\rho_{sp} = 1 - 6T/(n\{n^2 - 1\})$	—	—	—	0.9930

Table 14.12 provides the same calculations for the twins. As there are a few ties in this case, we cannot use Equation 14.8 but instead must use Equation 14.7.

14.8 PERMUTATION TESTS

14.8.1 Introducing Permutation Methods

The ranking procedures described in the present chapter have an advantage over parametric methods in that they do not depend on the underlying distributions of parent populations. As we will discuss in Section 14.9, ranking procedures are not sensitive to one or a few outlying observations. However, a disadvantage of ranking procedures is that they are less informative than corresponding parametric tests. Information is lost as a result of the rank transformations. For the sake of constructing a distribution-free method, we ignore the numerical values and hence the magnitude of differences among the observations. Note that if we observed the values 4, 5, and 6 we would assign them ranks 1, 2, and 3 respectively. On the other hand, had we observed the values 4, 5, and 10, we would still assign the ranks 1, 2, and 3, respectively. The fact that 10 is much larger than 6 is lost in the rankings.

Is there a way for us to have our cake and eat it too? Permutation tests retain the information in the numerical data but do not depend on parametric assumptions. They are computer-intensive techniques with many of the same virtues as the bootstrap.

TABLE 14.12. Aggressiveness Scores for 12 Identical Twins

Twin Set	Twin #1 1st Born Aggressiveness (rank)	Twin #2 2nd Born Aggressiveness (rank)	Rank Pair	Term $R(X_i)R(Y_i)$
1	86 (8)	88 (10)	(8, 10)	80
2	71 (3.5)	77 (7)	(3.5, 5)	17.5
3	77 (6.5)	76 (6)	(6.5, 6)	39
4	68 (1)	64 (1)	(1, 1)	1
5	91 (11.5)	96 (12)	(11.5, 12)	138
6	72 (5)	72 (4.5)	(5, 4.5)	22.5
7	77 (6.5)	65 (2.5)	(6.5, 2.5)	16.25
8	91 (11.5)	90 (11)	(11.5, 11)	126.5
9	70 (2)	65 (2.5)	(2, 2.5)	5
10	71 (3.5)	80 (8)	(3.5, 8)	28
11	88 (10)	81 (9)	(10, 9)	90
12	87 (9)	72 (4.5)	(9, 4.5)	40.5
Numerator for ρ_{sp}	—	—	—	604.25–507 = 97.25
Denominator for ρ_{sp}	—	—	—	11.90*10.86 = 129.2
ρ_{sp}	—	—	—	0.7527

In the late 1940s and early 1950s, research confirmed that under certain conditions, permutation methods can be nearly as powerful as the most powerful parametric tests. This observation is true as sample sizes become large [see, for example, Lehmann and Stein (1949) and Hoeffding (1952)]. Although permutation tests have existed for more than 60 years, their common usage has emerged only in the 1980s and 1990s. Late in the twentieth century, high-speed computing enabled one to determine the exact distributions of permutations under the null hypothesis. Permutation statistics generally have discrete distributions. Computation of all possible values of these statistics and their associated probabilities when the null hypothesis is true allows one to calculate critical values and p-values; the resulting tables are much like normal probability tables used for parametric Gaussian distributions

The concepts underlying permutation tests, also called randomization tests, go back to Fisher (1935). In the case of two populations, assume we have data from two distributions denoted as $X_1, X_2, \ldots, X_n$ for the first population, and $Y_1, Y_2, \ldots, Y_m$ for the second population. The test statistic is $T = \Sigma X_i$; we ask the question "How likely is it that we would observe the value T that we obtained if the Xs and the Ys really are independent samples from the same distribution?" This is our "null hypothesis": the two distributions are identical and the samples are obtained independently.

The first assumption for this test is that both samples are independent random samples from their respective parent populations. The second is that at least an interval measurement scale is being used. Under these conditions, and assuming the null hypothesis to be true, it makes sense to pool the data because each X and Y gives information about the common distribution for the two samples.

As it makes no difference whether we include an X or a Y in the calculation of T, any arrangement of the $n + m$ observations that assigns n to group one and m to group two is as probable as the other. Hence, under the null hypothesis, any assignment to the Xs of n out of the $n + m$ observations constitutes a value for T. Recall from Chapter 5 that there are exactly $C(n + m, n) = (n + m)!/[n!\, m!]$ ways to select n observations from pooled data to serve as the Xs.

Each arrangement leads to a potentially different value for T (some arrangements may give the same numerical values if the Xs and Ys are not all different values). The test is called a permutation test because we can think of the pooled observations as $Z_1, Z_2, \ldots, Z_n, Z_{n+1}, Z_{n+2}, \ldots, Z_{n+m}$, where the first n of Zs are the original Xs and the next m are the Ys. The other combinations can be obtained by a permutation of the indices from 1 to $n + m$, where the Xs are taken to be the first n indices after the permutation.

The other name for a permutation test—randomization test—comes about because each selection of ns assigned to the Xs can be viewed as a random selection of n of the samples. This condition applies when the samples are selected at random out of the set of $n + m$ values. Physically, we could mark each of the $n + m$ values on a piece of paper, place and mix them in a hat and then reach in and randomly draw out n of them without replacing any in the hat. Hence, permutation methods also are said to be sampling without replacement. Contrast this to a bootstrap sample that is selected by sampling a fixed number of times but always with replacement.

Since under the null hypothesis each permutation has the probability $1/C(n + m, n)$, in principle we have the null distribution. On the other hand, if the two populations really are different, than the observed T should be unusually low if the Xs tend to be smaller than the Ys and unusually large if the Xs tend to be larger than the Ys. The p-value for the test is then the sum of the probabilities for all permutations leading to values of T as extreme or more extreme (equal or larger or smaller) than the observed T.

So if k is the number of values as extreme as or more extreme than the observed T, the p-value is $k/C(n + m, n)$. Such a p-value can be one-sided or two-sided depending on how we define "more extreme." The process of determining the distribution of the test statistic (T) is in principle a very simple procedure. The problem is that we must enumerate all of these permutations and calculate T for each one to construct the corresponding permutation distribution. As n and m become large, the process of generating all of these permutations is a very computer-intensive procedure.

The basic idea of enumerating a multitude of permutations has been generalized to many other statistical problems. The problems are more complicated but the idea remains the same, namely, that a permutation distribution for the test can be calculated under the null hypothesis. The null distribution will not depend on the shape of the population distributions for the original observations or their scores.

Several excellent texts specialize in permutation tests. See, for example, Good (2000), Edgington (1995), Mielke and Berry (2001), or Manly (1997). Some books with the word "resampling" in the title include permutation methods and compare them with the bootstrap. These include Westfall and Young (1993), Lunneborg (2000), and Good (2001).

Another name for permutation tests is exact tests. The latter term is used because, conditioned on the observed data, the significance levels that are determined for the hypothesis test have a special characteristic: The significance levels satisfy the exactness property regardless of the population distribution of the pooled data.

In the 2×2 contingency table in Section 11.6, we considered an approximate chi-square test for independence. The next section will introduce an exact permutation test known as Fisher's exact test. This test can be used in a 2×2 table when the chi-square approximation is not very good.

14.8.2   Fisher's Exact Test

In a 2×2 contingency table, the elements are sometimes all random, but there are occasions when the row totals and the column totals are restricted in advance. In such cases, a permutation test for independence (or differences in group proportions), known as Fisher's exact test, is appropriate. The test is attributed to R. A. Fisher, who describes it in his design of experiments text (Fisher, 1935). However, as Conover (1999) points out, it was also discovered and presented in the literature almost simultaneously in Irwin (1935) and Yates (1934).

Fisher and others have argued for its more general use based on conditioning arguments. As Conover (1999) points out, it is very popular for all types of 2×2 tables because its exact p-values can be determined easily (by enumerating all the more extreme tables and their probabilities under the null hypothesis). As in the chapter on contingency tables, the null hypothesis is that if the rows represent two groups, then the proportions in the first column should be the same for each group (and, consequently, so should the proportions in the second column).

Consider N observations summarized in a 2×2 table. The row totals r and $N - r$ and the column totals c and $N - c$ are fixed in advance (or conditioned on afterwards). Refer to Table 14.13.

Because the values of r, c, and N are fixed in advance, the only quantity that is random is x, the entry in the cell corresponding to the intersection of Row 1 and Column 1. Now, x can vary from 0 up to the minimum of c and r. This limit on the value is due to the requirement that the row and column totals must always be r for the first row and c for the first column. Each different value of x determines a new distinct contingency table. Let us specify the null hypothesis that the probability p_1 of an observation in row 1, column 1 is the same as the probability p_2 of an observation in row 2,

TABLE 14.13.   Basic 2 × 2 Contingency Table for Fisher's Exact Test

	Column 1	Column 2	Row Totals
Row 1	x	$r - x$	r
Row 2	$c - x$	$N - r - c + x$	$N - r$
Column Totals	c	$N - c$	N

column 1. The null distribution for the test statistic T, defined to be equal to x, is the hypergeometric distribution. Equation 14.9 defines the test statistic T.

While not covered explicitly in previous chapters, the hypergeometric distribution is similar to discrete distributions that were discussed in Chapter 5. Remember that a discrete distribution is defined on a finite set of numbers. The hypergeometric distribution used for calculating test statistic for Fisher's exact test is given in Equation 14.9. Let T be the cell value for column 1, row 1 in a 2×2 contingency table with the constraints that the row one total is r and the column one total is c, with r and c less than or equal to the grand total N. Then for $x = 0, 1, \ldots, \min(r, c)$,

$$P(T = x) = \frac{C(r, x)C(N - r, c - x)}{C(N, c)} \tag{14.9}$$

and $P(T = x) = 0$ for all other values of x.

A one-sided p-value for Fisher's exact test is calculated as follows:

1. Find all 2×2 tables with the row and column totals of the observed table and with row 1, column 1 cell values equal to or smaller than the observed x.
2. Use the hypergeometric distribution from Equation 14.9 to calculate the probability of occurrence of these tables under the null hypothesis.
3. Sum the probabilities over all such tables.

The result at step (3) is the one-sided p-value. Two-sided and opposite one-sided p-values can be obtained according to a similar procedure. One needs to define the rejection region such that it is the area on one tail of the distribution that is comprised of probabilities that are as extreme as or more extreme than the significance level of the test. The second side or the opposite side would be the corresponding area on the opposite end of the distribution. The next example will illustrate how to carry out the procedure described above.

Example: Lady Tasting Tea

Fisher (1935) gave a now famous example of a lady who claims that she can tell simply by tasting tea whether milk or tea was poured into a cup first. Fisher used this example to demonstrate the principles of experimental design and hypothesis testing.

Let us suppose, as is described in Agresti (1990), page 61, that an experiment was conducted to test whether the lady simply is taking guesses versus the alternative that she has the skill to determine the order of pouring the two liquids. The lady is given eight cups of tea, four with milk poured first and four with tea poured first. The cups are numbered 1 to 8. The experimenter has recorded on a piece of paper which cup numbers had the tea poured first and which had the milk poured first.

The lady is told that four cups had milk poured first and four had tea poured first. Given this information, she will designate four of them for each group. This design is important because it forces each row and column total to be fixed (see Table

TABLE 14.14. Lady Tasting Tea Experiment: 2 × 2 Contingency Table for Fisher's Exact Test

Poured First	Milk Guessed as Poured First	Tea Guessed as Poured First	Row Totals
Milk	x	$4 - x$	4
Tea	$4 - x$	x	4
Column Totals	4	4	8

14.14). In this experiment, the use of Fisher's exact test is appropriate and uncontroversial. For other designs, the application of Fisher's exact test may be debatable even when there are some similarities to the foregoing example.

For this problem, there are only five contingency tables: (1) Correctly labeling all four cups with milk poured first and, hence, all with tea poured first; (2) incorrectly labeling one with milk poured first and, hence, one with tea poured first; (3) incorrectly labeling two with milk poured first (also two with tea poured first); (4) incorrectly labeling three with milk poured first (also three with tea poured first); and (5) incorrectly labeling all four with milk poured first (also all four with tea poured first).

Case (3) is the most likely under the null hypothesis, as it would be expected from random guessing. Cases (1) and (2) favor some ability to discriminate, and (4) and (5) indicate good discrimination but in the wrong direction. However, the sample size is too small for the test to provide very strong evidence for the lady's abilities, even in the most extreme cases in this example when she guesses three or four outcomes correctly.

Let us first compute the p-value when x is 3. In this case, it is appropriate to perform a one-sided test, as a significant test statistic would support the claim that she can distinguish the order of pouring milk and tea. We are testing the alternative hypothesis that the lady can determine that the milk was poured before the tea versus the null hypothesis that she cannot tell the difference in the order of pouring. Thus, we must evaluate two contingency tables, one for $x = 3$ and one for $x = 4$. The observed data are given in Table 14.15.

The probability associated with the observed table under the null hypothesis is $C(4, 3) \, C(4, 1)/C(8, 4) = (4 \; 4 \; 4!)/(8 \; 7 \; 6 \; 5) = 8/35 = 0.229$. The only table more extreme that favors the alternative hypothesis is the perfect table, Table 14.16.

TABLE 14.15. Lady Tasting Tea Experiment: Observed 2 × 2 Contingency Table for Fisher's Exact Test

Poured First	Milk Guessed as Poured First	Tea Guessed as Poured First	Row Totals
Milk	3	1	4
Tea	1	3	4
Column Totals	4	4	8

TABLE 14.16. Lady Tasting Tea Experiment: More Extreme 2 × 2 Contingency Table for Fisher's Exact Test

Poured First	Milk Guessed as Poured First	Tea Guessed as Poured First	Row Totals
Milk	4	0	4
Tea	0	4	4
Column Totals	4	4	8

The probability of this table under the null hypothesis is $1/C(8, 4) = 1/70 = 0.0142$. So the p-value for the combined tables is $0.229 + 0.014 = 0.243$. If we ran the tea drinking experiment and observed an x of 3, we would have an observed p-value of 0.243; this outcome would suggest that we cannot reject the null hypothesis that the lady is unable to discriminate between milk or tea poured first.

14.9   INSENSITIVITY OF RANK TESTS TO OUTLIERS

Outliers are unusually large or small observations that fall outside the range of most of the measurements for a specific variable. (Outliers in a bivariate scatter plot were illustrated in Chapter 12, Figure 12.4) Outliers impact the parametric tests that we have studied in the previous chapters of this text; for example, Z tests and t tests for evaluating the differences between two means; ANOVAs for evaluating the differences among three or more means; and tests for nonzero regression slopes and nonzero correlations. Rank tests are not sensitive to outliers because the rank transformation replaces the most extreme observations with the highest or lowest rank, depending on whether the outlier is in the upper or lower extreme of the distribution, respectively.

In illustration, suppose that we have a data set with 10 observations and a mean of 20, and that the next to the largest observation is 24 and the smallest is 16, but the largest observation is 30. To show that it is possible for this data set to have a mean of 20, we ask you to consider the following ten values: 16, 16.5, 16.5, 16.5, 17, 19.5, 21, 23, 24, 30. Note that the sum is 200 and hence the mean is 20. Clearly, the largest observation is an outlier because it differs from the mean by 10 more than the entire range (only 8) of the other 9 observations. The difference between the largest and second largest observation is 6. However, the ranks of the largest and second largest observations are 10 and 9, respectively. The difference in rank between the largest and second largest observation is always 1, regardless of the magnitude of the actual difference between the original observations prior to the transformation.

In conclusion, Chapter 14 has presented methods for analyzing data that do not satisfy the assumptions of the parametric techniques studied previously in this text. We called methods that are not dependent on the underlying distributions of parent populations (i.e., distribution-free methods) nonparametric techniques. Many of the nonparametric tests involved ranking data instead of using their actual measurements. As a result of ranking procedures, nonparametric tests lose information that is provided by parametric tests. The Wilcoxon rank-sum test (also known as the Mann–Whitney test) was used to evaluate the significance of differences between two independently selected samples. The Wilcoxon signed-rank test was identified as an analog to the paired t test. When there were three or more independent groups, the Kruskal–Wallis test was employed. Another nonparametric test discussed in this chapter was Spearman's rank order correlation coefficient. We also introduced permutation methods, with Fisher's exact test as an example.

14.10 EXERCISES

14.1 Apply the Wilcoxon rank-sum test to the following problem; we have modified the data from the pig blood loss experiment:

Pig Blood Loss Data (ml)

Control Group Pigs	Treatment Group Pigs
786	743
375	766
3446	655
1886	923
478	1916
587	897
434	3028
3764	1351
2281	902
2837	1378
Sample mean = 1687.40	Sample mean = 1255.90

Do the results differ from the standard two-sample t test with pooled variance? Are the p-values similar?

14.2 Apply the Wilcoxon rank-sum test in the following case to see if schizophrenia is randomly distributed across the seasons:

Season of Birth Among 100 Schizophrenic Patients

Season	Observed Number
Fall	20
Winter	35
Spring	20
Summer	25
Total	100

14.3   Using the following modification of the city data, apply the Wilcoxon signed-rank test to determine whether there is a difference in average temperature between the two cities. Compare your results to a paired t test.

Daily Temperatures for Two Cities and Their Paired Differences

Day	Washington Mean Temperature (°F)	New York Mean Temperature (°F)	Paired Difference #1 − #2
1 (January 15)	31	38	−7
2 (February 15)	35	33	2
3 (March 15)	40	37	3
4 (April 15)	52	45	7
5 (May 15)	70	65	5
6 (June 15)	76	74	2
7 (July 15)	93	89	4
8 (August 15)	91	85	6
9 (September 15)	74	69	5
10 (October 15)	55	51	4
11 (November 15)	26	25	1
12 (December 15)	26	24	2

14.4   Apply the sign test to the above example. Did the results change? Which test is more powerful, the sign test or the Wilcoxon signed-rank test? Why?

14.5   Suppose we compare four instructors for consistency of grading. Use the following table to apply the Kruskal–Wallis test to determine whether there is a difference among instructors.

Grade Counts for Students by Instructor

Grade	Instructor 1	2	3	4	Row Totals
A	4	10	6	20	40
B	14	6	7	10	37
C	17	9	8	5	39
D	6	7	6	5	24
F	2	6	1	10	19
Total # of students	43	38	28	50	159

14.6   Based on the temperature data in Exercise 14.3, use the day pairing to compute a Spearman rank order correlation between the two cities.

14.7   Use the modified aggressiveness scores for twins (given in the table below) to apply the Wilcoxon signed-rank test. What is the p-value?

Twin Set	Twin #1 (First Born) Aggressiveness	Twin #2 (Second Born) Aggressiveness	Paired Difference	Absolute Difference	Rank (sign)
1	85	88	−3	3	2(−)
2	71	78	−7	7	6 (−)
3	79	75	4	4	3.5 (+)
4	69	64	5	5	5 (+)
5	92	96	−4	4	3.5 (−)
6	72	72	0	0	—
7	79	64	15	15	11 (+)
8	91	89	2	2	1 (+)
9	70	62	8	8	7 (+)
10	71	80	−9	9	8 (−)
11	89	79	10	10	9 (+)
12	87	75	12	12	10 (+)

Source: modification of Example 1 page 355, Conover (1999).

14.8   Apply the sign test to the data in Exercise 14.7. Does the result change? What is the p-value?

14.9   Using the modified aggressiveness scores with the aid of the table below, determine Spearman's rank order correlation for the twins.

Aggressiveness Scores for 12 Sets of Identical Twins

Twin Set	Twin #1 (First Born) Aggressiveness (rank)	Twin #2 (Second Born) Aggressiveness (rank)	Rank Pair	Term $R(X_i) R(Y_i)$
1	85 (8)	88 (10)	(8, 10)	80
2	71 (3.5)	78 (7)	(3.5, 7)	24.5
3	79 (6.5)	75 (5.5)	(6.5, 5.5)	35.75
4	69 (1)	64 (2.5)	(1, 2.5)	2.5
5	92 (12)	96 (12)	(12, 12)	144
6	72 (5)	72 (4)	(5, 4)	20
7	79 (6.5)	64 (2.5)	(6.5, 2.5)	16.25
8	91 (11)	89 (11)	(11.5, 11)	126.5
9	70 (2)	62 (1)	(2, 1)	2
10	71 (3.5)	80 (9)	(3.5,9)	31.5
11	89 (10)	79 (8)	(10,8)	80
12	87 (9)	75 (5.5)	(9, 5.5)	49.5

14.10 Recall the Lady Tasting Tea example. Suppose that instead of being given four cups with milk poured first and four cups with tea poured first, the lady was given five cups with milk poured first and five cups with tea poured first. Suppose the outcome of the experiment was as shown in the table at the top of the next page.

Lady Tasting Tea Experiment:
Observed 2 × 2 Contingency Table for Fisher's Exact Test

Poured First	Milk Guessed as Poured First	Tea Guessed as Poured First	Row Totals
Milk	4	1	5
Tea	1	4	5
Column Totals	5	5	10

    a. Determine the more extreme tables.

    b. Do a two-sided Fisher's exact test at the 0.05 level of the null hypothesis that the lady is guessing randomly.

    c. Do a one-sided test at the 0.05 level.

    d. What is the p-value for the two-sided test?

    e. What is the p-value for the one-sided test?

    f. Which test makes more sense here, one-sided or two-sided?

14.11   ADDITIONAL READING

1. Agresti, A. (1990). *Categorical Data Analysis.* Wiley, New York

2. Conover, W. J. (1999). *Practical Nonparametric Statistics,* Third Edition. Wiley, New York

3. Edgington, E. S. (1995). *Randomization Tests,* Third Edition. Marcel Dekker, New York.

4. Fisher, R. A. (1935). *Design of Experiments.* Oliver and Boyd, London.

5. Good, P. I. (2000). *Permutation Tests: A Practical Guide to Resampling Methods for Testing Hypotheses,* Second Edition. Springer-Verlag, New York.

6. Good, P. I. (2001). *Resampling Methods: A Practical Guide to Data Analysis,* Second Edition. Birkhauser, Boston.

7. Hoeffding, W. (1952). The large-sample power of tests based on permutations of observations. *The Annals of Mathematical Statistics* **23,** 169–192.

8. Irwin, J. O. (1935). Tests of significance for differences between percentages based on small numbers. *Metron* **12,** 83–94.

9. Kendall, M. G. (1938). A new measure of rank correlation. *Biometrika* **30,** 81–93.

10. Lehmann, E. L. and Stein, C. (1949). On the theory of some nonparametric hypotheses. *The Annals of Mathematical Statistics* **20,** 28–45.

11. Lunneborg, C. E. (2000). *Data Analysis by Resampling: Concepts and Applications.* Duxbury Press, Pacific Grove, California.

12. Manly, B. F. J. (1997). *Randomization, Bootstrap and Monte Carlo Methods in Biology,* Second Edition. Chapman and Hall/CRC Press, London.

13. Mielke, Jr., P. W. and Berry, K. J. (2001). *Permutation Methods: A Distance Function Approach.* Springer-Verlag, New York.

14. Spearman, C. (1904). The proof and measurement of association between two things. *American Journal of Psychology* **15,** 72–101.

15. Westfall, P.H. and Young, S.S. (1993). *Resampling-Based Multiple Testing: Examples and Methods for p-Value Adjustment.* Wiley, New York.

16. Yates, F. (1934). Contingency tables involving small numbers and the χ^2 test. *J. Royal Statist. Soc.* **Supplement 1,** 217–235.

CHAPTER 15

Analysis of Survival Times

A substantial portion of the lecture was devoted to risks. . . .
He emphasized that one in a million is a very remote risk.
—Phillip H. Abelson, *Science,* Editorial, February 4, 1994

15.1 INTRODUCTION TO SURVIVAL DATA

In survival analysis, we follow patients over time, until the occurrence of a particular event such as death, relapse, recurrence, or some other event that represents a dichotomy. Of special interest to the practitioners of survival analysis is the construction of survival curves, which are based on the time interval between a procedure and an event.

Information from survival analysis is used frequently to assess the efficacy of clinical trials. Researchers follow patients during the trial in order to track events such as a recurrence of an illness, occurrence of an adverse event related to the treatment, or death. The term "survival analysis" came about because often mortality (death) was studied as the outcome; however, survival analysis can be applied more generally to many different types of events.

In a clinical trial, an investigator may want to compare a survival curve for a treatment group with one for a control group to determine whether the treatment is associated with increased longevity; one of the notable examples arises from the area of cancer treatment studies, which focus on five-year survival rates after treatment. A new, specialized area in survival analysis is the estimation of cure rates. The investigator may believe that a certain percentage of patients will be cured by a treatment and, thus, uses survival analysis to estimate the cure rate. Section 15.2.4 will cover cure rate models that use a modification to the survival curve.

Several characteristics of survival data make them different from most data we encounter: (1) patients are in the study for varying amounts of time; (2) because some patients experience the event, these are the ones who provide complete infor-

Introductory Biostatistics for the Health Sciences, by Michael R. Chernick
and Robert H. Friis. ISBN 0-471-41137-X. Copyright © 2003 Wiley-Interscience.

mation; and (3) the trial is eventually terminated and the patients who have not experienced the event are "right-censored." The term right-censored refers to the fact that we do not know how much longer patients who remained in the trial until its end would have gone event-free. The time to the event for them is at least the time from treatment to the end of the study. Right-censoring is the primary characteristic of survival data that makes the analysis unique and different from other methods previously covered in this text.

As noted in point (1) above, a feature of data from survival analyses is that patients typically do not enter the study at the same time. Clinical trials generally have an accrual period that could be six months or longer. Candidates for the study are found and a sufficient number enrolled during the accrual period until statistical power or precision requirements have been met.

Still another factor that produces varying amounts of observation time in the study has to do with the initiation of disease onset. Although the time of occurrence of the event is generally well defined and easily recognized, the onset of the clinical syndrome leading to the event may be ambiguous. Thus, what is called "the starting time" for the time to event is sometimes difficult to define. For example, if we are studying a chronic disease such as cancer, diabetes, or heart disease, the precise time of onset may be impossible to delineate.

A common substitute for date of onset is date of diagnosis. This alternative may be unreliable because of the considerable lag that often exists between the first occurrence of a disease and its diagnosis. This lag may be due to health service utilization patterns (e.g., lack of health insurance coverage, infrequent doctor visits, and delay in seeking health care) or the natural history of many chronic diseases (e.g., inapparent signs and symptoms of the early phases of disease). Some infections, such as HIV or hepatitis C, are associated with an extended latency period between lodgment of a virus and development of observable symptoms. Consequently, date of diagnosis is used as the best available proxy for date of onset.

With respect to point (2) above, some patients may be lost to follow-up. For example, they decide to drop out of the study because they leave the geographic area. Sometimes, statisticians treat this form of censoring differently from right censoring. Although start times vary on the actual time scale, in survival analysis we create a scale that ignores the starting time. We are interested only in the time interval from entry into the study (or treatment time, beginning when the patient is randomized into a treatment group) until the event or censoring occurs. Thus, we modify the time axis as if all patients start together.

We can use parametric models to describe patients' survival functions. These models are applicable when each patient is viewed as having a time to event that is similar to a random draw from some survival distribution whose form is known except for a few parameters (the exponential and Weibull distributions are examples of such parametric models). When the parametric form is difficult to specify, nonparametric techniques can be used to estimate the survival function. Details follow in the next section.

15.2   SURVIVAL PROBABILITIES

15.2.1   Introduction

Suppose we would like to estimate the survival of patients who are about to undergo a clinical procedure. From an existing set of survival and censoring times observed from patients who already have been in a clinical trial, we can estimate survival of new patients about to experience the procedure. For example, to accomplish this extrapolation, we could look at the survival history of patients with implanted defibrillators. We could try to predict the probability that a new patient planning to undergo the same implant procedure would survive for a specified length of time.

Sometimes, researchers are interested in a particular time interval, such as surviving for another five years (a common survival time). But often the time interval is the whole curve, which represents survival for x months or more, for $0 < x < L$, where L is some period (usually L is less than or equal to the length of the study, but if parametric methods are used, L can be longer). Altman (1991) provides an example of data expressed as survival time in months. (Refer to Table 15.1.)

The methods for predicting survival times are clever and account for the fact that some cases are censored. Researchers portray survival data in graphs or tables called life tables, survival curves, or Kaplan–Meier curves (described in detail in the next sections).

We will define the survival function and present ways of estimating it. Let $S(t)$ denote the survival function. $S(t) = P(X > t)$, where X is the survival time for a randomly selected patient. $S(t)$ represents the probability that a typically selected patient would survive a period of t units of time after entry into the study (generally after receiving the treatment). The methods described in Sections 15.2.2 and 15.2.3 use data similar to those given in Table 15.1 to estimate the survival curve $S(t)$ at various times t.

TABLE 15.1. Survival Times for Patients

Patient no.	Time at Entry (months)	Time at Death or censor (months)	Dead or Censored	Survival Time (months)
1	0.0	11.8	D	11.8
2	0.0	12.5	C	12.5*
3	0.4	18.0	C	17.6*
4	1.2	4.4	C	3.2*
5	1.2	6.6	D	5.4
6	3.0	18.0	C	15.0*
7	3.4	4.9	D	1.5
8	4.7	18.0	C	13.3*
9	5.0	18.0	C	13.0*
10	5.8	10.1	D	4.3

*Censored observations.
Source: adapted from Altman (1991), p. 367, Table 13.1, with permission.

We notice from Table 15.1 that patients are accrued during the first six months of the study. We infer this from the fact that the last (10th) patient was entered at 5.8 months into the study. Patients are then followed until the 18th month, when the trial is terminated. Note that the maximum time at death or censoring is 18 months.

Four patients died during the trial and six were known to be living at the end of the trial or were lost to follow-up prior to the completion of the trial. (Refer to the column labeled "Dead or Censored.") So the survival times for those six were censored. Patients 3, 6, 8, and 9 completed the trial and were censored at the 18 month time point; patients 2 and 4 were lost to follow-up; and the remaining patients (1, 5, 7, and 10) died.

The information in this table is all we need to construct a life table or a parametric (e.g., Weibull) or nonparametric (i.e., Kaplan–Meier) survival curve. In the next section, we will use the data from Table 15.1 to illustrate how to construct a life table.

15.2.2   Life Tables

Life tables give estimates for survival during time intervals and present the cumulative survival probability at the end of the interval. The key idea for estimating the cumulative survival for both life tables and the Kaplan–Meier curve is represented by the following result for conditional probabilities: Let $t_2 > t_1$. Let $P(t_2|t_1) = P(X > t_2|X > t_1)$, where X = survival time, t_1 = time at the beginning of the interval, and t_2 = the time at the end of the interval. That is, $P(t_2|t_1)$ is the conditional probability that a patient's survival time X is at least t_2, given that we have observed the patient surviving to t_1. Using this conditional probability, we have the following product relationship for a survival curve, $S(t)$, as shown by Equation 15.1:

$$S(t_2) = P(t_2|t_1)\, S(t_1) \qquad \text{for any } t_2 > t_1 \geq 0 \qquad (15.1)$$

where
S = survival time
t_1 = initial time
t_2 = latter time point

For the life table, the key is to use the data in Table 15.1 to estimate $P(t_2|t_1)$ at the endpoints of the selected intervals. Remember that $S(t)$ denotes the survival function. For the first interval from $[0, a]$, we know that for all patients $S(0) = 1$ and, accordingly, $S(a) = P(a|0)$; i.e., all patients are alive at the beginning of the interval and a portion of them survive until time a.

The life table method, also referred to as the Cutler–Ederer method (Cutler and Ederer, 1958), is called an actuarial method because it is the method most often used by actuaries to establish premiums for insuring customers.

Now we will construct a life table for the data in Table 15.1. We note from the last column that the survival times, including the censored times, range from 1.5 months to 17.6 months. We will group the data in three-month intervals giving us seven intervals, namely, $[0, 3)$, $[3, 6)$, $[6, 9)$, $[9, 12)$, $[12, 15)$, $[15, 18)$, and $[18, \infty)$. (See Table 15.2.) For each interval, we need to determine the number of subjects who died during that interval, the number withdrawn during the interval, the total number at risk at the beginning of the interval, and the average number at risk during the interval. From these quantities, we compute: (1) the estimated proportion who died during the interval, given that they survived the previous intervals; and (2) the estimated proportion who would survive during the interval given that they survived during the previous intervals.

Table 15.2 uses eight terms that may be unfamiliar to the reader. Following are the precise definitions of these eight elements for a life table:

- The first column is labeled "Time Interval." We denote the jth interval I_j.
- The number who die during the jth interval is D_j. (D_j counts all of the patients whose time of death occurs during the jth interval.)
- The number withdrawn during the jth interval is W_j. (W_j counts all of the patients whose censoring time occurs during the jth interval.)
- The number at risk at the start of the jth interval is N_j. (This is the number of subjects who entered into the study minus all deaths and all withdrawals that occurred prior to the jth interval.)
- The average number at risk in the jth interval $N_j' = N_j - W_j/2$. Referring to the second row of Table 15.2 under column N_j', $N_j' = N_j - W_j/2 = 9 - \frac{1}{2} = 8.5$. The term N_j' reflects an actuarial technique to account for the fact that W_j of the patients who were at risk at the beginning of the interval are no longer at risk at the end of the interval.
- N_j' represents the average number of patients at risk in the interval when the withdrawals occur uniformly over the interval. We use N_j' to improve the estimate of the probability of not surviving during the jth interval. We define $q_j = D_j/N_j'$ and assert that D_j/N_j' is better than using D_j/N_j or D_j/N_{j+1}, where N_{j+1} is the number at risk at the start of the $j + 1$ interval. We then define the estimate of the conditional probability of surviving during the interval given that the patient survived during the previous $j - 1$ intervals as p_j. The estimate for surviving past the jth interval is obtained by using the conditioning principle given in Equation 15.1. In Table 15.2 (second row), $q_j = D_j/N_j' = 2/8.5 = 0.235$.
- The estimated proportion surviving during the interval is p_j. From Table 15.2 (second row), $p_j = (N_j' - D_j)/N_j' = [(8.5 - 2)/8.5] = 0.765$.
- The cumulative survival estimate for the jth interval is denoted S_j and is defined recursively by $S_j = p_j S_{j-1}$.

The method of recursion allows one to calculate a quantity such as S_n by first calculating S_0 and then providing a formula that shows how to calculate S_1 from S_0. This same formula then can be used to calculate S_2 from S_1 and then S_3 from S_2 and so on until we get S_n from S_{n-1}. In the method of recursion, the equation is called a recursive equation. A calculation example will be given in the next section. Refer to Table 15.2 to see the terms that we defined in the list above.

TABLE 15.2. Life Table for Survival Times for Patients Using Data from Table 15.1 ($N = 38$)

Time Interval, I_j	Number of Deaths, D_j	Number of Withdrawals, W_j	Number at Risk, N_j	Average Number at Risk, N_j'	Estimated Proportion of Deaths, q_j	Estimated Proportion Surviving, p_j	Estimated Cumulative Survival, S_j
[0, 3)	1	0	10	10	0.1	0.9	0.9
[3, 6)	2	1	9	8.5	0.235	0.765	0.688
[6, 9)	0	0	6	6	0.0	1.0	0.688
[9, 12)	1	0	6	6	0.167	0.833	0.573
[12, 15)	0	3	5	3.5	0	1.0	0.573
[15, 18)	0	2	2	1	0	1.0	0.573
[18, ∞)	0	0	0	0	—	—	—

15.2.3   The Kaplan–Meier Curve

The Kaplan–Meier curve is a nonparametric estimate of the survival curve (see Kaplan and Meier, 1958). It is computed by using the same conditioning principle that we employed for the life table estimate in Section 15.2.2. Because the Kaplan–Meier curve is an estimator based on the products of conditional probabilities, it is also sometimes called the product-limit estimator.

The Kaplan–Meier curve starts out with $S(t) = 1$ for all t less than the first event time (such as a death at t_1). Then $S(t_1)$ becomes $S(0) (n_1 - d_1)/n_1$, where n_1 is the number at risk at time t_1 and d_1 is the number who die at time t_1. Referring to Table 15.2 (column S_j, first row), $S(t_1) = S(0) [(n_1 - d_1)/n_1] = 1[(10 - 1)/10] = 0.9$. We substitute N_j' for n_1 in the formula. At the next time of death t_2, $S(t_2) = S(t_1) (n_2 - d_2)/n_2$, where n_2 and d_2 are, respectively, the corresponding number of patients at risk and deaths at time t_2. In Table 15.2 (second row), $S(t_2) = S(t_1) [(n_2 - d_2)/n_2] = (0.9)[(8.5 -2)/8.5] = 0.688$. The estimate $S(t)$ stays constant at all times between events (i.e., deaths) but jumps down by the factor $(n_j - d_j)/n_j$ at the time t_j of the jth deaths. You can verify this fact for the S_j column in Table 15.2. We allow for the possibility of more than one death at the same instant of time. The number at risk drops at withdrawal times as well as at the times of death. Thus, we use N_j' instead of N_j to estimate n_j in the formula for $S(t)$.

The Kaplan–Meier estimates can be portrayed in a table similar to the life table (Table 15.2), except that the intervals will be the times between events. Table 15.3 shows the Kaplan–Meier estimate for the patient data used in the previous section to construct a life table. Note that the column labels are essentially the same as those in Table 15.2, with the following two exceptions: (1) the column labeled "Average Number at Risk, N_j'," has been eliminated; and (2) the "Estimated Cumulative Survival" becomes $S(t_j)$, a term that we defined in the foregoing paragraph.

In the row for t_1 under the column "Estimated Cumulative Survival" we obtain 0.9 by multiplying $S_0 = 1$ by $p_1 = 0.9$, where $p_1 = 1 - q_1$ and $q_1 = D_1/N_1 = 1/10 = 0.1$. In the row for t_2, $q_2 = D_2/N_2 = 1/8 = 0.125$. So $p_2 = 1 - q_2 = 0.875$ and, finally, $S_2 =$

TABLE 15.3. Kaplan–Meier Survival Estimates for Patients in Table 15.2

Time Interval, I_j	Number of Deaths, D_j	Number of Withdrawals, W_j	Number at Risk, N_j	Estimated Proportion of Deaths, q_j	Estimated Proportion Surviving, p_j	Estimated Cumulative Survival, $S(t_j)$
$t_1 = 1.5$	1	0	10	0.1	0.9	0.9
$t_2 = 4.3$	1	1	8	0.125	0.875	0.788
$t_3 = 5.4$	1	0	7	0.143	0.857	0.675
$t_4 = 11.8$	1	0	6	0.167	0.833	0.562
> 11.8	0	5	5	0	1.0	0.562

$p_2 S_1 = (0.875)(0.90) = 0.788$. The remaining rows involve the same calculations and the recurrence relation $S_k = p_k S_{k-1}$.

Approximate confidence intervals for the Kaplan–Meier curve at specific time points can be obtained by using the Greenwood formula for the standard error of the estimate and a normal approximation for the distribution of the Kaplan–Meier estimate. A simpler estimate is obtained based on the results in the paper by Peto et al. (1977).

In Greenwood's formula, Var(S_j) is estimated as $V_j = S_j^2 [\sum_{i=1}^{j} q_i/(N_i p_i)]$. Computationally, this is more easily calculated recursively as $V_j = S_j^2 [q_j/(N_j p_j) + V_{j-1}/S_{j-1}^2]$, where we define $S_0 = 1$ and $V_0 = 0$.

Although the Greenwood formula is computationally easy using the recursion equation, the Peto approximation is much simpler. Peto's estimate of variance is given by the formula $W_j = S_j^2 (1 - S_j)/N_j$. The simplicity of this formula is that it depends only on the survival probability estimate at time j and the number remaining at risk at time j, whereas Greenwood's formula depends on survival probability estimates, number at risk, and probability estimates of survival and death in preceding time intervals.

Peto's estimate has a heuristic interpretation. If we ignore the censoring and think of failure by time j as a binomial outcome, to expect N_j patients to remain at time j we should have started with approximately N_j/S_j patients. Think of this number (N_j/S_j) as an integer corresponding to the number of patients in a binomial experiment. Now the variance of a binomial proportion is $p(1 - p)/n$, where n is the sample size and p is the success probability. In our heuristic argument, $S_j = p$ and $N_j/S_j = n$. So the variance is $S_j(1 - S_j)/\{N_j/S_j\} = S_j^2(1 - S_j)/N_j$. We see that this variance is just Peto's formula.

The square root of these variance estimates (Greenwood and Peto) is the corresponding estimate of the standard error of the Kaplan–Meier estimate S_j at time j. Approximate confidence intervals then are obtained through a normal approximation that uses the normal distribution constants 1.96 for a two-sided 95% confidence interval or 1.645 for a two-sided 90% confidence interval. So the Greenwood 95% two-sided confidence interval at time j would be $[S_j - 1.96\sqrt{V_j}, S_j + 1.96\sqrt{V_j}]$ and for Peto it would be $[S_j - 1.96\sqrt{W_j}, S_j + 1.96\sqrt{W_j}]$. Greenwood's and Peto's meth-

---

**Display 15.1. Greenwood's Method for 95% Confidence
Interval of Kaplan–Meier Estimate**

$$[S_j - 1.96\sqrt{V_j}, S_j + 1.96\sqrt{V_j}]$$

where S_j = Kaplan–Meier survival probability estimate at the jth event time, and

$$V_j = S_j^2\left[\sum_{i=1}^{j} q_i/(N_i p_i)\right]$$

where q_i is the probability of death in event interval i, $p_i = 1 - q_i$ is the probability of surviving interval i, and N_i is the number of patients remaining at risk at the ith event time. Alternatively, V_j can be calculated by the recursion:

$$V_j = S_j^2[q_j/(N_j p_j) + V_{j-1}/S_{j-1}^2]$$

---

ods are exhibited in Displays 15.1 and 15.2. Because we have used several approximations, these confidence intervals are not exact, but only approximate.

Now we can construct 95% confidence intervals for our Kaplan–Meier estimates in Table 15.3. Let us compute the Greenwood and Peto intervals at time $t_3 = 5.4$. For the Greenwood method, we must determine V_3 first. We will do this using the recursive formula, first finding V_1, then V_2 from V_1, and finally V_3 from V_2. So $V_1 = S_1^2[q_1/(N_1 p_1)] = (0.9)^2 [0.1/(10(0.9)] = 0.9 (0.01) = 0.009$. Then $V_2 = S_2^2 [q_2/(N_2 p_2) + V_1/S_1^2] = (0.788)^2 [0.125/(8 (0.875)) + 0.009/(0.9)^2] = 0.621 [0.125/7 + 0.009/0.81] = 0.621(0.0179 + 0.0111) = 0.621(0.029) = 0.0180$. Finally, $V_3 = S_3^2[q_3/(N_3\ p_3) + V_2/S_2^2] = (0.675)^2 [0.143/\{7(0.857)\} + 0.018/(0.788)^2] = 0.4556 [0.143/6] = 0.0109$. So the 95% confidence interval is $[0.675 - 1.96\sqrt{0.0109}, 0.675 + 1.96\sqrt{0.0109}] = [0.675 - 0.2046, 0.675 + 0.2046] = [0.4704, 0.8796]$.

For the Peto interval, W_3 is simply $S_3^2(1 - S_3)/N_3 = (0.675)^2(0.325/7) = 0.4556$

**Display 15.2. Peto's Method for 95% Confidence
Interval of Kaplan–Meier Estimate**

$$[S_j - 1.96\sqrt{W_j}, S_j + 1.96\sqrt{W_j}]$$

where S_j = Kaplan–Meier survival probability estimate at the jth event time, and

$$W_j = S_j^2(1 - S_j)/N_j$$

where N_j is the number of patients remaining at risk at the jth event time.

(0.0464) = So the Peto interval is $[0.675 - 1.96\sqrt{0.0212}, 0.675 + 1.96\sqrt{0.0212}]$ = $[0.675 - 0.285, 0.675 + 0.285]$ = $[0.390, 0.960]$. Note that the Peto interval is wider and thus somewhat more conservative for the lower endpoint.

Some research [see Dorey and Korn (1987)] has shown that Peto's method can give better lower confidence bounds than Greenwood's, especially at long follow-up times in which the number of patients remaining at risk is small. The Greenwood interval tends to be too narrow in these situations; hence, the FDA sometimes recommends using Peto's method for the lower bound. We have seen how the Peto interval is wider than the Greenwood interval in the foregoing example. For more details about the Kaplan–Meier curve and life tables, see Altman (1991) and Lawless (1982).

As we can see from the example in Table 15.3, the Kaplan–Meier curve gives results similar to the life table method and is based on the same computational principle. However, the Kaplan–Meier curve takes step decreases at the actual time of events (e.g., deaths), whereas the life table method makes the jumps at the end of the group intervals.

The Kaplan–Meier curve is preferred to the life table when all the event times are known precisely. For example, the Kaplan–Meier method does a better job than the life table when dealing with withdrawals when all withdrawals prior to an event (such as death) are removed in determining the number of patients at risk. In contrast, the life table groups the events into time intervals; hence, it subtracts half the withdrawals in the interval in order to estimate the interval survival (or failure) probability.

However, there are many practical situations in which the event times are not known precisely but an interval for the event can be defined. For example, recurrence of some event may be detected at follow-up visits, which could be scheduled every three months. All that is really known is that the recurrence occurred between the last two follow-up visits. So a life table with a three-month grouping may be more appropriate than a Kaplan–Meier curve in such cases.

Although survival curves are very useful, some difficulties occur when not all the events are reported. Lack of completeness in reporting events is a common problem that medical device companies confront when they report on the reliability of their products using Kaplan–Meier estimates from passive databases (i.e., databases that depend on voluntary reporting of problems). Such databases are notorious for underreporting events and overestimating performance as estimated in the survival curve. Techniques have been proposed to adjust these curves to account for biases. However, no proposal is free from potential problems. See Chernick, Poulsen, and Wang (2002) for a look at the problem of overadjustment with an algorithm that has been suggested for pacemakers.

15.2.4   Parametric Survival Curves

If we give the survival function a specific functional form, we can estimate the survival curve based on just a few parameter estimates. We will illustrate this procedure with the negative exponential and Weibull distributions.

The negative exponential, a simple one-parameter family of probability distributions, models well the lifetime distributions for some products, such as electric light bulbs; i.e., it is useful in describing their time to failure.

The Weibull distribution is a two-parameter family of distributions that has been used even more widely than the negative exponential to model time to failure for manufactured products. The Weibull distribution shares one major characteristic with the normal distribution model; i.e., it is a limiting distribution. Each distribution is successful under certain circumstances.

Whereas the normal distribution is a limiting distribution for sums or averages of independent observations with the same distribution, the Weibull is a limiting distribution for the smallest value in a sample of independent observations with the same distribution.

Recall that in Chapter 7 we saw that as the sample size (n) increases, the sampling distribution of means becomes more and more similar to a normal distribution. Because the distribution continues to become close to the normal distribution as the sample size increases, we call the normal distribution a limiting distribution. Similarly, if we have a sample of size n, the probability distribution for the smallest value among the n observations approaches the Weibull distribution more closely as the sample size n increases. To obtain standard forms for the Weibull as we did with the normal distribution, we subtract a constant from the original statistic (e.g., minimum value in the sample) and then divide the result by another constant.

This procedure is analogous to $Z = (X - \mu)/(\sigma/\sqrt{n})$ for the standard normal distribution. The normal distribution works well when the variable of interest can be viewed as a sum. The Weibull works well when the variable of interest can be viewed as the smallest value.

For mortality, we can think of time to death as the time when an illness, exposure factor, or other occurrence causes a person to die. Mortality can be modeled in terms of many competing causes. For example, a person who dies in an automobile accident is no longer at risk of dying from coronary heart disease. A mortality model can sort these competing causes in order to determine which one occurs first. Suppose we specify the observed time of death that occurs for the first of these competing causes. We denote this time as the minimum of random times to death. In this particular situation, the Weibull model should fit well.

For the negative exponential distribution, the survival function $S(t) = e^{-\lambda t}$ for all $t \geq 0$. The single parameter λ is called the rate parameter, which is also equal to the so-called hazard function or instantaneous death rate. The term λ represents the limit of the probability of death in the next instant of time given survival up to time t. Its mathematical definition is given in the next paragraph.

In survival analysis, the distribution function $F(t)$ is defined as $F(t) = P(X \leq t) = 1 - S(t)$. For those who have studied differential equations, we note that the density function for continuous functions $F(t)$ is the first derivative of f and is denoted as $f(t)$. The hazard function $h(t)$ is defined as $h(t) = f(t)/S(t)$. We interpret $h(t)$ as the rate of occurrence of an event that happens in a small interval beyond t, given that it has not occurred by t.

For the negative exponential model, $F(t) = 1 - e^{-\lambda t}$ and $f(t) = \lambda e^{-\lambda t}$. So $h(t) =$

$\lambda e^{-\lambda t}/e^{-\lambda t} = \lambda$. The exponential model has the property of a constant hazard rate. This is sometimes called the lack of memory property because the rate does not depend on t. Note that hazard rates usually depend on the time t.

The negative exponential model can be used for studying light bulbs, which are no more likely to fail in the next five minutes when they have been on for one hundred hours than they are in the first five minutes after being installed. This unusual property is one of the reasons why, although good for modeling the life of light bulbs, the exponential is not a good model in general. For many products we expect the hazard rate to increase with age. Display 15.3, which is based on the survival function, defines the negative exponential model.

A common model for mortality is the so-called bathtub-shaped hazard rate function. At or near birth, the hazard rate is high, but once the baby survives for a few days the hazard rate drops significantly. For many years, the hazard rate stays flat (constant). But as the person ages, the hazard rate starts to increase sharply. This function would have the shape of a bathtub.

The Weibull model can be viewed also as a generalization of the negative exponential. It is determined by two parameters, λ and β, where λ refers to a rate parameter and β refers to the shape of the parameter distribution. The case $\beta = 1$ is the negative exponential (for reasons explained in the next paragraph). The model can be defined by its distribution $F(t)$, survival function $S(t)$, density function $f(t)$, or hazard function $h(t)$. The latter, $h(t)$, can be used to derive mathematically each of the other three functions: $F(t)$, $S(t)$, and $f(t)$. So we can describe the Weibull by its hazard function $h(t)$. (Refer to Display 15.4 for the Weibull model.)

The Weibull model can have an increasing hazard rate, a decreasing hazard rate, or in the special case of the negative exponential, a constant hazard rate. The Weibull does not exhibit a bathtub shape. To obtain the bathtub shape, we need a more complex parametric model. Such models are beyond the scope of this course.

We note that for $\beta > 1$, the hazard function is increasing in t; for $\beta = 1$, it is a constant function of t; and for $\beta < 1$ it is decreasing in t.

For complete data, likelihood methods are used to find the estimates of the parameters for survival distributions. Sometimes survival times are right-censored; the estimation problem becomes more complicated. Many fine texts, including Lawless (1982), provide methods for estimation (point estimates and confidence intervals) and testing model parameters.

For the negative exponential, the point estimate of λ is simply the number of

---

Display 15.3. Negative Exponential Survival Distribution

$$S(t) = \exp(-\lambda t)$$

where $t \geq 0$, and $\lambda > 0$ is the rate parameter. $F(t) = 1 - \exp(-\lambda t)$, $f(t) = \lambda \exp(-\lambda t)$, and $h(t) = \lambda$.

Display 15.4. Weibull Survival Distribution

$$h(t) = \lambda\beta(\lambda t)^{\beta-1}$$

where $t \geq 0$, $\lambda > 0$ is the rate parameter, and $\beta > 0$ is the shape parameter. $S(t) = \exp[-(\lambda t)^{\beta}]$ and $f(t) = \lambda\beta(\lambda t)^{\beta-1} \exp[-(\lambda t)^{\beta}]$.

---

events divided by the total time on test, where the total time on test is defined as the sum of the survival times for all the patients (time to censoring is used for the right-censored cases). Once the parameter λ has been estimated, the survival curve estimate is determined by plugging the estimate for λ into the formula. So if the estimate for λ is denoted λ_h and the estimate for the survival curve is $S_h(t)$, then $S_h(t) = e^{-\lambda h t}$.

Let us consider the data in Table 15.1 again. There are four events (deaths) at 11.8, 5.4, 1.5, and 4.3 months into the trial and six censored times at 3.2, 12.5, 17.6, 13.3, 15.0, and 13.0 months. The estimate λ_h is just the number of events/total time on test = $4/(11.8 + 5.4 + 1.5 + 4.3 + 3.2 + 12.5 + 17.6 + 13.3 + 15.0 + 13.0) = 4/97.6 = 0.041$. So $S_h(t) = \exp(-0.041t)$.

Refer to Table 15.4. The column labeled "Estimated Cumulative Survival" compares the survival estimates at the event time points, $S_h(t_j)$, for the negative exponential with the results for the Kaplan–Meier (KM) estimates (KM given in parentheses). The discrepancies between the negative exponential and the Kaplan–Meier estimates indicate that the exponential does not fit this model well. The discrepancy is particularly noticeable at time 5.4 months, when the parametric estimate is 0.801 and the Kaplan–Meier is 0.675. However, the sample size is small, and this discrepancy may not be statistically significant. Note that for the exponential model the estimates $S_h(t_j) = e^{-\lambda h_j}$. So, since $\lambda_h = 0.041$ at $t_1 = 1.5$, $S_h(t_1) = \exp[-0.041 (1.5)] = \exp(-0.0615) = 0.940$. At $t_2 = 4.3$, $S_h(t_2) = \exp[-0.041 (4.3)] = \exp(-0.1763) = 0.838$.

TABLE 15.4. Negative Exponential Survival Estimates for Patients in Table 15.2

Time Interval, I_j	Number of Deaths, D_j	Number of Withdrawals, W_j	Number at Risk, N_j	Estimated Proportion of Deaths, q_j	Estimated Proportion Surviving, p_j	Estimated Cumulative Survival, for Negative Exponential*, $S_h(t_j)$
$t_1 = 1.5$	1	0	10	0.1	0.9	0.940 (0.9)
$t_2 = 4.3$	1	1	8	0.125	0.875	0.838 (0.788)
$t_3 = 5.4$	1	0	7	0.143	0.857	0.801 (0.675)
$t_4 = 11.8$	1	0	6	0.167	0.833	0.616 (0.562)
18	0	5	5	0	1.0	0.478 (0.562)

*Kaplan–Meier estimates are shown in parentheses.

15.2.5 Cure Rate Models

Cure rate models can be estimated by using the same survival data described in the previous section. However, in producing survival curves, we usually assume that the cumulative survival probability $S(t)$ goes to zero as t approaches infinity. In cure rate models, we assume that some fraction of the patient population afflicted with a particular disease is actually cured, will not die, and will not experience a recurrence. This proportion is called the cure fraction or cure rate. With a Kaplan–Meier curve, a cure rate would show up as a nonzero asymptote to the curve. By that we mean that the survival probability curve will flatten out at a value p equal to the cure rate.

Berkson and Gage (1952) first discussed a mixture model that is the most popular and easy to understand cure rate model. It assumes that a certain fraction p of the entire population will be cured by the treatment and the remaining $1 - p$ fraction of the population will not be cured. Equation 15.2 defines the mixture model for the population survivor function $S(t)$ by using p and $1 - p$:

$$S(t) = p + (1 - p)S^*(t) \qquad (15.2)$$

Figure 15.1 shows a mixture survival curve with $S^*(t)$ representing an exponential survival curve with rate 1 event per year and p, the cure proportion, equal to 0.2. for any $t > 0$, where p is the cure fraction and $S^*(t)$ is the survival function for the uncured subpopulation.

The survivor function $S^*(t)$ can be estimated by parametric or nonparametric methods. Maller and Zhou (1996) provide extensive treatment of cure models using the frequentist approach. Ibrahim, Chen, and Sinha (2001) cover cure models from the Bayesian perspective and provide many additional references. We will not pursue this topic further.

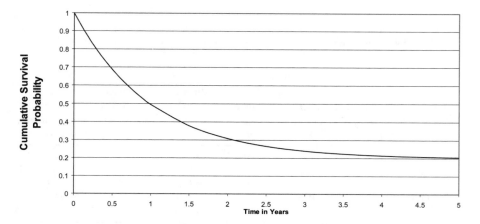

Figure 15.1. Exponential cure rate model with cure rate $p = 0.2$.

Although the concept of cure rates goes back to the 1950s, much of the research activity on this topic took place in the 1990s. Good algorithms for mixtures, such as the EM algorithm or a Markov chain Monte Carlo algorithm, became popular as recently as the 1980s and 1990s. Available at no charge, the software package Win-BUGS performs Gibbs sampling algorithms for Markov chain Monte Carlo applications. (See Chapter 16.)

15.3   COMPARING TWO OR MORE SURVIVAL CURVES—THE LOG RANK TEST

To compare two survival curves in a parametric family of distributions such as the negative exponential or the Weibull, we need to test only the hypothesis that the parameters are equal versus the alternative hypothesis that the parameters differ in some way. We will not go into the details of such parametric comparisons. However, nonparametric procedures look for differences in survival distributions based on the information in the Kaplan–Meier curves. In this section, we consider specific nonparametric tests for two or more survival curves.

The log rank test, a nonparametric procedure for comparing two or more survival functions, is a test of the null hypothesis that all the survival functions are the same, versus the alternative that at least one survival function differs from the rest. The idea is to compare the observed frequency of deaths or failures for each curve in various time intervals with what would be expected under the null hypothesis that all the curves are the same. Details can be found in the original paper [see Mantel (1966)] or in Lee (1992), pages 109–112.

Now we will describe a simple chi-square test that is very similar to the log rank test. For the chi-square test, we simply let O_1 be the observed number of deaths in group 1, O_2 the observed number in group 2, O_3 the observed number in group 3, and so on until all the groups have been enumerated.

A chi-square statistic is determined by computing the expected numbers E_1, E_2, E_3, etc., of deaths in each group. For this calculation to hold, all the groups need to come from the same population of survival times. Then, similar to other chi-square calculations (refer to Chapter 11), the statistic $\chi^2 = (O_1 - E_1)^2/E_1 + (O_2 - E_2)^2/E_2 + \ldots + (O_k - E_k)^2/E_k$ has approximately a chi-square distribution with $k - 1$ degrees of freedom when the null hypothesis is true. We will go through an example in detail in which $k = 2$, and the test statistic is then chi-square with 1 degree of freedom under the null hypothesis.

This simple calculation is taken from Lee (1992), Example 5.2, page 107. Suppose that ten female breast cancer patients are randomized to receive either cyclic administration of cyclophosphamide, methatrexate, and fluorouracil (CMF), or no additional treatment after a radical mastectomy. Five patients are randomized to the CMF treatment arm and five to the control arm.

We are interested in knowing whether time to relapse (time in remission) is lengthened by the treatment versus the null hypothesis that the treatment makes no difference. The results at the end of the trial are as follows: CMF patient remission times in months are 23, 16+, 18+, 20+, and 24+; the control group remission times are 15, 18, 19, 19, and 20. The plus sign (+) indicates that the data were right-censored, e.g., 16+ means right-censored at 16 months. The events without plus signs refer to remission, 1 case for the CMF group and all 5 cases for control group.

Table 15.5 shows the remission times (T), the number of remissions at remission time (d_1), the number at risk in group 1 (n_{1t}), the number at risk in group 2 (n_{2t}), expected frequency in group 1 (E_1), and expected frequency in group 2 (E_2). We will use these terms to compute a chi-square statistic. In order to complete the table, we list the remission times for the pooled data in ascending order. The remission times ranged from 15 to 23 months.

At each time t, the contribution to E_1 is $d_t n_{1t}/(n_{1t} + n_{2t})$ and, similarly, for E_2 it is $d_t n_{2t}/(n_{1t} + n_{2t})$. We know that the observed number of remissions is 1 for group 1 and 5 for group 2. As we see from the first column in the table, the remission times are at times 15, 18, 19, 20, and 23 with two remissions at 19. As described previously, the events without the plus signs are the cases in which the patients relapsed and the time is the time in remission. For the CMF group we saw that the only such event was at 23 months for one patient. For the control group we note that five such events occurred at times 15, 18, 19, 19, and 20. So $\chi^2 = (O_1 - E_1)^2/E_1 + (O_2 - E_2)^2/E_2 = (1 - 3.75)^2/4.75 + (5 - 2.25)^2/2.25 = 1.592 + 3.361 = 4.953$. From the chi-square distribution with 1 degree of freedom, we see that this result is statistically significant at the 0.05 level ($0.05 > p > 0.01$). Note that with 1 degree of freedom the critical value for $p = 0.05$ is 3.841 and for $p = 0.01$ it is 6.635. Since 4.953 lies between these values we can conclude that the p-value is between 0.01 and 0.05. Thus, we may conclude that there are significantly shorter remission times in the control group.

Now let's consider an example from the treatment of prostate cancer. A procedure called cryoablation is used to remove tumors from the prostate gland. Researchers assigned each patient to one of three risk groups (i.e., risk of recurrence) based on measures of severity of the disease prior to the procedure. Then, the researchers followed the patients for up to eight years.

The three categories of risk were designated as low, moderate, and high. Ka-

TABLE 15.5. Computation of Expected Numbers for Chi-square Test

Remission Time, T	Remissions at Remission Time, d_t	Number at Risk in Group 1 (CMF), n_{1t}	Number at Risk in Group 2 (Control), n_{2t}	Expected Frequency in Group 1, E_1	Expected Frequency in Group 2, E_2
15	1	5	5	0.5	0.5
18	1	4	4	0.5	0.5
19	2	3	3	1.0	1.0
20	1	3	1	0.75	0.25
23	1	2	0	1.0	0
Total	—	—	—	3.75	2.25

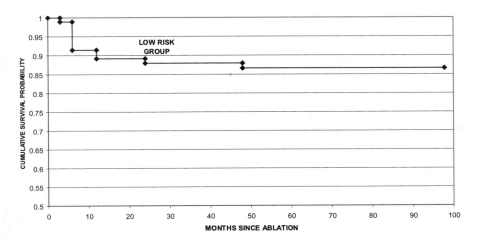

Figure 15.2. Cryoablation biochemical-free survival PSA > 1 criterion.

plan–Meier survival curves were generated for each risk group; the log rank test was used to compare these survival curves. Failure was defined as having a prostate-specific antigen lab test result above 1.0 ng/mL. Figures 15.2, 15.3, and 15.4 present the Kaplan–Meier curves.

The curves are very similar. However, the total sample size was only 561, with 94 patients in the low risk group, 178 in the medium risk group, and 289 in the high-risk group. The *p*-value for the log rank test was 0.2597, indicating that the curves were not statistically significantly different.

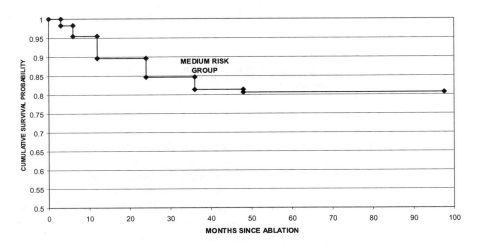

Figure 15.3. Cryoablation biochemical-free survival PSA > 1 criterion.

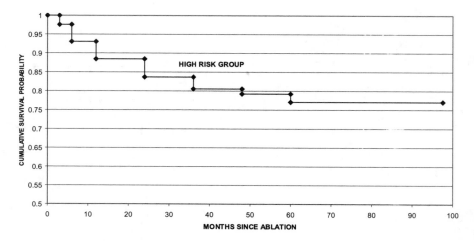

Figure 15.4. Cryoablation biochemical-free survival PSA > 1 criterion.

With this final example, we conclude Chapter 15. You have seen that analyses of survival times yield much useful information regarding the survival of patients and estimation of cure rates. In the next chapter, we will identify computer software programs that can be used for survival analyses. Chapter 16 also will present a variety of software packages that are applicable to many of the statistical techniques covered in this text.

15.4   EXERCISES

15.1   Give definitions of the following terms in your own words and indicate when it is appropriate to use each of them.
   a. Life tables
   b. The Kaplan–Meier curve
   c. The negative exponential survival distribution
   d. The Weibull distribution
   e. Cure rate models
   f. Log rank test

15.2   For a negative exponential survival function $S(t)$, recall that $S(t) = \exp(\lambda t)$, where λ is the rate parameter or hazard rate function. Consider the conditional probability that the survival time is $T > t_2$, given that we know $T > t_1$, where $t_1 < t_2$. Denote by $S(t_2|t_1)$ the conditional probability of survival beyond t_2, given that the patient survives beyond t_1, i.e., $P[T > t_2|T > t_1]$. Show that $S(t_2|t_1) = \exp[\lambda(t_2 - t_1)]$. The term $\exp[\lambda(t_2 - t_1)]$ is called the lack of memory property of the negative exponential lifetime model because the survival at time t_1 has the same distribution as the survival at time 0; if $\tau = t_2$

$- t_1$, the probability of surviving τ units of time is the same at 0 as it is at t_1, namely $\exp(\lambda\tau)$. The probability of surviving depends only on τ and not on the time t_1 that we are conditioning on.

15.3 If the survival function $S(t) = 1 - t/b$ for $0 \le t \le b$ for a fixed positive constant b, calculate the hazard function $h(t)$ for $0 \le t \le b$. Recall that $F(t) = 1 - S(t)$ and $f(t)$ is the derivative of F with respect to t. By definition, $h(t) = f(t)/S(t)$. What is the lowest value for the hazard rate? Is there a highest value for the hazard rate? (Hint: Choose M large. If there exists a $c < b$ such that $h(c)$ is greater than M and M is arbitrary, then there is no highest value for the hazard function.)

15.4 If the survival times in months for one group are $\{7.5, 12, 16, 33^+, 55, 61\}$ and $\{31, 60, 65, 76^+, 80^+, 92\}$ for the second group, apply the chi-square test to see if the survival curves are significantly different from one another. Recall that the notation of a plus as a superscript on the number indicates censoring at the denoted time, namely at 33 months for the case in group 1 and at 76 and 80 months for the cases in group 2. Test at the 0.01 significance level. Does the result seem obvious just from looking at the data?

15.5 Suppose the survival times (in months since transplant) for eight patients who received bone marrow transplants are 3.0, 4.5, 6.0, 11.0, 18.5, 20.0, 28.0, and 36.0. Assume no censoring.
   a. What is the median survival time?
   b. What is the mean survival time?
   c. Using 5 months as the interval, construct a life table for these data.

15.6 Using the data in Exercise 15.5,
   a. Calculate a Kaplan–Meier curve for the survival distribution.
   b. Fit a negative exponential survival model to the data.
   c. Compare the fitted exponential to the Kaplan–Meier curve at the eight event times.
   d. Based on the comparison in c, would you say the exponential is a good fit?

15.7 Again, we use the data from Exercise 15.5, but we assume that 6.0, 18.5, and 28 are censor times.
   a. Estimate the median survival time.
   b. Why would an estimate of the mean survival time based on averaging all the times be inappropriate?
   c. Using 5 months as an interval, construct a life table for the data.

15.8 Using the data in Exercise 15.7, construct a Kaplan–Meier estimate of the survival distribution.

15.9 Again using the data in Exercise 15.7, fit a negative exponential model. Compare it to the Kaplan–Meier curve at the event times 3, 4.5, 11.0, 20.0, and 36.0 months, and decide whether or not the negative exponential provides a good fit.

15.10 Using a chi-square test, formally test the goodness of fit of the negative exponential distribution obtained in Exercise 15.9. Test at the 0.05 level of significance.

15.11 Listed below in units of months are the survival and censor times (censoring denoted by a superscripted plus sign) for six males and six females.
Males: 1, 3, 4$^+$, 9, 11, 17
Females: 1, 3$^+$, 6, 9, 10, 11$^+$
  a. Calculate a Kaplan–Meier curve for the males.
  b. Calculate a Kaplan–Meier curve for the females.
  c. Apply a chi-square test to determine if the two survival curves differ from one another.

15.12 For the data in Exercise 15.11:
  a. Compute the mean survival time for males using all the observations (including the censoring times).
  b. Repeat part a for the females.
  c. Compute the mean survival times for males and females, respectively, using only the uncensored times.
  d. Which estimate makes more sense if censoring can be considered to occur at random?

15.5 ADDITIONAL READING

1. Altman, D. G. (1991). *Practical Statistics for Medical Research.* Chapman and Hall, London.
2. Chernick, M. R., Poulsen, E. G., and Wang, Y. (2002). Effects of bias adjustment on actuarial survival curves. *Drug Information Journal* **36,** 595–609.
3. Cutler, S. J. and Ederer, F. (1958). Maximum utilization of the life table method in analyzing survival. *Journal of Chronic Diseases* **8,** 699–712.
4. Dorey, F. J. and Korn, E. L. (1987). Effective sample size for confidence intervals for survival probabilities. *Statistics in Medicine* **6,** 679–687.
5. Kaplan, E. L. and Meier, P. (1958). Nonparametric estimation from incomplete observations. *Journal of the American Statistical Association* **53,** 457–481.
6. Ibrahim, J. G., Chen, M.-H., and Sinha, D. (2001). *Bayesian Survival Analysis.* Springer-Verlag, New York.
7. Lawless, J. F. (1982). *Statistical Models and Methods for Lifetime Data.* Wiley, New York.

8. Lee, E. T. (1992). *Statistical Methods for Survival Data Analysis,* Second Edition. Wiley, New York.

9. Maller, R. and Zhou, X. (1996). *Survival Analysis with Long-Term Survivors.* Wiley, New York.

10. Mantel, N. (1966). Evaluation of survival data and two new rank order statistics arising in its consideration. *Cancer Chemotherapy Reports* **50,** 163–170.

11. Peto, R., Pike, M. C., Armitage, P., Breslow, N. E., Cox, D. R., Howard, S. V., Mantel, N., McPherson, K., Peto, J., and Smith, P. G. (1977). Design and analysis of randomized clinical trials requiring prolonged observation of each patient, Part II. *British Journal of Cancer* **35,** 1–39.

CHAPTER 16

Software Packages for Statistical Analysis

Teaching data analysis is not easy, and the time allowed is always far from sufficient.

—John W. Tukey, The Future of Data Analysis,
Annals of Mathematical Statistics **33,** 1, 11, 1962

16.1 GENERAL-PURPOSE PACKAGES

Software packages for statistical analysis have evolved over the past three decades from those designed primarily for mainframe applications to software directed toward personal computer users. Examples of statistical packages include BMDP, SPSS, SAS, Splus, Minitab, and a wide variety of other programs. Wilfred Dixon and his colleagues in statistics at the University of California, Los Angeles, produced one of the earliest successful statistical packages, known as BMDP. This package for mainframe computers was so successful in the 1960s and 1970s that eventually BMDP Inc. was founded to handle the production and sale of the software.

BMDP handled summary statistics, hypothesis testing and confidence intervals, regression, and analysis of variance. The demand for additional statistical routines from biostatisticians led Dixon and his colleagues at UCLA to develop multivariate routines for cluster analysis and classification, as well as survival analysis and time series methods.

However, in the 1980s and 1990s microcomputers and, subsequently, personal computers supplanted mainframes. Because BMDP was slow to make adjustments, the business eventually failed. SPSS Inc. bought the software package for distribution and development in the United States. BMDP's branch in Cork, Ireland eventually developed into an offshoot company, Statistical Solutions, which still has a license to market and distribute BMDP software in Europe.

Statistical Packages for the Social Sciences (SPSS) was originally a software package developed in the late 1960s at Stanford University to help solve problems in the social sciences. Norman H. Nie, C. Hadlai (Tex) Hull, Dale Bent, and three Stanford University graduate students were the originators. SPSS incorporated in 1975 and established headquarters in Chicago, where the company, headed by Nie as Chairman of the Board, remains today.

A very popular package in the social sciences, SPSS provides standard regression and analysis of variance programs. In addition, it emphasizes multivariate methods that are important to social scientists, e.g., factor analysis, cluster analysis, classification, time series methods, and categorical data analysis. Initially, SPSS suffered because it valued marketing more highly than good numerical algorithms, whereas BMDP excelled at the use of good, stable numerical methods. In recent years SPSS Inc. has improved its algorithms.

SPSS has grown into a large corporation that acquired several major software packages during the period 1994–1999. For example, SPSS bought the rights to BMDP in the United States and bought another good statistical package, SYSTAT, that was developed by Leland Wilkinson. The firm has developed data mining software products in addition to the standard array of statistical tools. As a result of its acquisitions and software enhancements, the company is now in competition with other major statistical software and data analysis vendors such as SAS. To learn about SPSS and all its products, including SYSTAT, go to their website: www.spss.com.

Academics at North Carolina State University developed the Statistical Analysis System, (SAS) in the late 1960s. Like BMDP, SAS was a software tool devised to handle statistical research problems at a university. SAS became so successful that in 1976 NCSU faculty member James Goodnight, in an agreement with the university, gained the commercial rights to the software and formed the company that is now called the SAS Institute Inc. SAS software has become the most successful statistical software package of all, due in part to Goodnight's and the other founders' ability to anticipate the demands of the marketplace. The SAS Institute has produced excellent numerical algorithms and has been at the forefront in designing software with topnotch data management capabilities. Because of it's capabilities. SAS is the software of choice for major businesses and the entire pharmaceutical industry. As the personal computer came along, SAS developed PC SAS with a user-friendly Windows interface.

SAS software is divided into modules. The statistics module, called STAT, provides procedures for doing the standard parametric and nonparametric procedures including analysis of variance, regression, classification and clustering, and survival analysis. Specialized procedures such as time series analysis and statistical quality control have their own modules. We demonstrate SAS output in examples in this text because of SAS's dominant use in industry. SAS is also a programming language that enables you to produce statistical analyses to meet your particular needs and to manipulate your data sets in ways to enhance the analysis.

SAS now invests a lot of its development money in data mining. Their data mining package, Enterprise Miner, is one of the best packages currently available. Another advantage of SAS is its capability to transport data files in various formats and convert them to SAS data sets without tremendous effort on the part of the user. To learn the latest information about SAS, you can go to its website: www.sas.com.

S is a statistical language that was developed by AT&T Bell Laboratories in the 1970s and 1980s. It was designed to be an object-oriented language conducive to interactive data analysis and research. It is particularly suited for interactive graphics.

In the mid 1980s, R. Douglas Martin and other faculty members at the University of Washington formed a software company called Statistical Sciences. The company's purpose was to create a user-friendly front end for S. The founders called their software Splus. The package has been tremendously popular at universities and other research institutions because it provides state-of-the-art statistical tools with a user-friendly interface so that the user does not have to be knowledgeable about the S language. The company was later bought by Mathsoft and has now changed its name to Insightful Corp.

Splus software is known for its interactive capability. It includes the latest developments in time series, outlier detection, density estimation, nonparametric regression, and smoothing techniques including LOESS and spline function curve estimates. Insightful Corp. also has developed classification and regression tree algorithms and a module for group sequential design and analysis. To learn the latest about Splus and other products, go to Insightful's website: www.insightful.com.

Minitab is another general-purpose statistical package. It was designed to facilitate teaching statistical methods by using computers. Established in 1972, Minitab is used widely in educational applications. The company's founding statisticians were experts in statistical quality control methods. Consequently, the company prides itself on the usefulness and appropriateness of its quality control tools. Minitab is also a very user-friendly product with good documentation. To learn more about Minitab, go to their website at www.minitab.com.

Other good general-purpose software packages on the market today include STATA and NCSS. Their websites, which provide detailed information on their products, are www.stata.com and www.ncss.com, respectively. NCSS also produces a fine program for determining statistical power and sample size (both discussed in Section 16.3.)

For a detailed account of software packages that are useful in biostatistics, refer to the article "Software" by Arena and Rockette (2001). In addition to providing detailed discussion of the tools, the authors provide a very useful and extensive table that gives the title of each package, its emphasis relevant to clinical trials, and the name of the current vendor that sells it (including websites and mailing addresses). This list is very extensive and includes special-purpose as well as general-purpose software.

Bayesian and other statistical techniques are benefiting greatly from the Markov chain Monte Carlo computational algorithms. Refer to Robert and Casella (1999) for an excellent reference on this subject. Spiegelhalter and his colleagues at the MRC Biostatistics Unit in Cambridge, England, developed a software tool called BUGS, which stands for Bayesian inference using Gibbs sampling. Gibbs sampling is a particular type of Markov chain Monte Carlo algorithm, as is the Metropolis–Hastings algorithm. BUGS is also used in Bayesian survival analysis methods, as recently described by Ibrahim, Chen, and Sinha (2001). BUGS, with documentation, can be downloaded at no cost from the Internet (http://www.mrc-bsu.cam.ac.uk/bugs/).

At present, the most commonly used version of BUGS is WinBUGS. This attractive version is menu-driven for the Windows operating system. WinBUGS is well described with many examples in Congdon (2001). Both the Markov chain Monte Carlo algorithm and the Metropolis–Hastings algorithm can be implemented through WinBUGS. Diagnostic software for convergence of Markov chains, called CODA (Convergence Diagnostics and Output Analysis), by Martin Plummer can be downloaded at http://www-fis.iarc.fr/coda/. Brian Smith has produced another, more recent package, which is available at http://www.public-health.uiowa.edu/boa/.

16.2 EXACT METHODS

Among the class of nonparametric techniques is a group of methods called permutation, or randomization, methods. The methods have the advantage that conditioned on some aspect of the data at hand, they have a significance level that is exactly the specified level. The conditioning we refer to is conditioning on the marginal totals in a 2×2 table. In a two-sample problem, we condition on observing the combined observations without regard to which population they came from.

For the parametric techniques that we have studied in this course, achieving the correct significance level is simply a matter of finding the correct critical value(s) in a table of the sampling distribution under the null hypothesis. For more complicated testing situations in which nonparametric methods are used or approximate distributions are applied, the test may not be exact. For example, many bootstrap testing procedures provide useful nonparametric tests but they are not exact over the entire range of distributions that we consider under the null hypothesis. For such hypothesis tests that have a large set of possible distributions for the population being sampled, this exactness property is not obtainable.

We saw that Fisher's exact test, an alternative to the chi-square test for a 2×2 contingency table, is one example of an exact permutation test. Cytel Corp. is one of the few companies that produce software specializing in exact methods. Cyrus Mehta, Cytel's president, began to develop the corporation's main products, StatXact and LogXact, in 1987. Cytel provides the most extensive and best algorithms for performing exact probability calculations. The software programs employ fast algorithms based on network optimization algorithms that were originally developed for operations research problems. Cytel's current products are described on their website at www.cytel.com. The latest version of StatXact includes sample size and power calculations.

16.3 SAMPLE SIZE DETERMINATION

Originally, none of the general-purpose statistical packages contained software to help statisticians determine sample size requirements. As you have seen, sample size requirements are important for researchers and pharmaceutical and medical device companies to assess the economic feasibility of a particular study, such as a phase III clinical trial for establishing the efficacy and safety of a drug.

To fill this void, Janet Elashoff of UCLA and the Cedars Sinai Medical Center wrote a small-business innovative research proposal to develop such software. The result was a statistical package called nQuery Advisor. This highly innovative product provided useful and correct results for a variety of important sample size estimation problems, a very user-friendly interface, and verbal interpretations for the resulting tables. The tool was so successful that a company, Statistical Solutions, decided to market the software. Now in version 4, the product has undergone several improvements since its introduction.

nQuery Advisor now has several competitors. Some of the competitors that provide sample size determination include StatXact, UnifyPow, Power and Precision, and PASS 2000. Version 4 of StatXact introduced sample size determination for exact binomial tests. Version 5, which is much more extensive, includes multinomial tests and a more user-friendly menu for the sample size options.

The SAS Institute is planning to produce a sample size estimation package and may buy the rights to UnifyPow. Chernick and Liu (2002) compare these various packages with respect to the way they determine the power function for the case of the single proportion test against a hypothesized value.

We list the user manuals for these products in the reference section of this chapter. Each product has its own web site. They are as follows: www.cytel.com for StatXact, www.ncss.com for PASS 2000, www.statsolusa.com for nQuery Advisor, www.PowerAnalysis.com for Power and Precision, and www.bio.ri.ccf.org/Unifypow/ for UnifyPow.

Other sample size packages are PASS 2000 by NCSS, EaSt by Cytel, and $S +$ SeqTrial by Insightful. These three packages are designed to handle what are called group sequential designs. Sequential methods are a special topic in statistics that is not within the scope of this text.

Group sequential designs allow the sample size to depend on the results of intermediate analyses. We mention them here because the fixed sample size problems that we have been discussing in the text are special cases of the more general problem of sample size estimation. The group sequential software can be made to solve fixed sample size problems by setting the number of interim stages in the design to 1.

16.4   WHY YOU SHOULD AVOID EXCEL

The Microsoft product Excel is a very popular and useful spreadsheet program. Excel provides random number generators and functions to generate means, standard deviations, and minima and maxima of a set of numbers in a spreadsheet. It also has a data analysis toolkit as an add-on option. The toolkit provides many standard statistical tools, including regression and analysis of variance.

Many universities, particularly business schools, have considered using Excel for routine statistical analyses and as a tool to teach statistics to undergraduate classes. However, statisticians have discovered numerical instabilities in many of the algorithms. In some versions of Excel, even calculations of means and standard deviations could be incorrect because of blank rows or columns treated as zero in value instead of being ignored. The pseudorandom number generators that are used in Excel are also known to be faulty. Microsoft has not fixed many of the problems that have been pointed out to them. For all of these reasons, we think it is better to export Excel data files to other packages such as SAS before doing even routine statistical analyses.

Academic institutions are tempted to use Excel for statistical analyses. Nowadays, PCs are owned and used by the schools themselves as well as most of the community. Excel is automatically preinstalled in most of the computers sold to universities and their students. Some universities have site licenses for the distribution of well-known software products. We recommend that you use Excel for typical spreadsheet applications and for graphics such as bar charts, pie charts, and scatter plots but not for statistical analyses.

16.5   REFERENCES

1. Arena, V. C. and Rockette, H. E. (2001). "Software" in *Biostatistics in Clinical Trials,* Redmond, C. and Colton, T. (editors), pp. 424–437. Wiley, New York.
2. Borenstein, M., Rothstein, H., Cohen, J., Schoefeld, D., Berlin, J., and Lakatos, E. (2001). *Power and Precision™.* Biostat Inc., Englewood, New Jersey.
3. Chernick, M. R. and Liu, C. Y. (2002). "The Saw-toothed Behavior of Power versus Sample Size and Software Solutions: Single Binomial Proportion using Exact Methods." *The American Statistician* **56**, 149–155.
4. Congdon, P. (2001). *Bayesian Statistical Modelling,* Wiley, New York.
5. CYTEL Software Corp. (1998). *StatXact4 for Windows: Statistical Software for Exact Nonparametric Inference User Manual.* CYTEL: Cambridge, Massachusetts.
6. Elashoff, J. D. (2000). *nQuery Advisor® Release 4.0 Users Guide.* Statistical Solutions: Boston.
7. Hintze, J. L. (2000). *PASS User's Guide: PASS 2000 Power Analysis and Sample Size for Windows.* NCSS Inc., Kaysville.
8. Ibrahim, J. G., Chen, M.-H., and Sinha, D. (2001) *Bayesian Survival Analysis.* Springer-Verlag, New York.
9. O'Brien, R. G. and Muller, K.E. (1993). "Unified Power Analysis for t-Tests through Multivariate Hypotheses" in *Applied Analysis of Variance in Behavioral Science,* Edwards, L. K. (editor), pp. 297–344. Marcel Dekker, New York.

Postscript

You have now completed the course and if you have studied carefully and learned as instructed you should now appreciate these ten commandments of statistical inference.*

    I. Thou shalt not hunt statistical significance with a shotgun.

    II. Thou shalt not enter the valley of the methods of inference without an experimental design.

    III. Thou shalt not make statistical inference in the absence of a model.

    IV. Thou shalt honor the assumptions of the model.

    V. Thou shalt not adulterate the model to obtain significant results.

    VI. Thou shalt not covet thy colleague's data.

    VII. Thou shalt not bear false witness against the control group.

    VIII. Thou shalt *not* worship the 0.05 significance level.

    IX. Thou shalt not apply large sample approximations in vain.

    X. Thou shalt not infer causal relationships from statistical significance.

*Michael F. Driscoll, The Ten Commandments of Statistical Inference, *The American Mathematical Monthly, 84, 8,* 628, 1977.

APPENDIX A

Percentage Points, F-Distribution ($\alpha = 0.05$)

n \ m	1	2	3	4	5	6	7	8	9	10	12	15	20	24	30	40	60	120	∞
1	161.4	199.5	215.7	224.6	230.2	234.0	236.8	238.9	240.5	241.9	243.9	245.9	248.0	249.1	250.1	251.1	252.2	253.3	254.3
2	18.51	19.00	19.16	19.25	19.30	19.33	19.35	19.37	19.38	19.40	19.41	19.43	19.45	19.45	19.46	19.47	19.48	19.49	19.50
3	10.13	9.55	9.28	9.12	9.01	8.94	8.89	8.85	8.81	8.79	8.74	8.70	8.66	8.64	8.62	8.59	8.57	8.55	8.53
4	7.71	6.94	6.59	6.39	6.26	6.16	6.09	6.04	6.00	5.96	5.91	5.86	5.80	5.77	5.75	5.72	5.69	5.66	5.63
5	6.61	5.79	5.41	5.19	5.05	4.95	4.88	4.82	4.77	4.74	4.68	4.62	4.56	4.53	4.50	4.46	4.43	4.40	4.36
6	5.99	5.14	4.76	4.53	4.39	4.28	4.21	4.15	4.10	4.06	4.00	3.94	3.87	3.84	3.81	3.77	3.74	3.70	3.67
7	5.59	4.74	4.35	4.12	3.97	3.87	3.79	3.73	3.68	3.64	3.57	3.51	3.44	3.41	3.38	3.34	3.30	3.27	3.23
8	5.32	4.46	4.07	3.84	3.69	3.58	3.50	3.44	3.39	3.35	3.28	3.22	3.15	3.12	3.08	3.04	3.01	2.97	2.93
9	5.12	4.26	3.86	3.63	3.48	3.37	3.29	3.23	3.18	3.14	3.07	3.01	2.94	2.90	2.86	2.83	2.79	2.75	2.71
10	4.96	4.10	3.71	3.48	3.33	3.22	3.14	3.07	3.02	2.98	2.91	2.85	2.77	2.74	2.70	2.66	2.62	2.58	2.54
11	4.84	3.98	3.59	3.36	3.20	3.09	3.01	2.95	2.90	2.85	2.79	2.72	2.65	2.61	2.57	2.53	2.49	2.45	2.40
12	4.75	3.89	3.49	3.26	3.11	3.00	2.91	2.85	2.80	2.75	2.69	2.62	2.54	2.51	2.47	2.43	2.38	2.34	2.30
13	4.67	3.81	3.41	3.18	3.03	2.92	2.83	2.77	2.71	2.67	2.60	2.53	2.46	2.42	2.38	2.34	2.30	2.25	2.21
14	4.60	3.74	3.34	3.11	2.96	2.85	2.76	2.70	2.65	2.60	2.53	2.46	2.39	2.35	2.31	2.27	2.22	2.18	2.13
15	4.54	3.68	3.29	3.06	2.90	2.79	2.71	2.64	2.59	2.54	2.48	2.40	2.33	2.29	2.25	2.20	2.16	2.11	2.07
16	4.49	3.63	3.24	3.01	2.85	2.74	2.66	2.59	2.54	2.49	2.42	2.35	2.28	2.24	2.19	2.15	2.11	2.06	2.01
17	4.45	3.59	3.20	2.96	2.81	2.70	2.61	2.55	2.49	2.45	2.38	2.31	2.23	2.19	2.15	2.10	2.06	2.01	1.96
18	4.41	3.55	3.16	2.93	2.77	2.66	2.58	2.51	2.46	2.41	2.34	2.27	2.19	2.15	2.11	2.06	2.02	1.97	1.92
19	4.38	3.52	3.13	2.90	2.74	2.63	2.54	2.48	2.42	2.38	2.31	2.23	2.16	2.11	2.07	2.03	1.98	1.93	1.88
20	4.35	3.49	3.10	2.87	2.71	2.60	2.51	2.45	2.39	2.35	2.28	2.20	2.12	2.08	2.04	1.99	1.95	1.90	1.84
21	4.32	3.47	3.07	2.84	2.68	2.57	2.49	2.42	2.37	2.32	2.25	2.18	2.10	2.05	2.01	1.96	1.92	1.87	1.81
22	4.30	3.44	3.05	2.82	2.66	2.55	2.46	2.40	2.34	2.30	2.23	2.15	2.07	2.03	1.98	1.94	1.89	1.84	1.78
23	4.28	3.42	3.03	2.80	2.64	2.53	2.44	2.37	2.32	2.27	2.20	2.13	2.05	2.01	1.96	1.91	1.86	1.81	1.76
24	4.26	3.40	3.01	2.78	2.62	2.51	2.42	2.36	2.30	2.25	2.18	2.11	2.03	1.98	1.94	1.89	1.84	1.79	1.73
25	4.24	3.39	2.99	2.76	2.60	2.49	2.40	2.34	2.28	2.24	2.16	2.09	2.01	1.96	1.92	1.87	1.82	1.77	1.71
26	4.23	3.37	2.98	2.74	2.59	2.47	2.39	2.32	2.27	2.22	2.15	2.07	1.99	1.95	1.90	1.85	1.80	1.75	1.69
27	4.21	3.35	2.96	2.73	2.57	2.46	2.37	2.31	2.25	2.20	2.13	2.06	1.97	1.93	1.88	1.84	1.79	1.73	1.67
28	4.20	3.34	2.95	2.71	2.56	2.45	2.36	2.29	2.24	2.19	2.12	2.04	1.96	1.91	1.87	1.82	1.77	1.71	1.65
29	4.18	3.33	2.93	2.70	2.55	2.43	2.35	2.28	2.22	2.18	2.10	2.03	1.94	1.90	1.85	1.81	1.75	1.70	1.64
30	4.17	3.32	2.92	2.69	2.53	2.42	2.33	2.27	2.21	2.16	2.09	2.01	1.93	1.89	1.84	1.79	1.74	1.68	1.62
40	4.08	3.23	2.84	2.61	2.45	2.34	2.25	2.18	2.12	2.08	2.00	1.92	1.84	1.79	1.74	1.69	1.64	1.58	1.51
60	4.00	3.15	2.76	2.53	2.37	2.25	2.17	2.10	2.04	1.99	1.92	1.84	1.75	1.70	1.65	1.59	1.53	1.47	1.39
120	3.92	3.07	2.68	2.45	2.29	2.17	2.09	2.02	1.96	1.91	1.83	1.75	1.66	1.61	1.55	1.50	1.43	1.35	1.25
∞	3.84	3.00	2.60	2.37	2.21	2.10	2.01	1.94	1.88	1.83	1.75	1.67	1.57	1.52	1.46	1.39	1.32	1.22	1.00

Source: *Handbook of Tables for Probability and Statistics,* William H. Beyer (editor). Cleveland, Ohio: The Chemical Rubber Co., 1966, p. 242.

APPENDIX B

Studentized Range Statistic

Upper 5% Points

v \ n	2	3	4	5	6	7	8	9	10
1	17.97	26.98	32.82	37.08	40.41	43.12	45.40	47.36	49.07
2	6.08	8.33	9.80	10.88	11.74	12.44	13.03	13.54	13.99
3	4.50	5.91	6.82	7.50	8.04	8.48	8.85	9.18	9.46
4	3.93	5.04	5.76	6.29	6.71	7.05	7.35	7.60	7.83
5	3.64	4.60	5.22	5.67	6.03	6.33	6.58	6.80	6.99
6	3.46	4.34	4.90	5.30	5.63	5.90	6.12	6.32	6.49
7	3.34	4.16	4.68	5.06	5.36	5.61	5.82	6.00	6.16
8	3.26	4.04	4.53	4.89	5.17	5.40	5.60	5.77	5.92
9	3.20	3.95	4.41	4.76	5.02	5.24	5.43	5.59	5.74
10	3.15	3.88	4.33	4.65	4.91	5.12	5.30	5.46	5.60
11	3.11	3.82	4.26	4.57	4.82	5.03	5.20	5.35	5.49
12	3.08	3.77	4.20	4.51	4.75	4.95	5.12	5.27	5.39
13	3.06	3.73	4.15	4.45	4.69	4.88	5.05	5.19	5.32
14	3.03	3.70	4.11	4.41	4.64	4.83	4.99	5.13	5.25
15	3.01	3.67	4.08	4.37	4.59	4.78	4.94	5.08	5.20
16	3.00	3.65	4.05	4.33	4.56	4.74	4.90	5.03	5.15
17	2.98	3.63	4.02	4.30	4.52	4.70	4.86	4.99	5.11
18	2.97	3.61	4.00	4.28	4.49	4.67	4.82	4.96	5.07
19	2.96	3.59	3.98	4.25	4.47	4.65	4.79	4.92	5.04
20	2.95	3.58	3.96	4.23	4.45	4.62	4.77	4.90	5.01
24	2.92	3.53	3.90	4.17	4.37	4.54	4.68	4.81	4.92
30	2.89	3:49	3.85	4.10	4.30	4.46	4.60	4.72	4.82
40	2.86	3.44	3.79	4.04	4.23	4.39	4.52	4.63	4.73
60	2.83	3.40	3.74	3.98	4.16	4.31	4.44	4.55	4.65
120	2.80	3.36	3.68	3.92	4.10	4.24	4.36	4.47	4.56
∞	2.77	3.31	3.63	3.86	4.03	4.17	4.29	4.39	4.47

Introductory Biostatistics for the Health Sciences, by Michael R. Chernick and Robert H. Friis. ISBN 0-471-41137-X. Copyright © 2003 Wiley-Interscience.

Upper 5% Points (*cont.*)

v \ n	11	12	13	14	15	16	17	18	19	20
1	50.59	51.96	53.20	54.33	55.36	56.32	57.22	58.04	58.83	59.56
2	14.39	14.75	15.08	15.38	15.65	15.91	16.14	16.37	16.57	16.77
3	9.72	9.95	10.15	10.35	10.53	10.69	10.84	10.98	11.11	11.24
4	8.03	8.21	8.37	8.52	8.66	8.79	8.91	9.03	9.13	9.23
5	7.17	7.32	7.47	7.60	7.72	7.83	7.93	8.03	8.12	8.21
6	6.65	6.79	6.92	7.03	7.14	7.24	7.34	7.43	7.51	7.59
7	6.30	6.43	6.55	6.66	6.76	6.85	6.94	7.02	7.10	7.17
8	6.05	6.18	6.29	6.39	6.48	6.57	6.65	6.73	6.80	6.87
9	5.87	5.98	6.09	6.19	6.28	6.36	6.44	6.51	6.58	6.64
10	5.72	5.83	5.93	6.03	6.11	6.19	6.27	6.34	6.40	6.47
11	5.61	5.71	5.81	5.90	5.98	6.06	6.13	6.20	6.27	6.33
12	5.51	5.61	5.71	5.80	5.88	5.95	6.02	6.09	6.15	6.21
13	5.43	5.53	5.63	5.71	5.79	5.86	5.93	5.99	6.05	6.11
14	5.36	5.46	5.55	5.64	5.71	5.79	5.85	5.91	5.97	6.03
15	5.31	5.40	5.49	5.57	5.65	5.72	5.78	5.85	5.90	5.96
16	5.26	5.35	5.44	5.52	5.59	5.66	5.73	5.79	5.84	5.90
17	5.21	5.31	5.39	5.47	5.54	5.61	5.67	5.73	5.79	5.84
18	5.17	5.27	5.35	5.43	5.50	5.57	5.63	5.69	5.74	5.79
19	5.14	5.23	5.31	5.39	5.46	5.53	5.59	5.65	5.70	5.75
20	5.11	5.20	5.28	5.36	5.43	5.49	5.55	5.61	5.66	5.71
24	5.01	5.10	5.18	5.25	5.32	5.38	5.44	5.49	5.55	5.59
30	4.92	5.00	5.08	5.15	5.21	5.27	5.33	5.38	5.43	5.47
40	4.82	4.90	4.98	5.04	5.11	5.16	5.22	5.27	5.31	5.36
60	4.73	4.81	4.88	4.94	5.00	5.06	5.11	5.15	5.20	5.24
120	4.64	4.71	4.78	4.84	4.90	4.95	5.00	5.04	5.09	5.13
∞	4.55	4.62	4.68	4.74	4.80	4.85	4.89	4.93	4.97	5.01

Source: *Handbook of Tables for Probability and Statistics,* William H. Beyer (editor). Cleveland, Ohio: The Chemical Rubber Co., 1966, *p.* 286.

APPENDIX C

Quantiles of the Wilcoxon Signed-Rank Test Statistic

	$W_{0.005}$	$W_{0.01}$	$W_{0.025}$	$W_{0.05}$	$W_{0.10}$	$W_{0.20}$	$W_{0.30}$	$W_{0.40}$	$W_{0.50}$	$\dfrac{n(n+1)}{2}$
$n = 4$	0	0	0	0	I	3	3	4	5	10
5	0	0	0	1	3	4	5	6	7.5	15
6	0	0	1	3	4	6	8	9	10.5	21
7	0	1	3	4	6	9	11	12	14	28
8	1	2	4	6	9	12	14	16	18	36
9	2	4	6	9	11	15	18	20	22.5	45
10	4	6	9	11	15	19	22	25	27.5	55
11	6	8	11	14	18	23	27	30	33	66
12	8	10	14	18	22	28	32	36	39	78
13	10	13	18	22	27	33	38	42	45.5	91
14	13	16	22	26	32	39	44	48	52.5	105
15	16	20	26	31	37	45	51	55	60	120
16	20	24	30	36	43	51	58	63	68	136
17	24	28	35	42	49	58	65	71	76.5	153
18	28	33	41	48	56	66	73	80	85.5	171
19	33	38	47	54	63	74	82	89	95	190
20	38	44	53	61	70	83	91	98	105	210
21	44	50	59	68	78	91	100	108	115.5	231
22	49	56	67	76	87	100	110	119	126.5	253
23	55	63	74	84	95	110	120	130	138	276
24	62	70	82	92	105	120	131	141	150	300
25	69	77	90	101	114	131	143	153	162.5	325
26	76	85	99	111	125	142	155	165	175.5	351
27	84	94	108	120	135	154	167	178	189	378
28	92	102	117	131	146	166	180	192	203	406
29	101	111	127	141	158	178	193	206	217.5	435
30	110	121	138	152	170	191	207	220	232.5	465
31	119	131	148	164	182	205	221	235	248	496
32	129	141	160	176	195	219	236	250	264	528
33	139	152	171	188	208	233	251	266	280.5	561
34	149	163	183	201	222	248	266	282	297.5	595

Introductory Biostatistics for the Health Sciences, by Michael R. Chernick and Robert H. Friis. ISBN 0-471-41137-X. Copyright © 2003 Wiley-Interscience.

	$W_{0.005}$	$W_{0.01}$	$W_{0.025}$	$W_{0.05}$	$W_{0.10}$	$W_{0.20}$	$W_{0.30}$	$W_{0.40}$	$W_{0.50}$	$\dfrac{n(n+1)}{2}$
35	160	175	196	214	236	263	283	299	315	630
36	172	187	209	228	251	279	299	317	333	666
37	184	199	222	242	266	295	316	335	351.5	703
38	196	212	236	257	282	312	334	353	370.5	741
39	208	225	250	272	298	329	352	372	390	780
40	221	239	265	287	314	347	371	391	410	820
41	235	253	280	303	331	365	390	411	430.5	861
42	248	267	295	320	349	384	409	431	451.5	903
43	263	282	311	337	366	403	429	452	473	946
44	277	297	328	354	385	422	450	473	495	990
45	292	313	344	372	403	442	471	495	517.5	1035
46	308	329	362	390	423	463	492	517	540.5	1081
47	324	346	379	408	442	484	514	540	564	1128
48	340	363	397	428	463	505	536	563	588	1176
49	357	381	416	447	483	527	559	587	612.5	1225
50	374	398	435	467	504	550	583	611	637.5	1275

Source: Conover, W. J. (1999). *Practical Nonparametric Statistics,* 3rd Ed., pp. 545–546. Wiley, New York.

APPENDIX D

χ^2 Distribution

For various degrees of freedom (df), the tabled entries represent the values of x^2 above which a proportion p of the distribution falls.

df	\multicolumn{7}{c}{p}
	0.99	0.95	0.90	0.10	0.05	0.01	0.001
1	$.0^3 157$	.00393	.0158	2.706	3.841	6.635	10.827
2	.0201	.103	.211	4.605	5.991	9.210	13.815
3	.115	.352	.584	6.251	7.815	11.345	16.266
4	.297	.711	1.064	7.779	9.488	13.277	18.467
5	.554	1.145	1.610	9.236	11.070	15.086	20.515
6	.872	1.635	2.204	10.645	12.592	16.812	22.457
7	1.239	2.167	2.833	12.017	14.067	18.475	24.322
8	1.646	2.733	3.490	13.362	15.507	20.090	26.125
9	2.088	3.325	4.168	14.684	16.919	21.666	27.877
10	2.558	3.940	4.865	15.987	18.307	23.209	29.588
11	3.053	4.575	5.578	17.275	19.675	24.725	31.264
12	3.571	5.226	6.304	18.549	21.026	26.217	32.909
13	4.107	5.892	7.042	19.812	22.362	27.688	34.528
14	4.660	6.571	7.790	21.064	23.685	29.141	36.123
15	5.229	7.261	8.547	22.307	24.996	30.578	37.697
16	5.812	7.962	9.312	23.542	26.296	32.000	39.252
17	6.408	8.672	10.085	24.769	27.587	33.409	40.790
18	7.015	9.390	10.865	25.989	28.869	34.805	42.312
19	7.633	10.117	11.651	27.204	30.144	36.191	43.820
20	8.260	10.851	12.443	28.412	31.410	37.566	45.315
21	8.897	11.591	13.240	29.615	32.671	38.932	46.797
22	9.542	12.338	14.041	30.813	33.924	40.289	48.268
23	10.196	13.091	14.848	32.007	35.172	41.638	49.728
24	10.856	13.848	15.659	33.196	36.415	42.980	51.179
25	11.524	14.611	16.473	34.382	37.652	44.314	52.620

Introductory Biostatistics for the Health Sciences, by Michael R. Chernick and Robert H. Friis. ISBN 0-471-41137-X. Copyright © 2003 Wiley-Interscience.

df	p						
	0.99	0.95	0.90	0.10	0.05	0.01	0.001
26	12.198	15.379	17.292	35.563	38.885	45.642	54.052
27	12.879	16.151	18.114	36.741	40.113	46.963	55.476
28	13.565	16.928	18.939	37.916	41.337	48.278	56.893
29	14.256	17.708	19.768	39.087	42.557	49.588	58.302
30	14.953	18.493	20.599	40.256	43.773	50.892	59.703

Source: Adapted from Table IV of R. A. Fisher and F. Yates (1974). *Statistical Tables for Biological, Agricultural, and Medical Research,* 6th Ed., Longman Group, Ltd., London. (Previously published by Oliver & Boyd, Ltd., Edinburgh). Used with permission of the authors and publishers.

Table of the Standard Normal Distribution

Z	0.00	0.01	0.02	0.03	0.04	0.05	0.06	0.07	0.08	0.09
0.0	0.0000	0.0040	0.0080	0.0120	0.0160	0.0199	0.0239	0.0279	0.0319	0.0359
0.1	0.0398	0.0438	0.0478	0.0517	0.0557	0.0596	0.0636	0.0675	0.0714	0.0753
0.2	0.0793	0.0832	0.0871	0.0910	0.0948	0.0987	0.1026	0.1064	0.1103	0.1141
0.3	0.1179	0.1217	0.1255	0.1293	0.1331	0.1368	0.1406	0.1443	0.1480	0.1517
0.4	0.1554	0.1591	0.1628	0.1664	0.1700	0.1736	0.1772	0.1808	0.1844	0.1879
0.5	0.1915	0.1950	0.1985	0.2019	0.2054	0.2088	0.2123	0.2157	0.2190	0.2224
0.6	0.2257	0.2291	0.2324	0.2357	0.2389	0.2422	0.2454	0.2486	0.2517	0.2549
0.7	0.2580	0.2611	0.2642	0.2673	0.2704	0.2734	0.2764	0.2794	0.2823	0.2852
0.8	0.2881	0.2910	0.2939	0.2967	0.2995	0.3023	0.3051	0.3078	0.3106	0.3133
0.9	0.3159	0.3186	0.3212	0.3238	0.3264	0.3289	0.3315	0.3340	0.3365	0.3389
1.0	0.3413	0.3438	0.3461	0.3485	0.3508	0.3531	0.3554	0.3577	0.3599	0.3621
1.1	0.3643	0.3665	0.3686	0.3708	0.3729	0.3749	0.3770	0.3790	0.3810	0.3830
1.2	0.3849	0.3869	0.3888	0.3907	0.3925	0.3944	0.3962	0.3980	0.3997	0.4015
1.3	0.4032	0.4049	0.4066	0.4082	0.4099	0.4115	0.4131	0.4147	0.4162	0.4177
1.4	0.4192	0.4207	0.4222	0.4236	0.4251	0.4265	0.4279	0.4292	0.4306	0.4319
1.5	0.4332	0.4345	0.4350	0.4370	0.4382	0.4394	0.4406	0.4418	0.4429	0.4441
1.6	0.4452	0.4463	0.4474	0.4484	0.4495	0.4505	0.4515	0.4525	0.4535	0.4545
1.7	0.4554	0.4564	0.4573	0.4582	0.4591	0.4599	0.4608	0.4616	0.4625	0.4633
1.8	0.4641	0.4649	0.4656	0.4664	0.4671	0.4678	0.4686	0.4693	0.4699	0.4706
1.9	0.4713	0.4719	0.4726	0.4732	0.4738	0.4744	0.4750	0.4756	0.4761	0.4767
2.0	0.4772	0.4778	0.4783	0.4788	0.4793	0.4798	0.4803	0.4808	0.4812	0.4817
2.1	0.4821	0.4826	0.4830	0.4834	0.4838	0.4842	0.4846	0.4850	0.4854	0.4857
2.2	0.4861	0.4864	0.4868	0.4871	0.4875	0.4878	0.4881	0.4884	0.4887	0.4890
2.3	0.4893	0.4896	0.4898	0.4901	0.4904	0.4906	0.4909	0.4911	0.4913	0.4916
2.4	0.4918	0.4920	0.4922	0.4925	0.4927	0.4929	0.4931	0.4932	0.4934	0.4936
2.5	0.4938	0.4940	0.4941	0.4943	0.4945	0.4946	0.4948	0.4949	0.4951	0.4952
2.6	0.4953	0.4955	0.4956	0.4957	0.4959	0.4960	0.4961	0.4962	0.4963	0.4964
2.7	0.4965	0.4966	0.4967	0.4968	0.4969	0.4970	0.4971	0.4972	0.4973	0.4974
2.8	0.4974	0.4975	0.4976	0.4977	0.4977	0.4978	0.4979	0.4979	0.4980	0.4981
2.9	0.4981	0.4982	0.4982	0.4983	0.4984	0.4984	0.4985	0.4985	0.4986	0.4986
3.0	0.4987	0.4987	0.4987	0.4988	0.4988	0.4989	0.4989	0.4989	0.4990	0.4990

Source: Public domain.

Introductory Biostatistics for the Health Sciences, by Michael R. Chernick and Robert H. Friis. ISBN 0-471-41137-X. Copyright © 2003 Wiley-Interscience.

Percentage Points, Student's t Distribution

n \ F	0.90	0.95	0.975	0.99	0.995
1	3.078	6.314	12.706	31.821	63.657
2	1.886	2.920	4.303	6.965	9.925
3	1.638	2.353	3.182	4.541	5.841
4	1.533	2.132	2.776	3.747	4.604
5	1.476	2.015	2.571	3.365	4.032
6	1.440	1.943	2.447	3.143	3.707
7	1.415	1.895	2.365	2.998	3.499
8	2.397	1.860	2.306	2.896	3.355
9	1.383	1.833	2.262	2.821	3.250
10	1.372	1.812	2.228	2.764	3.169
11	1.363	1.796	2.201	2.718	3.106
12	1.356	1.782	2.179	2.681	3.055
13	1.350	1.771	2.160	2.650	3.012
14	1.345	1.761	2.145	2.624	2.977
15	1.341	1.753	2.131	2.602	2.947
16	1.337	1.746	2.120	2.583	2.921
17	1.333	1.740	2.110	2.567	2.898
18	1.330	1.734	2.101	2.552	2.878
19	1.328	1.729	2.093	2.539	2.861
20	1.325	1.725	2.086	2.528	2.845
21	1.323	1.721	2.080	2.518	2.831
22	1.321	1.717	2.074	2.508	2.819
23	1.319	1.714	2.069	2.500	2.807
24	1.318	1.711	2.064	2.492	2.797
25	1.316	1.708	2.060	2.485	2.787
26	1.315	1.706	2.056	2.479	2.779
27	1.314	1.703	2.052	2.473	2.771
28	1.313	1.701	2.048	2.467	2.763
29	1.311	1.699	2.045	2.462	2.756
30	1.310	1.697	2.042	2.457	2.750

(*continued*)

Introductory Biostatistics for the Health Sciences, by Michael R. Chernick
and Robert H. Friis. ISBN 0-471-41137-X. Copyright © 2003 Wiley-Interscience.

n \ F	0.90	0.95	0.975	0.99	0.995
40	1.303	1.684	2.021	2.423	2.704
60	1.296	1.671	2.000	2.390	2.660
120	1.289	1.658	1.980	2.358	2.617
∞	1.282	1.645	1.960	2.326	2.576

Source: *Handbook of Tables for Probability and Statistics,* William H. Beyer (editor). Cleveland, Ohio: The Chemical Rubber Co., 1966, *p.* 226.

APPENDIX G

Answers to Selected Exercises

Chapter 1

1.6 Cross-sectional studies are studies on a population at a fixed point in time. Many surveys are cross-sectional. They are used to measure current thinking or the opinion at a particular time that interests the investigator. An opinion poll on candidates in an election just before (a day or two) election might be used to predict the winner. Such a poll taken a few months before the election could be used by a particular candidate to gauge further campaign strategy.

1.8 a. Clinical trials are studies over time that follow patients to determine the safety and effectiveness of a particular experimental treatment. In clinical trials, patients are usually randomized to various treatment groups (at least two). One group may be given a placebo or an active control treatment for comparison. Blinding is often done and double-blinding is often preferred.

    b. Controlled trials are trials that include randomization and a control group. Uncontrolled trials are missing either randomization or the control or both.

    c. Controls are important to get objective comparison, to avoid bias and/or adjust for a "placebo effect."

    d. Blinding is a technique that keeps the patient and often the investigator from knowing which treatment the patient is getting. It is implemented through randomization codes that are used to assign the treatments to the patients but are not known to the investigator or the patient. At the end of the trial, these codes are used to match the patients to their treatments for the statistical analysis.

    e. Here are some outcomes that are measured in clinical trials:

      1. Patient satisfaction with the treatment
      2. Patient reported quality of life questions
      3. Comparison of glycemic control for diabetic patients between a new treatment and an active control
      4. Adverse events occurring during the trial
      5. Ability of a diabetes drug to lower cholesterol as well as control glucose levels
      6. Acute success rate for an ablation procedure with an experimental catheter and procedure compared to a control catheter and standard treatment.

7. Six-month capture threshold comparison of patients with a pacemaker with steroid-eluting leads compared to control group patients with a pacemaker that has a nonsteroid lead

8. Comparison of survival times for AIDS patients getting a new therapy versus AIDS patients getting standard treatment

Chapter 2

2.9 From Table 2.1, start in the first column and the third row and proceed across the row to generate the random numbers, going back to the first column on the next row when a row is completed. Placing a zero and a decimal point in front of the first digit of the number (we will do this throughout), we get for the first random number 0.69386. This random number picks the row. We multiply 0.69386 by 50, getting 34.693. We will always round up. This will give us integers between 1 and 50. So we take row 35. Now the next number in the table is used for the column. It is 0.71708. Since there are 8 columns, we multiply 0.71708 by 8 to get 5.7366 and round up to get 6. Now, the first sample from the table is (35, 6), the value in row 35 column 6. We look this up in Table 2.2 and find the height to be 61 inches.

For the second measurement, we take the next pair of numbers, 0.88608 and 0.67251. After the respective multiplications we have row 45 and column 6. We compare (45, 6) to our list, which consists only of (35, 6). Since this pair does not repeat a pair on the list, we accept it. The list is now (35, 6) and (45, 6) and the samples are, respectively, 61 and 65.

For the third measurement the next pair of random numbers is 0.22512 and 0.00169, giving the pair (12, 1). Since this pair is not on the list, we accept and the list becomes (35, 6), (45, 6), and (12, 1), with corresponding measurements 61, 65, and 59.

The next pair is 0.02887 and 0.84072, giving the pair (2, 7). This is accepted since it does not appear on the list. The resulting measurement is 63.

The next pair is 0.91832 and 0.97489 giving the pair (46, 8). Again, we accept. The corresponding measurement is 59.

We are half way to the result. The list of pairs is (35, 6), (45, 6), (12, 1), (2, 7), and (46, 8), corresponding to the sample measurements 61, 65, 59, 63, and 59.

The next pair of random numbers is 0.68381 and 0.61725 (note at this point we had to move to row 4 column 1). The pair is (35, 5). This again is not on the list and the corresponding measurement is 66.

The next pair of random numbers is 0.49122 and 0.75836 corresponding to the pair (25, 7). This is not on the list so we accept it and the corresponding sample measurement is 55.

The next pair of random numbers is 0.58711 and 0.52551 corresponding to the pair (8, 5). This pair is again not on our list so we accept it. The sample measurement is 65.

The next pair of random numbers is 0.58711 and 0.43014, corresponding to the pair (30, 4). This pair is again not on our list so we accept it. The sample measurement is 64.

The next pair of random numbers is 0.95376 and 0.57402, corresponding to the pair (48, 5). This pair is again not on our list so we accept it. The sample measurement is 57.

We now have 10 samples. Since we only took 10 out of 400 numbers (50 rows by 8 columns), our chances of a rejection on any sample was small and we did not get one.

The resulting 10 pairs are (35, 6), (45, 6), (12, 1), (2,7), (46,8), (35, 5), (25,7), (8, 5), (30, 4) and (48, 5) and the corresponding sample of ten measurements is 61, 65, 59, 63, 59, 66, 55, 65, 64, and 57.

Despite the complicated mechanism we used to generate the sample, this constitutes what we call a simple random sample since each of the 400 samples has probability 1/400 of being selected first and each of the remaining 399 has probability 1/399 of being selected second, given they weren't chosen first, etc.

2.11   a. The original sample is 61, 55, 52, 59, 62, 66, 63, 60, 67, and 64. We then index these samples 1–10. Index 1 corresponds to 61, 2 to 55, 3 to 52, 4 to 59, 5 to 62, 6 to 66, 7 to 63, 8 to 60, 9 to 67, and 10 to 64. We use a table of random numbers to pick the index. We will do this by running across row 21 of Table 2.1 to generate the 10 indices. The random numbers on row 21 are:

22011   71396   95174   43043   68304   36773   83931   43631   50995   68130

This we interpret as 0.22011, 0.71396, 0.95174, 0.43043, 0.68304, 0.36773, 0.83931, 0.43631, 0.50995, and 0.68130. To get the index, we multiply these numbers by 10 and round up to the next integer. The resulting indices are, respectively, 3, 8, 10, 5, 7, 4, 9, 5, 6, and 7. We see that indices 5 and 7 each repeated once and indices 1 and 2 did not occur. The corresponding sample is 52, 60, 64, 62, 63, 59, 67, 62, 66, and 63.

   b. The name we give to sampling with replacement n times from a sample of size n is bootstrap sampling. The sample we obtained we call a bootstrap sample.

2.13   a. A population is a complete list of all the subjects you are interested in. For Exercise 2.9, it consisted of the 400 height measurements for the female clinic patients. The sample is the chosen subset of the population, often selected at random. In this case it consisted of a random sample of 10 measurements corresponding to the female patients in specific rows and columns of the table. The resulting 10 pairs were (35, 6), (45, 6), (12, 1), (2,7), (46,8), (35, 5), (25,7), (8, 5), (30, 4), and (48, 5) and the corresponding sample of 10 measurements were 61, 65, 59, 63, 59, 66, 55, 65, 64, and 57.

   b. For the bootstrap sampling plan in Exercise 2.11, the population is the same set of 400 height measurements in Table 2.2. The original sample is a subset of size 10 taken from this population in a systematic fashion, as described in Exercise 2.11. The bootstrap sample is then obtained by sampling with replacement from this original sample of size 10. The resulting bootstrap sample is a sample of size 10 that may have some of the original sample values repeated one or more times depending on the result of the random drawing. As shown in our solution, the indices 5 and 7 repeated once each.

2.14 a. This method of sampling is systematic sampling. It specifically is a periodic method.

b. Because of the cyclic nature of the sampling scheme, there is a danger of bias. If the data is also cyclic with the same period we could be sampling only the peak values (or only the trough values). In that case, the sample estimate of the mean would be biased on the high side if we sampled the peaks and on the low side if we sampled the troughs.

Chapter 3

3.7 Since the range is from 0.7 to 23.3 and we are to choose 9 intervals, we choose to divide the data into 9 equal width intervals from 0 to 24.3, each of length 2.7. Data points at an interval boundary are included in the higher of the two intervals.

Class Interval	Measurement Class	Frequency	Relative Frequency
1	0–2.7	19	0.38
2	2.7–5.4	17	0.34
3	5.4–8.1	10	0.20
4	8.1–10.8	2	0.04
5	10.8–13.5	0	0.0
6	13.5–16.2	1	0.02
7	16.2–18.9	0	0.0
8	18.9–21.6	0	0.0
9	21.6–24.3	1	0.02
Total	—	50	1.0

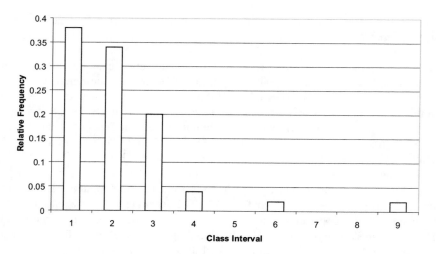

Relative Frequency Histogram for Exercise 3.7.

The mean is 4.426 and the median is 3.90.

3.9 The numbers range from 0.7 to 23.3, so the stem and leaf plot looks as follows:

```
 0   7777
 1   00125566
 2   0011235789
 3   25999
 4   01234889
 5   045
 6   1579
 7   66
 8   02
 9   0
10   6
11
12
13
14   1
15
16
17
18
19
20
21
22
23   3
```

3.10 The median is 5. The lower quartile is 4 and the upper quartile is 7. The smallest value is 2 and the largest 9.

Chapter 4

4.1 Measures of location are statistical estimates that describe the center of a probability distribution. Some measures are more appropriate than others, depending on the shape of the distribution.

a. The arithmetic mean is the "center of gravity" for the distribution. It is simply the sum of the observations divided by the number of observations. It is an appropriate measure for symmetric distributions like the normal distribution.

b. The median is the middle value. For an odd number of samples, that is, if $n = 2m + 1$, an odd number, the median is the $m + 1$ value when ordered from smallest to largest. If $n = 2m$, an even number, then the median is the average of the m and $m + 1$ values ordered from smallest to largest. Approximately half the values are below and half are above the median.

c. The mode is the most frequently occurring value (or values if more than one value tie for most frequent). For a density function, the mode is the peak in the density (i.e., the top of the mountain).

d. A unimodal distribution is one that has a density with only one peak. A bimodal distribution is one with a density that has two peaks (not necessarily equal). Mutimodal distributions have two or more peaks.

e. Skewed distributions are distributions that are not symmetric. A right or positively skewed distribution has a long trailing tail to the right. A left or negatively skewed distribution has the distribution concentrated to the right with the longer tail to the left.

f. The geometric mean for a sample of size n is the nth root of the product of the observations. The log of the geometric mean is the arithmetic mean of the logarithms. Cosequently, the geometric mean is appropriate for the lognormal distribution and distribution with shape similar to the lognormal.

g. The harmonic mean of a sample is the reciprocal of average of the reciprocal of the observations.

4.9   The first data set is odd since it contains 5 values $\{8, 7, 3, 5, 3\}$. Ordering the data from smallest to largest, we get the sequence 3, 3, 5, 7, 8. The third observation in this sequence is the median. Hence, the median is 5. The second data set is even since it contains 6 values $\{7, 8, 3, 6, 10, 10\}$. Ordering them from smallest to largest we get 3, 6, 7, 8, 10, 10. In this sequence, the third observation is the one just below the middle and the fourth is the observation just above. So by the definition of sample median, the median is the average of these observations $(7 + 8)/2 = 7.5$.

4.13   a.   First the sample mean is calculated as $(3 + 3 + 3 + 3 + 3)/5 = 3$. Next calculate the squared deviations $(3 - 3)^2 = 0$, $(3 - 3)^2 = 0$, $(3 - 3)^2 = 0$, $(3 - 3)^2 = 0$, and $(3 - 3)^2 = 0$. Add up the terms and divide by $n - 1 = 4$ to get 0 for S^2. The sample standard deviation is the square root of the answer is $\sqrt{0} = 0$. The shortcut formula is

$$S^2 = \frac{\Sigma x_i^2 - nm^2}{n - 1}$$

where m is the sample mean and n is the sample size. $\Sigma x_i^2 = 3^2 + 3^2 + 3^2 + 3^2 + 3^2 = 45$. $nm^2 = 5(3)^2 = 45$. So $S^2 = (45 - 45)/4 = 0$.

In the second case, the sample mean is $(5 + 7 + 9 + 11)/4 = 32/4 = 8$. Next calculate the squared deviations $(5 - 8)^2 = 9$, $(7 - 8)^2 = 1$, $(9 - 8)^2 = 1$, and $(11 - 8)^2 = 9$. Add up the terms and divide by $n - 1 = 3$ to get $20/3 = 6.67$ for S^2. The sample standard deviation is the square root of the answer is $\sqrt{6.67} = 2.58$. The shortcut formula is

$$S^2 = \frac{\Sigma x_i^2 - nm^2}{n - 1}$$

where m is the sample mean and n is the sample size. $\Sigma x_i^2 = 5^2 + 7^2 + 9^2 + 11^2 = 276$. $nm^2 = 4(8)^2 = 256$. So $S^2 = (276 - 256)/3 = 20/3 = 6.67$.

In the last example, we have just 2 observations, 33 and 49. The mean is 41. Next calculate the squared deviations $(33 - 41)^2 = 64$ and $(4 9 - 41)^2 = 64$. Add up the terms and divide by $n - 1 = 1$ to get 128 for S^2. The sample standard deviation is the square root of the answer, $\sqrt{128} = 11.31$. The shortcut formula is

$$S^2 = \frac{\Sigma x_i^2 - nm^2}{n - 1}$$

where m is the sample mean and n is the sample size. $\Sigma x_i^2 = 33^2 + 49^2 = 3490$. $nm^2 = 2(41)^2 = 3362$. So $S^2 = (3490 - 3362)/1 = 128$.

b. For the first sample, all the values were the same. So there is no variation and the variance is zero.

4.15 In this problem, we use the home run sluggers data to compare some measures of dispersion. Recall that the data are as follows:

McGwire: 49, 32, 33, 39, 22, 42, 9, 9, 39, 52, 58, 70, 65, 32
Sosa   4, 15, 10, 8, 33, 25, 36, 40, 36, 66, 63, 50
Bonds   16, 25, 24, 19, 33, 25, 34, 46, 37, 33, 42, 40, 37, 34, 49
Griffey   16, 22, 22, 27, 45, 40, 17, 49, 56, 56, 48, 40

a. The sample ranges are $70 - 9 = 61$ for McGwire, $66 - 4 = 62$ for Sosa, $49 - 16 = 33$ for Bonds, and $56 - 16 = 40$ for Griffey.

b. We use the shortcut formula to calculate the standard deviations. Recall that

$$S^2 = \frac{\Sigma x_i^2 - nm^2}{n - 1}$$

For McGwire, the $\Sigma x_i^2 = (49)^2 + (32)^2 + (33)^2 + (39)^2 + (22)^2 + (42)^2 + (9)^2 + (9)^2 + (39)^2 + (52)^2 + (58)^2 + (70)^2 + (65)^2 + (32)^2 = 2401 + 1024 + 1089 + 1521 + 484 + 1764 + 81 + 81 + 1521 + 2704 + 3364 + 4900 + 4225 + 1024 = 26183$, and since $m = (49 + 32 + 33 + 39 + 22 + 42 + 9 + 9 + 39 + 52 + 58 + 70 + 65 + 32)/14 = 551/14 = 39.357$, $nm^2 = 14(39.357)^2 = 21685.786$. So $S^2 = (26183 - 21685.786)/13 = 345.94$ and $S = \sqrt{345.94} = 18.6$.

For Sosa, the $\Sigma x_i^2 = (4)^2 + (15)^2 + (10)^2 + (8)^2 + (33)^2 + (25)^2 + (36)^2 + (40)^2 + (36)^2 + (66)^2 + (63)^2 + (50)^2 = 16 + 225 + 100 + 64 + 1089 + 625 + 1296 + 4356 + 3969 + 2500 = 14240$, and since $m = (4 + 15 + 10 + 8 + 33 + 25 + 36 + 40 + 36 + 66 + 63 + 50)/12 = 386/12 = 32.167$, $nm^2 = 12(32.167)^2 = 12416.333$. So $S^2 = (14240 - 12416.333)/11 = 165.79$ and $S = \sqrt{165.79} = 12.9$.

For Bonds, the $\Sigma x_i^2 = (16)^2 + (25)^2 + (24)^2 + (19)^2 + (33)^2 + (25)^2 + (34)^2 + (46)^2 + (37)^2 + (33)^2 + (42)^2 + (40)^2 + (37)^2 + (34)^2 + (49)^2 = 256 + 625 + 576 + 361 + 1089 + 625 + 1156 + 2116 + 1369 + 1089 + 1764 + 1600 + 1369 + 1156 + 2401 = 17552$, and since $m = (16 + 25 + 24 + 19 + 33 + 25 + 34 + 46 + 37 + 33 + 42 + 40 + 37 + 34 + 49)/15 = 494/15 = 32.933$, $nm^2 = 15(32.933)^2 = 16269.0667$. So $S^2 = (17552 - 16269.0667)/14 = 91.64$ and $S = \sqrt{91.64} = 9.57$.

Finally, for Griffey, the $\Sigma x_i^2 = (16)^2 + (22)^2 + (22)^2 + (27)^2 + (45)^2 + (40)^2 + (17)^2 + (49)^2 + (56)^2 + (56)^2 + (48)^2 + (40)^2 = 256 + 484 + 484 + 729 + 2025 + 1600 + 289 + 2401 + 3136 + 3136 + 2304 + 1600 = 18444$, and since $m = (16 + $

22 + 22 + 27 + 45 + 40 + 17 + 49 + 56 + 56 + 48 + 40)/12 = 438/12 = 36.5, nm^2 = 12(36.5)² = 15987. So S^2 = (18444 − 15987)/11 = 223.36 and $S = \sqrt{223.36}$ = 14.95.

c. For McGwire, since m = 39.357, the sum of absolute deviations is |49 − 39.357| + |32 − 39.357| + |33 − 39.357| + |39 − 39.357| + |22 − 39.357| + |42 − 39.357| + |9 − 39.357| + |9 − 39.357| + |39 − 39.357| + |52 − 39.357| + |58 − 39.357| + |70 − 39.357| + |65 − 39.357| + |32 − 39.357| = 9.643 + 7.357 + 6.357 + 0.357 + 17.357 + 2.643 + 30.357 + 30.357 + 0.357 + 12.643 + 18.643 + 30.643 + 25.643 + 7.357 = 169.357. Divide by the sample size n = 14 to get 12.097 for the sample mean absolute deviation.

Now, for Sosa, since m = 32.167, the sum of absolute deviations is |4 − 32.167| + |15 − 32.167| + |10 − 32.167| + |8 − 32.167| + |33 − 32.167| + |25 − 32.167| + |36 − 32.167| + |40 − 32.167| + |36 − 32.167| + |66 − 32.167| + |63 − 32.167| + |50 − 32.167| = 28.167 + 17.167 + 22.167 + 24.167 + 0.833 + 7.167 + 3.833 + 7.833 + 3.833 + 33.833 + 30.833 + 17.833 = 197.667. Divide by the sample size n = 12 to get 16.472 for the sample mean absolute deviation.

Now, for Bonds, since m = 32.167, the sum of absolute deviations is |16 − 32.933| + |25 − 32.933| + |24 − 32.933| + |19 − 32.933| + |33 − 32.933| + |25 − 32.933| + |34 − 32.933| + |46 − 32.933| + |37 − 32.933| + |33 − 32.933| + |42 − 32.933| + |40 − 32.933| + |37 − 32.933| + |34 − 32.933| + |49 − 32.933| = 16.933 + 7.933 + 8.933 + 13.933 + 0.067 + 7.933 + 1.067 + 13.067 + 4.067 + 0.067 + 9.067 + 4.067 + 1.067 + 16.067 = 104.268. Divide by the sample size n = 14 to get 7.448 for the sample mean absolute deviation.

Now, for Griffey, since m = 36.5, the sum of absolute deviations is |16 − 36.5| + |22 − 36.5| + |22 − 36.5| + |27 − 36.5| + |45 − 36.5| + |40 − 36.5| + |17 − 36.5| + |49 − 36.5| + |56 − 36.5| + |56 − 36.5| + |48 − 36.5| + |40 − 36.5| = 20.5 + 14.5 + 14.5 + 9.5 + 8.5 + 3.5 + 19.5 + 12.5 + 19.5 + 19.5 + 11.5 + 3.5 = 157. Divide by the sample size n = 12 to get 13.083 for the sample mean absolute deviation.

By all measures, we see apparent differences in variability among these players, even though their home run averages tend to be similar in the range from 32 to 40. Bonds seems to be the most consistent (i.e., has the smallest variability based on all three measures). Oddly, this might change when the 2001 season is added in since he hit a record 73 home runs that year, which is 24 more than his previous high of 49 in the 2000 season.

Chapter 5

5.1 The probability of no females and 4 males is the same as getting 4 heads in a row tossing a fair coin or (1/2)⁴ = 1/16 = 0.0625. To get one female we could have the sequence FMMM, which has probability 1/16 also, but there are C_1^4 = 4!/(1! 3!) = 4 ways of arranging 1 female and 3 males. These 4 mutually exclusive cases each have probability 1/16. taking the sum the probability is 4/16 = 1/4 = 0.250 for 1 female. For 2 females and 2 males there are C_2^4 = 4!/(2! 2!) = 6 ways of getting 2 males and 2 females. So the probability is 6/16 = 3/8 = 0.375. For 3 females, we again have 4 ways of getting 3 females and 1 male, so the probability is 0.250 for 3

Notice that in the sum the terms $k = 0$ and $k = 1$ are both 0, so we can take the sum from $k = 2$ to n. Let $m = n - 2$ and $j = k - 2$. Substituting j and m in the equation above we get

$$\sum \frac{k(k-1)n!}{k!(n-k)!}p^k(1-p)^{n-k} = \sum \frac{n!}{(k-2)!(n-k)!}p^k(1-p)^{n-k}$$

$$= \sum \frac{n!}{j![n-(j+2)]!}p^{j+2}(1-p)^{n-(j+2)}.$$

The sum on the right side of the above equation goes from $j = 0$ to $j = m = n - 2$. By factoring our $n(n-1)p^2$ from the summation we get for the right side,

$$n(n-1)p^2 \sum \frac{(n-2)!}{j!(n-2-j)!}p^j(1-p)^{n-2-j}$$

but this sum equals 1 by equation (1) applied with $m = n - 2 > 0$. Note equation (1) holds trivially for $n - 2 = 0$. So $m = 0$ is also acceptable. So for any $n \geq 2$, Var$(X) = np + n(n-1)p^2 - n^2p^2 = np + n^2p^2 - np^2 - n^2p^2 = np - np^2 = np(1-p)$ For $n = 10$ and $p = 1/2$, the mean is 5 and the variance is $10(1/2)(1/2) = 5/2 = 2.5$. Note that the proof does not include the case $n = 1$, a single Bernoulli trial. In that case, we compute the variance directly, namely, Var$(X) = E[X - E(X)]^2$ and $E(X) = 0(1 - p) + 1(p) = p$. So Var$(X) = E(X - p)^2 = (1-p)(0-p)^2 + (p)(1-p)^2 = (1-p)p^2 + p(1-p)^2 = p(1-p)(p+1-p) = p(1-p) = np(1-p)$, since $n = 1$.

Chapter 6

6.7 a. $P(Z > 2.33) = 0.5 - P(0 < Z < 2.33) = 0.5 - 0.4901 = 0.0099$.

b. $P(Z < -2.58) = P(Z > 2.58) = 0.5 - P(0 < Z < 2.58) = 0.5 - 0.4951 = 0.0049$.

c. From the table of the standard normal distribution, we see that we want to find the probability that $Z > 1.65$ or $Z < -1.65$ or $p = P(Z < -1.65) + P(Z > 1.65)$. By symmetry $P(Z < -1.65) = P(Z > 1.65)$. So $p = 2P(Z > 1.65)$. We also know that $P(Z > 1.65) = 0.5 - P(0 < Z < 1.65)$. So $p = 1 - 2P(0 < Z < 1.65)$. We look up $P(0 < Z < 1.65)$ in the table for the normal distribution and find it is 0.4505. So $p = 1 - 0.9010 = 0.099$.

d. From the table of the standard normal distribution we see that we want to find the probability that $Z > 1.96$ or $Z < -1.96$ or $p = P(Z < -1.96) + P(Z > 1.96)$. By symmetry $P(Z < -1.96) = P(Z > 1.96)$. So $p = 2P(Z > 1.96)$. We also know that $P(Z > 1.96) = 0.5 - P(0 < Z < 1.96)$. So $p = 1 - 2P(0 < Z < 1.96)$. We look up $P(0 < Z < 1.96)$ in the table for the normal distribution and find it is 0.4750. So $p = 1 - 0.95 = 0.05$.

e. From the table of the standard normal distribution we see that we want to find the probability that $Z > 2.33$ or $Z < -2.33$ or $p = P(Z < -2.33) + P(Z > 2.33)$. By symmetry $P(Z < -2.33) = P(Z > 2.33)$. So $p = 2P(Z > 2.33)$. We also know that $P(Z > 2.33) = 0.5 - P(0 < Z < 2.33)$. So $p = 1 - 2P(0 < Z < 2.33)$. We look up $P(0 < Z < $

2.33) in the table for the normal distribution and find it is 0.4901. So $p = 1 - 0.9802 = 0.0198$.

6.9   a. We want $P(Z < \#) = 0.9920$. We know that since the probability is greater than 0.5 # is greater than 0. So $P(Z < \#) = 0.5 + P(0 < Z < \#) = 0.9920$. So to determine # we solve $P(0 < Z < \#) = 0.9920 - 0.5 = 0.4920$. We look it up and find that 0.4920 corresponds to # = 2.41.

b. We want $P(Z > \#) = 0.0005$. # is in the upper-right tail of the distribution so $P(Z > \#) = 0.5 - P(0 < Z < \#)$. We find # by solving $P(0 < Z < \#) = 0.5 - 0.0005 = 0.4995$. Our table only goes to 3.09 and we see that $P(0 < Z < 3.09) = 0.4990 < 0.4995$. So #>3.09.

c. We want $P(Z < \#) = 0.0250$. This is in the lower tail so # < 0. $P(Z < \#) = P(Z > -\#) = 0.5 - P(0 < Z < -\#)$. So $P(0 < Z < -\#) = 0.5 - 0.025 = 0.475$. The table tells us that $-\# = 1.96$. Therefore $\# = -1.96$.

d. We want $P(Z < \#) = 0.6554$. Since the probability is greater than 0.5 we know # > 0. $P(Z < \#) = 0.5 + P(0 < Z < \#)$. So $P(0 < Z < \#) = 0.6554 - 0.5 = 0.1554$. Solving for # by table look-up we see that # = 0.40.

e. We want $P(Z > \#) = 0.0049$. Again, we are in the right tail. So # > 0. $P(Z > \#) = 0.5 - P(0 < Z < \#)$. We must therefore determine # that satisfies $P(0 < Z < \#) = 0.5 - 0.0049 = 0.4951$. We see that # = 2.58.

6.10   To standard we take the score and subtract the sample mean and then divide by the sample standard deviation. Call the raw score W and the standardized score Z. Then since the sample mean is 65 and the sample standard deviation is 7, we set $Z = (W - 65)/7$.

a. $W = 40$. So $Z = (40 - 65)/7 = -25/7 = -3.57$.

b. $W = 50$. So $Z = (50 - 65)/7 = -15/7 = -2.14$.

c. $W = 60$. So $Z = (60 - 65)/7 = -5/7 = -0.714$.

d. $W = 70$. So $Z = (70 - 65)/7 = 5/7 = 0.714$.

e.   We want to determine the probability that $W > 75$. $Z = (75 - 65)/7 = 10/7 = 1.43$. $P(Z > 1.43) = 0.50 - P(0 < Z < 1.43)$. So $P(0 < Z < 1.43) = 0.5 - 0.4236 = 0.0764$.

6.12   The population has a mean blood glucose level of 99 with a standard deviation of 12. So we normalize by setting $Z = (X - 99)/12$.

a. $P(X > 120) = P(Z > 21/12) = P(Z > 1.75) = 0.5 - P(0 < Z < 1.75) = 0.5 - 0.4599 = 0.0401$.

b. $P(70 < X < 100) = P(-29/12 < Z < 1/12) = P(-20/12 < Z < 0) + P(0 < Z < 1/12) = P(0 < Z < 20/12) + P(0 < Z < 1/12) = P(0 < Z < 1.67) + P(0 < Z < 0.08) = 0.4525 + 0.0319 = 0.4844$.

c. $P(X < 83) = P(Z < -16/12) = P(Z < -1.33) = P(Z > 1.33) = 0.5 - P(0 < Z < 1.33) = 0.5 - 0.4082 = 0, 0918$.

d. $P(X > 110) + P(X < 70) = P(Z > 11/12) + P(Z < -29/12) = 0.5 - P(0 < Z < 11/12) + P(Z > 29/12) = 0.5 - P(0 < Z < 0.92) + 0.5 - P(0 < Z < 2.42) = 1 - 0.3212 - 0.4922 = 1 - 0.8134 = 0.1866$.

e. If X is outside two standard deviations of the mean Z is either >2 or <-2. So we want to know $P(Z > 2) + P(Z < -2) = 2P(Z > 2) = 2[0.5 - P(0 < Z < 2)] = 1.0-2P(0 < Z < 2) = 1 - 2(0.4772) = 0.0456$.

6.17   a. The mean remaining life for 25-year-old American males is normal with mean 50 and standard deviation 5. We want the proportion of this population that will live past 75. So we seek $P(X > 50)$ since a 75 year old has lived 50 years past 25. To cover to a standard normal, we note that if Z is standard normal it has the distribution of $(X - 50)/5$. So $P(X > 50) = P[(X - 50)/5 > 0] = P(Z > 0) = 0.50$.
   b. For the age of 85 we want $P(X > 60)$. $P(X > 60) = P((X - 50)/5 > (60 - 50)/5)$ $= P(Z > 2) = 0.5 - P(0 < Z < 2) = 0.5 - 0.4772 = 0.0228$.
   c. We seek $P(X > 65) = P(Z > 15/5) = P(Z > 3) = 0.5 - P(0 < Z < 3) = 0.5 - 0.4987 = 0.0013$.
   d. We want $P(X < 40) = P(Z < (40 - 50)/5) = P(Z < -2) = P(Z > 2) = 0.5 - P(0 < Z < 2). = 0.5 - 0.4772 = 0.0228$.

Chapter 7

7.2   Since the population distribution is normal, the sample mean also has a normal distribution. Its mean is also 100 but the standard deviation is $10/\sqrt{n}$, where n is the sample size. As n increases, the standard error of the mean decreases at a rate of $1/\sqrt{n}$.
   a. In this case, $n = 4$ and so $\sqrt{n} = 2$ or the standard deviation is $10/2 = 5$.
   b. In this case, $n = 9$ and so $\sqrt{n} = 3$ or the standard deviation is $10/3 = 3.33$.
   c. In this case, $n = 16$ and so $\sqrt{n} = 4$ or the standard deviation is $10/4 = 2.50$.
   d. In this case, $n = 25$ and so $\sqrt{n} = 5$ or the standard deviation is $10/5 = 2.0$.
   e. In this case, $n = 36$ and so $\sqrt{n} = 6$ or the standard deviation is $10/6 = 1.67$.

7.4   The population is normal with mean 11.93 and standard deviation 3 . So the standard error of the mean is $3/\sqrt{n}$. Since $n = 9$, the standard error of the mean is $3/3 = 1.0$.
   a. To find the probability that the sample mean is between 8.93 and 14.93, we first normalize it. The sample mean has a mean of 11.93 and a standard deviation of 1. So $Z = (W - 11.93)/1$ and $P(8.93 < W < 14.93) = P(-3 < Z < 3) = 2P(0 < Z < 3) = 2 (0.4987) = 0.9974$.
   b. To find the probability that the sample mean is below 7.53, we normalize first. $Z = (W - 11.93)$ and $P(W < 7.53) = P(Z < -4.4) = P(Z > 4.4) = 0.5 - P(0 < Z < 4.4) < 0.5 - 0.04990 = 0.0001$.
   c. To find the probability that the sample mean is above 16.43, we normalize first. $Z = (W - 11.93)$ and $P(W > 16.43) = P(Z > 1.5) = 0.5 - P(0 < Z < 1.5) < 0.5 - 0.4332 = 0.0668$.

7.5   We repeat the calculations in 7.4 but with a sample size of 36. . So the standard error of the mean is $3/\sqrt{n}$. Since $n = 36$, the standard error of the mean is $3/6 = 0.5$.

a. To find the probability that the sample mean is between 8.93 and 14.93, we first normalize it. The sample mean has a mean of 11.93 and a standard deviation of 1. So $Z = (W - 11.93)/0.5 = 2(W - 11.93)$ and $P(8.93 < W < 14.93) = P(-6 < Z < 6) = 2P(0 < Z < 6) > 2(0.4990) = 0.9980$.

b. To find the probability that the sample mean is below 7.53, we normalize first. $Z = 2(W - 11.93)$ and $P(W < 7.53) = P(Z < -8.8) = P(Z > 8.8) = 0.5 - P(0 < Z < 8.8) < 0.5 - 0.04990 = 0.0001$.

c. To find the probability that the sample mean is above 16.43, we normalize first. $Z = 2(W - 11.93)$ and $P(W > 16.43) = P(Z > 3.0) = 0.5 - P(0 < Z < 3.0) < 0.5 - 0.4987 = 0.0013$.

7.7 X is normal with mean 180.18 cm and standard deviation 4.75 cm. Find the probability that the sample mean is greater than 184.93 cm when

a. The sample size $n = 5$. The mean for the sampling distribution of the sample average is 180.18 and it has a standard error of $4.75/\sqrt{5} = 4.75/2.24 = 2.12$. $P(X > 184.93) = P(Z > 4.75/2.12) = P(Z > 2.24) = 0.5 - P(0 < Z < 2.24) = 0.5 - 0.4875 = 0.0125$.

b. The sample size is 10, the mean for the sampling distribution of the sample average is 180.18, and it has a standard error of $4.75/\sqrt{10} = 4.75/3.16 = 1.50$. $P(X > 184.93) = P(Z > 1.50) = 0.5 - P(0 < Z < 1.50) = 0.5 - 0.4332 = 0.0668$.

c. The sample size is 20, the mean for the sampling distribution of the sample average is 180.18 and it has a standard error of $4.75/\sqrt{20} = 4.75/4.47 = 1.06$. $P(X > 184.93) = P(Z > 1.06) = 0.5 - P(0 < Z < 1.06) = 0.5 - 0.3554 = 0.1446$.

7.11 a. The observed data have a variance that is the same from one observation to the next; the sample average has a different distribution with a variance that is smaller by a factor of $1/n$. It has the same mean, and if the samples do not have a normal distribution the sample mean will by the central limit theorem have a distribution that is closer to the normal than the population distribution.

b. The population standard deviation is the square root of the population variance. The standard error of the mean is the standard deviation for the sampling distribution of the sample average. For random samples, it differs from the population standard deviation by a factor of $1/\sqrt{n}$.

c. The standard error of the mean is used to create a standard normal or a t statistic for testing a hypothesis about a population mean based on a random sample. It is also used to construct confidence intervals for means when a random sample is available.

d. The population standard deviation should be used to characterize the population distribution. It is used when you want to make statements about probabilities associated with individual outcomes such as the probability that a randomly selected patient will have a measurement between the values A and B.

7.13 The normalized statistic has Student's t distribution with 5 degrees of freedom. The normalized statistic $t = (X - 28)/(2.83/\sqrt{6})$, where X is the sample mean. We ignore the fact that for our particular sample $X = 26$. We are only interested in the proportion of such estimates that would fall below 24 (our particular one did not since 26 > 24). We take 24 for X since the probability that the sample mean falls below 24 is the same with unknown variance as the probability that $t < (24–28)/(2.83/\sqrt{6}) = -4/1.155 = -3.46$. We look up t with 5 degrees of freedom and find that $P(t < -3.46) = P(t > 3.46) < 1 - 0.99 = 0.01$ since $P(t > 3.365)1 - P(t < 3.365) = 1 - 0.99 = 0.01$ for t with 5 degrees of freedom. We use the one-tailed probability.

Chapter 8

8.2   A point estimate is a single value intended to approximate a population para-meter. An unbiased estimate is an estimate or a function of observed random vari-ables that has the property that the average of its sampling distribution is equal to the population parameter, whatever that value might be. Unbiasedness is a desirable property but the key for an estimator is accuracy. Unbiased estimators with small variance are desirable but an unbiased estimator with a large variance is not if other estimates can be found that are more accurate. The mean square error is a measure of accuracy. It penalizes an estimate for both bias and variance. An estimate with small mean square error tends to be close to the true parameter value.

8.7   The bootstrap principle states that we can approximate the sampling distribu-tion of a point estimate by mimicking the random sample we observe to compute the estimate. The bootstrap estimates are obtained by sampling with replacement from the observed data. Bootstrap sampling mimics the random sampling of the original data. The original sample replaces the population and the bootstrap sample replaces the original sample. The bootstrap estimates are obtained by applying the function of the observations to the bootstrap sample. The distribution of these bootstrap esti-mates is used as an approximation to the sampling distribution for the estimate.

8.8   The bootstrap confidence intervals are obtained by generating bootstrap sam-ples by the Monte Carlo approximation. The histogram of values of the bootstrap estimates can then be used to generate confidence intervals. One of the simplest of bootstrap confidence intervals is called Efron's percentile method. It constructs a $100(1 - \alpha)\%$ confidence interval by taking the lower endpoint to be the $100(\alpha/2)$ percentile and the upper endpoint to be the $100(1 - \alpha/2)$ percentile.

8.10   We need to find C, the 97.5 percentage point from the t distribution with $n - 1$ degrees of freedom such that $Cs/\sqrt{n} \le d$. Here $d = 1.2$ and $S = 9.4$. So we need to find the smallest n such that $n \ge C^2 S^2/d^2 = C^2(61.36)$. From the table of Student's t distribution, we see the results in the following table:

$df = n - 1$	C	$C^2(61.36)$
9	2.2622	314.01
29	2.0452	256.66
100	1.984	241.53
200	1.9719	238.59

From the table, we see that $n > 235$, since for $n = 235$, $C > 1.96$ and $(1.96)^2(61.36) = 235.72$. Also, $C < 1.9719$ for $n = 235$, so for $n = 235$, $235.72 < C^2(61.36) < 238.59$. Now 239 is clearly large enough.

8.14 Since the mean score is 55 and the standard deviation is 5, we want to find n so that the half-width of a 99% confidence interval for the population mean has a half-width d no greater than 0.4. Again, n must satisfy $n \geq C^2S^2/d^2 = C^2(156.25)$, where C is the 99.5 percentile of a t distribution with $n - 1$ degrees of freedom. We use the following table:

$df = n - 1$	C	$C^2(156.25)$
29	2.7564	1187.14
200	2.6006	1056.74
1000	2.5758	1036.68
1036	2.5758	1036.68

After $df = 200$, the value of C is close enough to the limiting normal value that we use the limiting value of 2.5758. We see that we need $df = 1036$ or $n = 1037$ to meet our requirement. For a 95% confidence interval with the same mean and standard deviation, we would require a smaller n for the same $d = 0.4$ since the constant C is smaller—1.96 compared to 2.5758. We reduce the sample size by lowering the level of confidence. We still require $n \geq C^2S^2/d^2 = C^2(156.25)$ but now since $C = 1.96$, we have $n > 600.25$ or $n = 601$.

8.16 a. We have assumed that the standard deviation is known to be 2.5. A 95% confidence interval for 36 construction workers would then be $[16 - (1.96)(2.5)/\sqrt{36}, 16 + (1.96)(2.5)/\sqrt{36}] = [15.1833, 16.8167]$.
  b. Had n been 49, we just replace $\sqrt{36} = 6$ by $\sqrt{49} = 7$. This gives $[16 - (1.96)(2.5)/7, 16 + (1.96)(2.5)/7] = [15.3, 16.7]$.
  c. Now if $n = 64$ we replace 7 by $8 = \sqrt{64}$ to get $[16 - (1.96)(2.5)/8, 16 + (1.96)(2.5)/8] = [15.3875, 16.6125]$.
  d. As we see from a through c we kept the level the same and we found that the width continued to decrease as the sample size increased. With each new interval being contained in the previous one (since the mean and standard deviation did not change). This just illustrates that the width of the interval, which is a constant divided by the square root of the sample size, decreases because the square root of the sample size increases as the sample size increases.
  e. The halfwidth of the interval in c is $0.6125 = (1.96)(2.5)/8$.

Chapter 9

9.3 H_0: The mean $\mu = 11.2$ versus the alternative H_A: The mean $\mu \neq 11.2$. This is a two-sided test.

9.5 H_0: The mean difference $\mu_1 - \mu_2 = 0$ versus the alternative H_A: The mean difference $\mu_1 - \mu_2 \neq 0$.

9.9   The sample size is 5, the population variance is known to be 5, and the data is normally distributed. Under the null hypothesis, the mean is 0. We want to find the critical value C such that $P(-C < X < C) = 0.95$, where X is the sample mean. Under the null hypothesis, $Z = X/(\sqrt{5}/\sqrt{5}) = X$ since the standard deviation is $\sqrt{5}$ and the standard error of the mean is the standard deviation divided by $\sqrt{n}$ where the sample size n is in this case 5. Since Z is standard normal and $Z = X$ from the table, we see that $C = 1.96$.

9.10   In this case, the true mean is 1 and the critical value C is 1.96, as determined in Exercise 9.9. The power of the test is the probability that $X > 1.96$ or $X < -1.96$ under the alternative that the mean is 1 instead of 0. Under this alternative, X has a normal distribution with mean equal to 1 and standard error equal to 1. So under the alternative a standard normal $Z = X - 1$. $P(X > 1.96) = P(Z > 0.96) = 0.5 - P(0 < Z < 0.96) = 0.5 - 0.3315 = 0.1685$. Now $P(X < -1.96) = P(Z < -2.96) = P(Z > 2.96) = 0.5 - P(0 < Z < 2.96) = 0.5 - 0.4985 = 0.0015$. So the power of the test is 0.1685 + 0.0015 = 0.17.

9.11   In this case, the true mean is 1.5 and the critical value C is 1.96 as determined in Exercise 9.9. The power of the test is the probability that $X > 1.96$ or $X < -1.96$ under the alternative that the mean is 1.5 instead of 0. Under this alternative, X has a normal distribution with mean equal to 1.5 and standard error equal to 1. So under the alternative a standard normal $Z = X - 1.5$. $P(X > 1.96) = P(Z > 0.46) = 0.5 - P(0 < Z < 0.46) = 0.5 - 0.1772 = 0.3228$. Now $P(X < -1.96) = P(Z < 3.46) = P(Z > 3.46) = 0.5 - P(0 < Z < 3.46) < 0.5 - 0.4990 = 0.001$. So the power of the test is approximately 0.3228 + 0.001 = 0.3238.

9.19   a. $n = 12$, $\alpha = 0.05$ one-tailed to the right: $t = 1.7939$ $(df = 11)$
    b. $n = 12$, $\alpha = 0.01$ one-tailed to the right: $t = 2.718$ $(df = 11)$
    c. $n = 19$, $\alpha = 0.05$ one-tailed to the left: $t = -1.7341$ $(df = 18)$
    d. $n = 19$, $\alpha = 0.05$ two-tailed: $t = -1.7341$ and $t = 1.7341$ $(df = 18)$
    e. $n = 28$, $\alpha = 0.05$ one-tailed to the left: $t = -1.7033$ $(df = 27)$
    f. $n = 41$, $\alpha = 0.05$ two-tailed: $t = -1.6839$ and $t = 1.6839$ $(df = 40)$
    g. $n = 8$, $\alpha = 0.10$ two-tailed: $t = -2.3646$ and $t = 2.3646$ $(df = 7)$
    h. $n = 201$, $\alpha = 0.001$ two-tailed: $t = -3.3400$ and $t = 3.3400$ $(df = 200)$

9.22   A meta-analysis is a procedure for drawing statistical inference based on combining information from several independent studies. It is often done because studies are conducted that individually do not have sufficient power to reject a null hypothesis but several such studies could do so if their information could be pooled together. This can be done when the same or similar hypotheses are tested and the subjects are selected and analyzed in similar ways.

9.26   Sensitivity is the probability that the clinical test declares the patient as having the disease (a positive test result), given that he or she does in fact have the disease. If p is the sensitivity, $1 - p$ is the type II error since the null hypothesis is the hypothesis that the patient does not have the disease and $1 - p$ is the conditional probability of not declaring the patient to have the disease given that he does have it. Specificity is the probability that a clinical test declares the patient well (a negative test result), given that he or she does not have the disease. If p is the specificity, $1 - p$ is the type I error since $1 - p$ is the conditional probability of declaring the patient has the disease when he does not.

Chapter 10

10.2 $Z' = (W_1 - W_2)/\sqrt{[W_c(1 - W_c)/n_1 + W_c(1 - W_c)/n_2]}$, where $W_c = (X_1 + X_2)/(n_1 + n_2)$ and $X_1 = 12$, the number with peripheral neuropathy out of $n_1 = 35$ in the control group of diabetic patients and $X_2 = 3$, out of the 11 patients taking an oral agent to prevent hyperglycemia, so $n_2 = 11$. Z' is approximately standard normal under the null hypothesis. $W_c = 15/46 = 0.3261$. $W_1 = 12/35 = 0.3429$ and $W_2 = 3/11 = 0.2727$. So $Z' = 0.07/\sqrt{0.3261(0.6739)/35 + 0.2727(0.7273)/11} = 0.07/0.1559 = 0.4490$. In this case, the p-value (two-sided) is approximately $2(0.5 - 0.1736) = 0.6528$. So we cannot detect a significant difference between these two proportions.

10.6 The number of Latin American patients with edentulism is $x = 34$. The sample size is $n = 100$. The confidence level $1 - \alpha = 0.90$. The formula for the confidence interval is by Clopper–Pearson [$\{1 + (100 - 34 + 1)F(0.95:200 - 68 + 2, 68)/34\}^{-1}$, $\{1 + (100 - 34)/\{35F(0.95:68 + 2, 2(100 - 34)\}^{-1}] = [1/\{1 + 67F(0.95:134, 68)/34\}$, $1/\{1 + 66/(35F(0.95:70, 132))\}]$. $F(0.95:134, 68) \approx 1.45$ and $F(0.95:70, 132) \approx 1.42$. So the interval is [0.259, 0.430]

10.8 The sample proportion $p = 171/402 = 0.425$. We are testing the hypothesis that $p = 0.39$ against the alternative $p > 0.39$ that the proportion overweight in the lower social class in Britain is higher than for the general British population. Take $Z = (0.425 - 0.39)/\{\sqrt{(0.39)}\sqrt{(0.61)}/\sqrt{402}\} = 0.035/0.02433 = 1.439$. This is nonsignificant. For a one-sided test at the 0.01 significance level, the critical $Z = 2.33$.

Chapter 11

11.3

	Normal Glycemic Control	Abnormal Glycemic Control	Total
Treated Patients	120 = 0.60(200)	80 = 0.40(200)	200
Control Group Patients	30 = 0.15(200)	170 = 0.85(200)	200
Total	150	250	400

Yes if the treatment was ineffective we would see independence in the 2×2 table and approximatelyonly approximately 37.5% or 75 students would have normal control in each group. We would expect 37.5% or about 75 to be normal on one test and the same 75 on the other. So the expected table would be as follows:

	Normal Glycemic Control	Abnormal Glycemic Control	Total
Treated Patients	75 = 0.375(200)	125 = 0.625(200)	200
Control Group Patients	75 = 0.375(200)	125 = 0.625(200)	200
Total	150	250	400

$$\text{Chi-square} = \frac{(120-75)^2}{75} + \frac{(80-125)^2}{125} + \frac{(30-75)^2}{75} + \frac{(170-125)^2}{125}$$

$$= 27 + 16.2 + 27 + 16.2 = 86.4.$$

Since we are looking at a chi-square statistic with 1 degree of freedom, we should clearly reject independence in favor of the conclusion that the treatment is effective.

11.4   We recall that the chi-square test applies to testing independence between two groups. The expected frequencies are the row total times the column total divided by the total sample size. So in the survey, the participants' health as self-reported versus having smoked 100 or more cigarettes or not in their lifetime should have about the same distribution in each column. So in the first row, for example, $E = 632(369)/1489 = 156.62$ for the participants who smoked 100 or more cigarettes and $E = 857(369)/1489 = 212.38$ for those that smoked less than 100 cigarettes. Continuing in this way the table looks as follows:

Health Status	Smoked 100 or More Cigarettes, Observed (Expected)	Did Not Smoke 100 or More Cigarettes, Observed (Expected)
Excellent	142 (156.62)	227 (212.38)
Very good/ good	368 (358.81)	475 (485.19)
Fair/poor	122 (117.57)	155 (159.43)
Total	632	857

Summing $(O - E)^2/E$ we get $1.36 + 1.01 + 0.026 + 0.214 + 0.167 + 0.123 = 2.9$. Since this table has 3 rows and 2 columns, the degrees of freedom for the chi-square is $(R-1)(C-1) = 2(1) = 2$. Checking the 5% critical value in the chi-square table, we see that $C = 5.991$, and since $2.9 < 5.991$, we cannot reject the null hypothesis that the distribution of health status for is the same for those that smoked 100 or more cigarettes compared with those that did not smoke 100 or more cigarettes. Although it may be surprising that the distributions are so similar, it only indicates that they perceive their health similarly. Their actual health status by other measures could be considerably different.

11.7   The approach is the same as in 11.4 except that $R = 2$ and $C = 2$. So the chi-square statistic will have only 1 degree of freedom. First we must construct the table as follows:

	Hypoglycemic, Observed	Not Hypoglycemic, Observed	Total
Elevated Diastolic BP	370 = 37% of 1000		500 = 50% 0f 1000
Diastolic BP Not Elevated			
Total	450 = 45% of 1000		1000

This is what we are given for the table. We can fill in the remaining cells by sub-traction since we know the totals for the first row, the first column, and the grand total:

	Hypoglycemic, Observed	Not Hypoglycemic, Observed	Total
Elevated Diastolic BP	370 = 37% of 1000	130 = 500 − 370	500 = 50% of 1000
Diastolic BP Not Elevated	80 = 450 − 370	420 = 500 − 80	500 = 1000 − 500
Total	450 = 45% of 1000	550 = 1000 − 450	1000

Now we compute the expected numbers and compute the chi-square statistic:

	Hypoglycemic, Observed (Expected)	Not Hypoglycemic, Observed (Expected)	Total
Elevated Diastolic BP	370 (225)	130 (275)	500
Diastolic BP Not Elevated	80 (225)	420 (275)	500
Total	450	550	1000

Inspection of the table shows a very poor fit. Computing chi-square we have $(145)^2/225 + (145)^2/275 + (145)^2/225 + (145)^2/275 = 93.44 + 76.45 + 93.44 + 76.45 = 339.79$. The critical value at the 1% level for a chi-square with 1 degree of free-dom is $C = 6.635$. So clearly we reject the null hypothesis. There is a strong rela-tionship between elevated diastolic blood pressure and hypoglycemia for this popu-lation.

Chapter 12

12.3   We assume that X and Y have a bivariate normal distribution. Then the re-gression $E(Y|X)$ is linear. Then the product moment correlation has an interpreta-tion as a parameter of the bivariate normal distribution that represents the strength of the linear relationship. Even if X and Y do not have the bivariate normal distri-bution, if we can assume that $Y = \alpha + \beta X + \varepsilon$, where ε is a random variance with mean 0 and variance σ^2 independent of X, then the sample product moment cor-relation is still a measure of the strength of the linear relationship between X and Y.

12.7   The scatter plot and the regression line are given in the following figure:

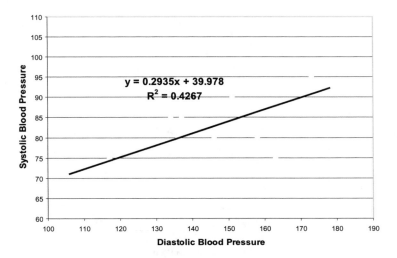

Systolic blood pressure versus diastolic blood pressure.

$r = \sqrt{0.4267} = 0.6532$. Recall that $[b - T_{1-\alpha/2}SE(b), b + T_{1-\alpha/2}SE(b)]$ where is the $100(1 - \alpha/2)$ percentile for Student's t distribution with $n - 2$ degrees of freedom. This interval is a $100(1 - \alpha)\%$ confidence interval for β. Here we require α to be 0.05. So $T_{1-\alpha/2} = 1.679$ since the degrees of freedom equals 46. To get $SE(b)$ recall that $SSE = \Sigma(y - \hat{Y})^2$, $S_{y.x} = \sqrt{SSE/n} - 2$, and $SE(b) = S_{y.x}/\sqrt{\Sigma(x - \bar{x})}$. Now $SSE = 1516.30$, so $SSE/(n - 2) = 1516.30/46 = 32.96$. So $S_{y.x} = 5.7413$ and $\sqrt{\Sigma(x - \bar{x})^2} = 114.4595$. So $SE(b) = 5.7413/114.4595 = 0.05016$. Hence the confidence interval is $[b - T_{1-\alpha/2}SE(b), b + T_{1-\alpha/2}SE(b)] = [0.2935 - 1.679(0.05016), 0.2935 + 1.679(0.05016)] = [0.2093, 0.3777]$. Recall that testing the significance of a linear relationship is the same as testing that the slope parameter is zero, which in turn is equivalent to testing whether the correlation r is zero. Recall the t test as follows:

$$t_{df} = \frac{r}{\sqrt{1 - r^2}}\sqrt{n - 2}$$

where $df = n - 2$ and $n = $ number of pairs. Here $n = 48$ and

$$r = \frac{\Sigma XY - \dfrac{(\Sigma X)(\Sigma Y)}{n}}{\sqrt{[\Sigma X^2 - (\Sigma X)^2/n][\Sigma Y^2 - (\Sigma Y)^2/n]}} = 0.6532$$

So $t = 0.6532\sqrt{46}/\sqrt{1 - 0.4267} = 4.4302/0.75717 = 5.851$ Comparing this to a t with 46 degrees of freedom we find the critical T at the 5% level (two-sided) is 1.679, Since 5.475 is larger than 1.679, we reject the null hypothesis.

12.9   The scatter plot and the regression line are given in the following figure:

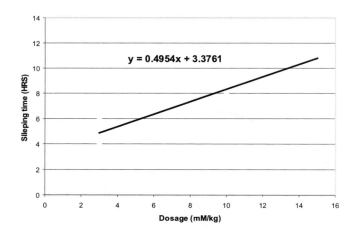

Sleeping Time versus Dosage.

   b. $y = 0.4954x + 3.3761$

   c. Recall that $[b - T_{1-\alpha/2}SE(b), b + T_{1-\alpha/2}SE(b)]$ where is the $100(1 - \alpha/2)$ percentile for Student's t distribution with $n - 2$ degrees of freedom. This interval is a $100(1 - \alpha)\%$ confidence interval for β. Here we require α to be 0.05. So $T_{1-\alpha/2} = 2.3646$ since the degrees of freedom equals 7. To get $SE(b)$ recall that $SSE = \Sigma(y - \hat{Y})^2$, $S_{y.x} = \sqrt{SSE/n - 2}$, and $SE(b) = S_{y.x}/\sqrt{\Sigma(x - \bar{x})^2}$. Now $SSE = 12.49541$, so $SSE/(n - 2) = 12.48541/7 = 1.78363$. So $S_{y.x} = 1.33553$ and $\sqrt{\Sigma(x - \bar{x})^2} = 14.7648$. So $SE(b) = 1.33553/14.7648 = 0.09045$. Hence the confidence interval is $[b - T_{1-\alpha/2}SE(b), b + T_{1-\alpha/2}SE(b)] = [0.4954 - 2.3646(0.09045), 0.4954 + 2.3646(0.09045)] = [0.2815, 0.7093]$.

   d. Recall that testing the significance of a linear relationship is the same as testing that the slope parameter is zero, which in turn is equivalent to testing whether the correlation r is zero. Recall the t test as follows:

$$t_{df} = \frac{r}{\sqrt{1 - r^2}}\sqrt{n - 2}$$

where $df = n - 2$ and n = number of pairs. Here $n = 9$ and $r = \Sigma XY - (\Sigma X)(\Sigma Y)/n/\sqrt{[\Sigma X^2 - (\Sigma X)^2/n][\Sigma Y^2 - (\Sigma Y)^2/n]} = \{780 - (84)(72)/9\}/\{\sqrt{1002} - (84)^2/9\sqrt{642} - (72)^2/9\} = 108/\{\sqrt{218}\sqrt{66}\} = 108/119.95 = 0.9004$. So $t = 0.9004\sqrt{7}/\sqrt{1 - 0.8107} = 5.475$. Comparing this to a t with 7 degrees of freedom, we find the critical T at the 5% level (two-sided) is 2.3646. Since 5.475 is larger than 2.3646, we reject the null hypothesis.

   e. $y = 0.4954(12) + 3.3761 = 9.3209$.

12.17 The sample multiple correlation coefficient R^2 in a multiple regression problem represents the percentage of the variation in Y that is explained by the predictor variables through the linear regression equation. A value of 1 indicates a perfect linear fit to the data. A value close to 1 indicates a good fit.

12.18 The drop in R^2 from 0.75 to 0.71 indicates that the addition of the fifth variable only explains an additional 4% of the variance in Y. This may not be explaining enough of the variation to include this variable in the model. Depending on the sample size this may or may not be statistically significant

12.21 Stepwise regression is a method for added and deleting variables in a stepwise fashion based on which variable in the equation is weakest and which from the list of possible entrants is strongest based on criteria such as "F to enter" and "F to exit." It is used to help pick a good subset of the variables for inclusion in the model.

12.23 An example of a logistic regression problem would be the military triage problem. In the case where a soldier is wounded and is in shock, the chances of his survival depends on the severity of his injury, which can be determined by several measurements including blood pressure. The army may in combat be faced with too many severely wounded soldiers to be able to treat all of them. When having to choose which patients to treat, the army wants to know the chance of survival. A logistic regression equation can predict the chance of survival of a patient based on vital signs. The equation can be developed based on historical data for shock trauma patients. In logistic regression, the outcome variable Y is binary. The patient survives or dies. A logit transformation is applied to the response before creating a linear relationship with the predictors. Ordinary least squares is no longer available as a simple analytic method for obtaining the regression parameters. The predictor variables can be continuous or discrete as in an ordinary multiple regression equation. Because the outcome variable is binary, its expected value is a proportion that represents the probability of the outcome associated with the value 1.

Chapter 13

13.1 Complete the following ANOVA table:

Source of Variation	Sum of Squares	Degrees of Freedom	Mean Square	F Ratio
Between	300			
Within	550	15		
Total		21		

Source of Variation	Sum of Squares	Degrees of Freedom	Mean Square	F Ratio
Between	300	6	50	1.364
Within	550	15	36.67	—
Total	850	21	—	—

13.3   Since we are looking at more than one pair of mean differences, there are multiple hypothesis tests, each having its own type I error. We want to control simultaneously the type I errors that we could make. Tukey's method guarantees that the probability of making a type I error on any of the tests is controlled to be less than α. A simple α-level t test on two or more mean differences would not provide such a control.

13.11   We construct an ANOVA table based on the data in the table below:

Machine Liquid Weight of Cans in Ounces

	Machine A	Machine B	Machine C	Machine D	Total
	Value (SS Term)	Value (SS Term)	Value (SS Term)	Value (SS Term)	(SS)
	12.05 (0.000144)	11.98 (0.0016)	12.04 (0.000784)	12.00 (0.0004)	
	12.07 (0.001024)	12.05 (0.0009)	12.03 (0.000324)	11.97 (0.0001)	
	12.04 (0.000004)	12.06 (0.0016)	12.03 (0.000324)	11.98 (0.0000)	
	12.04 (0.000004)	12.02 (0.0000)	12.00 (0.000144)	11.99 (0.0001)	
	11.99 (0.002304)	11.99 (0.0009)	11.96 (0.002704)	11.96 (0.0004)	
Means	12.038 (0.00348)	12.02 (0.005)	12.012 (0.00428)	11.98 (0.0010)	(0.01376)

From above, the within-group sum of squares is 0.01376. The grand mean is 12.0125. So the between-group sum of squares is $5\{(12.038 - 12.0125)^2 + (12.02 - 12.0125)^2 + (12.012 - 12.0125)^2 + (11.98 - 12.0125)^2\} = 5(0.00065025 + 0.00005625 + 0.00000025 + 0.00105625) = 5(0.001763) = 0.008815$.

Source of Variation	Sum of Squares	Degrees of freedom (df)	Mean Square	F ratio
Between	0.008815	3	$MS_b = 0.008815/3$ $= 0.00293833$	$F = 0.00293833/0.00086$ $= 3.42$
Within	0.01376	16	$MS_w = 0.01376/16$ $= 0.00086$	—
Total	0.022575	19	—	—

The result is significant at the 5% level since the critical f with 3 and 16 degrees of freedom is 3.24. So Tukey's test is appropriate. Recall that $HSD = q(\alpha, k, N - k) \sqrt{MS_w/n}$ where n is the number of observations per group, k is the number of groups, $N = kn$ is the total sample size, and $q(\alpha, k, N - k)$ is gotten from Tukey's table for the studentized range. In this case $k = 4$, $n = 5$, $N = 20$, and $MS_w = 0.00086$. So $HSD = q(\alpha, 4, 16)\, 0.01311$. We take $\alpha = 0.05$ and from the table get $q = 4.05$. So $HSD = 0.0531$. So we can reject the hypothesis that the two means are equal if their differences are 0.0531 or more. The mean differences are 0.018 for A minus B, 0.026 for A minus C, 0.058 for A minus D, 0.008 for B minus C, 0.040 for B minus D and 0.032 for C minus D. Note that only A minus D gives a value greater than HSD. So we conclude that D is less than A but cannot be confident about a difference between any other pairs.

Chapter 14

14.1 First let us look at the two sample t test. The control group mean is 1687.4 and the treatment group mean is 1255.9. The pooled estimate of the standard deviation is 1073.075.

The t statistic is $(\overline{X}_c - \overline{X}_t)/(S_p\sqrt{2/n})$, where n is the sample size in each group. Since $n = 10$, $S_p = 1073.75$, and the mean difference is 614.325, $t = 0.8992$. This is not significant for a t with 18 degrees of freedom. Now consider the Wilcoxon test. We may see different results because the distributions are very nonnormal. Consider the following table:

Control Group Pigs Value (Pooled Rank)	Treatment Group Pigs Value (Pooled Rank)
786 (8)	743(6)
375 (1)	766 (7)
3446 (19)	655 (5)
1886 (14)	923 (11)
478 (3)	1916 (15)
587 (4)	897 (9)
434 (2)	3028 (18)
3764 (20)	1351 (12)
2281 (16)	902 (10)
2837 (17)	1378 (13)
Sample Mean = 1687.4	Sample Mean = 1255.9
Rank sum = 104	Rank sum = 106

The rank sum for the first sample is 104 and the rank sum for the control group and the treatment group is 106. They are virtually the same. Both tests lead to the same conclusion. The two-sided p-value for the t test is close to 0.40. For the Wilcoxon test it is 0.97 for the two-sided p-value and 0.38 for the t test (based on SAS results). The p-values are similar.

14.3 We consider the following table:

Daily Temperatures for Two Cities and Their Paired Differences

Day	Philadelphia Mean Temperature (°F) (rank)	New York Mean Temperature (°F) (rank)	Paired Difference #1–#2	Absolute Difference	Rank of Absolute difference (sign)
1 (January 15)	31	38	−7	7	11.5 (−)
2 (February 15)	35	33	2	2	3 (+)
3 (March 15)	40	37	3	3	5 (+)
4 (April 15)	52	45	7	7	11.5 (+)
5 (May 15)	70	65	5	5	8.5 (+)
6 (June 15)	76	74	2	2	3 (+)

(continued)

Day	Philadelphia Mean Temperature (°F) (rank)	New York Mean Temperature (°F) (rank)	Paired Difference #1–#2	Absolute Difference	Rank of Absolute difference (sign)
7 (July 15)	93	89	4	4	6.5 (+)
8 (August 15)	91	85	6	6	10 (+)
9 (September 15)	74	69	5	5	8.5 (+)
10 (October 15)	55	51	4	4	6.5 (+)
11 (November 15)	26	25	1	1	1 (+)
12 (December 15)	26	24	2	2	3 (+)

For the paired t test, we have a mean difference of 2.833. The standard deviation of the differences is $S = 3.589$ and the t statistic is $t = 2.833/1.036 = 2.734$. This is a Student t with 11 degrees of freedom under the null hypothesis. For a two-sided 0.02 significance level, the critical t is 2.718. So since $2.734 > 2.718$, the p-value is less than 0.02.

The sum of the negative ranks is only 11.5, whereas the sum of the positive ranks is 66.5. If the null hypothesis were true, we would expect these ranks to be approximately equal at around 39. The null hypothesis is clearly rejected in this case. We get an approximate p-value by using the normal approximation, $Z = (11.5-39)/\sqrt{(2n + 1)(39)/6}$, where $n = 12$ is the number of pairs. So $Z = -27.5/\sqrt{25(39)/6} = -27.5/12.75 = -2.157$. This is a one-sided p-value of $0.5 - 0.4845 = 0.0155$ or two-sided $p = 0.031$. This agrees closely with the result for the paired t test.

14.9 We use the following table:

Aggressiveness Scores for 12 Identical Twins

Twin Set	Twin #1 1st born Aggressiveness (rank) [square of rank]	Twin #2 2nd born Aggressiveness (rank) [square of rank]	Rank Pair	Term $R(X_i)R(Y_i)$
1	85 (8) [64]	88 (10) [100]	(8, 10)	80
2	71 (3.5) [12.25]	78 (7) [49]	(3.5,7)	24.5
3	79 (6.5) [42.25]	75 (5.5) [30.25]	(6.5, 5.5)	35.75
4	69 (1) [1]	64 (2.5) [6.25]	(1, 2.5)	2.5
5	92 (12) [144]	96 (12) [144]	(12, 12)	144
6	72 (5) [25]	72 (4) [16]	(5, 4)	20
7	79 (6.5) [42.25]	64 (2.5) [6.25]	(6.5, 2.5)	16.25
8	91 (11) [121]	89 (11) [121]	(11.5, 11)	126.5
9	70 (2) [4]	62 (1) [1]	(2, 1)	2
10	71 (3.5) [12.25]	80 (9) [81]	(3.5,9)	31.5
11	89 (10) [100]	79 (8) [64]	(10,8)	80
12	87 (9) [81]	75 (5.5) [30.25]	(9, 5.5)	49.5
Total [sum of squared ranks]	[649]	[649]		612.5

Recall that the rank correlation is given by the following formula:

$$\rho_{sp} = \frac{\displaystyle\sum_{i=1}^{n} R(X_i)R(Y_i) - n\left(\frac{n+1}{2}\right)^2}{\left[\displaystyle\sum_{i=1}^{n} R(X_i)^2 - n\left(\frac{n+1}{2}\right)^2\right]^{1/2}\left[\displaystyle\sum_{i=1}^{n} R(Y_i)^2 - n(n + \left(\frac{n+1}{2}\right)^2\right]^{1/2}} \qquad (14.7)$$

where n is the number of ranked pairs, $R(X_i)$ is the rank of X_i, and $R(Y_i)$ is the rank of Y_i.

The numerator is $612.5 - 12 (13/2)^2 = 612.5 - 507 = 105.5$. The terms in the denominator are $(649 - 507)^{1/2}$ and $(649 - 507)^{1/2}$. So $\rho_{sp} = 105.5/(649 - 507) = 105.5/142 = 0.743$ a strong positive relationship.

Chapter 15

15.2 $S(t_2|t_1) = P\{T > t_2|T > t_1\} = P\{T > t_2 \cap T > t_1\}/P\{T > t_1\}$. Since $t_2 > t_1$, the event $T > t_2$ is contained in the event $T > t_1$. Therefore $P\{T > t_2 \cap T > t_1\} = P\{T > t_2\}$. So $S(t_2|t_1) = P\{T > t_2\}/P\{T > t_1\} = \exp(\lambda t_2)/\exp(\lambda t_1) = \exp(\lambda t_2 - \lambda t_1) = \exp[\lambda(t_2 - t_1)]$.

15.4 We get the expected and observed numbers for the chi-square test from the following table:

Event Time, T	Number of Events at Event Time (d_i)	Number at Risk in Group 1 (n_{1t})	Number at Risk in Group 2 (n_{2t})	E_1	E_2
7.5	1	6	6	0.5000	0.5000
12	1	5	6	0.4545	0.5455
16	1	4	6	0.4000	0.6000
31	1	3	6	0.3333	0.6667
55	1	2	5	0.2857	0.7143
60	1	1	5	0.1667	0.8333
61	1	1	4	0.2000	0.8000
65	1	0	4	0.0000	1.0000
92	1	0	1	0.0000	1.0000
Total	—	—	—	2.3402	6.6598

Now for the chi-square, we have the observed number of 5 events for group 1 and 5 events for group 2. So $\chi^2 = (5 - 2.3402)^2/2.3402 + (5 - 6.6598)^2/6.6598 = 3.437$. This does not quite reach the 5% level of significance. The distributions do appear to differ by inspection, but the sample size is small (only 5 events in each group).

15.6 a. We generate the Kaplan–Meier curve using the following table:

Time Interval	Number of Deaths, D_j	Number of Withdrawals, W_j	Number at Risk, n_j	Estimated Proportion of Deaths, q_j	Estimated Proportion Surviving, p_j	Estimated Cumulative Survival, $S(t_j)$
$t_1 = 3.0$	1	0	8	0.125	0.875	0.875
$t_2 = 4.5$	1	0	7	0.143	0.857	0.750
$t_3 = 6.0$	1	0	6	0.167	0.833	0.625
$t_4 = 11.0$	1	0	5	0.200	0.800	0.500
$t_5 = 18.5$	1	0	4	0.250	0.750	0.375
$t_6 = 20.0$	1	0	3	0.333	0.667	0.250
$t_7 = 28.0$	1	0	2	0.500	0.500	0.125
$t_8 = 36.0$	1	0	1	1.000	0.000	0.000

b and c. For the negative exponential, $S(t) = \exp(-\lambda t)$ and we estimate time between failures $1/\lambda$ from the data as total time on test divided by the total number deaths $= (3.0 + 4.5 + 6.0 + 11.0 + 18.5 + 20.0 + 28.0 + 36.0)/8 = 127/8 = 15.875$. So the estimate for $\lambda = 1/15.875 = 0.063$.

Time Interval	Number of Deaths, D_j	Number of Withdrawals, W_j	Number at Risk, n_j	Estimated Proportion of Deaths, q_j	Estimated Proportion Surviving, p_j	Estimated Cumulative Survival $S_h(t_j)$ for Negative Exponential and (KM)
$t_1 = 3.0$	1	0	8	0.125	0.875	0.828 (0.875)
$t_2 = 4.5$	1	0	7	0.143	0.857	0.753 (0.750)
$t_3 = 6.0$	1	0	6	0.167	0.833	0.685 (0.625)
$t_4 = 11.0$	1	0	5	0.200	0.800	0.500 (0.500)
$t_5 = 18.5$	1	0	4	0.250	0.750	0.312 (0.375)
$t_6 = 20.0$	1	0	3	0.333	0.667	0.284 (0.250)
$t_7 = 28.0$	1	0	2	0.500	0.500	0.171 (0.125)
$t_8 = 36.0$	1	0	1	1.000	0.000	0.104 (0.000)
$TTT = 15.875$						

d. This exponential model seems to reasonably fit the data.

15.8 Here we change the events at times 6.0, 18.5, and 28.0 to censored times rather than event times. The corresponding Kaplan–Meier table looks as follows:

Time Interval	Number of Deaths, D_j	Number of Withdrawals, W_j	Number at Risk, n_j	Estimated Proportion of Deaths, q_j	Estimated Proportion Surviving, p_j	Estimated Cumulative Survival, $S(t_j)$
$t_1 = 3.0$	1	0	8	0.125	0.875	0.875
$t_2 = 4.5$	1	0	7	0.143	0.857	0.750
$t_3 = 11.0$	1	1	5	0.200	0.800	0.600
$t_4 = 20.0$	1	1	3	0.333	0.667	0.400
$t_5 = 36.0$	1	1	1	0.500	0.500	0.200

Index

Introductory Biostatistics for the Health Sciences, by Michael R. Chernick and Robert H. Friis. ISBN 0-471-41137-X. Copyright © 2003 Wiley-Interscience.